From Eating Disorders to Dysfunctional Eating Attitudes and Behaviors Continuum

The Core of Body Perceptions

Editors

Johana Monthuy-Blanc

Montreal Mental Health University Institute Research Center
Montréal, QC, Canada
and
Department of Education Sciences,
Université du Québec à Trois-Rivières
Trois-Rivières, QC, Canada
and
Department of Psychiatry and Addiction Medicine
Université de Montréal
Montréal, QC, Canada

Giulia Corno

Department of Psychoeducation and Psychology,
Université du Québec en Outaouais
Gatineau, QC, Canada
and
Centre Intégré de Santé et des Services Sociaux de l'Outaouais,
Gatineau, QC, Canada
and
Montreal Mental Health University Institute Research Center
Montréal, QC, Canada

CRC Press
Taylor & Francis Group
Boca Raton London New York

CRC Press is an imprint of the
Taylor & Francis Group, an **informa** business
A SCIENCE PUBLISHERS BOOK

Cover credit: Visuallys/Équipe Visuallys IA Hiver-Printemps 2023 avec Midjourney.

First edition published 2027
by CRC Press
2385 NW Executive Center Drive, Suite 320, Boca Raton FL 33431

and by CRC Press
4 Park Square, Milton Park, Abingdon, Oxon, OX14 4RN

CRC Press is an imprint of Taylor & Francis Group, LLC

Library of Congress Cataloging-in-Publication Data (applied for)

ISBN: 978-1-032-68497-0 (hbk)
ISBN: 978-1-032-71811-8 (pbk)
ISBN: 978-1-032-71812-5 (ebk)

DOI: 10.1201/9781032718125

Typeset in Times New Roman
by Prime Publishing Services

Preface

Johana Monthuy-Blanc[1,2,3,*] and *Giulia Corno*[1,4,5]

1. Context of the book

1.1 Eating disorders as life-threatening psychosomatic conditions

For some individuals, eating is associated with shared satisfaction and embodied pleasure; for others, eating is intertwined with concealed suffering. These latter individuals are those diagnosed with feeding and eating disorders, commonly known as eating disorders. Few mental health conditions render the connection between "mind and body" as tangible and intense as eating disorders (Onnis 2009). In this sense, the classic definition by Fairburn and Harrison (2003) remains highly relevant: eating disorders are conceptualized as "a severe and persistent disturbance in eating behavior associated with distressing thoughts and emotions, which significantly impairs physical health and psychosocial functioning" (p. 408). This definition underscores that eating disorders fundamentally disrupt a vital, innate physiological function: eating and drinking. Consequently, eating disorders fall within the domain of psychosomatic disorders (from the Greek *psyché*, the mind, and *soma*, the body, Knapp 1985). This somatoform nature generates two ambivalent reactions: fascination toward individuals who control, or attempt to control, an essential physiological need required to survive, and a sense of urgency among caregivers and close others (including peer supporters), who attempt to protect the individual from

[1] Montreal Mental Health University Institute Research Center, 7401, rue Hochelaga, H1N 3MG, Montréal, QC, Canada.

[2] Department of Education Sciences, Université du Québec à Trois-Rivières, 3351, boulevard des Forges Blv, G9A 5H7, Trois-Rivières, QC, Canada.

[3] Department of Psychiatry and Addiction Medicine, Université de Montréal Pavillon Roger-Gaudry 2900, boulevard Édouard-Montpetit, bureau S-750 Montréal (Québec) H3T 1J4.

[4] Department of Psychoeducation and Psychology, Université du Québec en Outaouais, 283, boulevard Alexandre-Taché, J8X 3X7, Gatineau, QC, Canada.

[5] Centre Intégré de Santé et des Services Sociaux de l'Outaouais, 909, boulveard de la Vérendrye Ouest Blvd, J8P 7H2, Gatineau, QC, Canada.

Email: giulia.corno@uqo.ca

* Corresponding author: johana.monthuy-blanc@uqtr.ca

the consequences of this unmet physiological need. This raises a central question: how does one survive, mentally and physically, an eating disorder? Two primary causes of mortality are implicated: suicide and cardiac failure (Van Son et al. 2010). These life-threatening outcomes make eating disorders the deadliest mental health conditions in contemporary diagnostic classifications (Jie et al. 2022).

1.2 Eating disorders: Ancient disorders with contemporary relevance

This intertwined relationship between "mind and body," which destabilizes the act of eating, helps explain both the long-standing scholarly attention to eating disturbances and their early inclusion in diagnostic nosology. Notably, in the first edition of the DSM (American Psychiatric Association 1952), anorexia nervosa did not yet appear as a distinct psychiatric entity but was subsumed under the overarching category of *Psychophysiologic Autonomic and Visceral Disorders*, where it was interpreted as a psychophysiological gastrointestinal reaction (Bhattacharya et al. 2022). Historically, eating disorders can be traced through at least four major periods (excluding antiquity). First, during the Middle Ages (5th–15th centuries), extreme self-starvation motivated by ascetic practices, such as deprivation of worldly pleasures, was interpreted as an expression of purity and religious devotion, exemplified by the "holy anorexia" of Catherine of Siena (Guitton 2011). In contrast, episodes of food frenzy (that led to binge eating today) followed by self-induced vomiting were viewed as behaviors associated with wealth in times of widespread famine (Gordon 2001). Second, throughout the modern and contemporary periods (15th–20th centuries), biographers documented symptoms resembling or explicitly describing eating disorders among prominent historical figures such as Mary, Queen of Scots (16th century), Empress Elisabeth of Austria ("Sissi"; 19th century), Marilyn Monroe, and Audrey Hepburn (20th century; Raimbault and Eliacheff 2001). Third, the 17th century marked a decisive turning point with Richard Morton's (1694) first clinical description of anorexia as a psychological disorder (Pearce 2004), giving rise to the now widely used term anorexia nervosa. Finally, in the 20th century, anorexia nervosa and bulimia nervosa were formally recognized as mental disorders through the work of Meyer and Feldman (1965) and Russell (1979). During this period, the core features of bulimia nervosa, such as irresistible urges to binge eat, intense fear of weight gain, and body-related concerns shared with anorexia nervosa, were highlighted.

Around the same time, Hilde Bruch (1961, 1962, 1973, 1978) conceptualized eating disorders as perceptual and cognitive disturbances, notably describing "a paralyzing sense of ineffectiveness" (Bruch 1962, p. 191), as well as distorted physical self-perceptions emphasizing deficits in interoceptive awareness. In 1979, Stunkard identified binge-eating episodes among individuals with overweight, paving the way for binge-eating disorder, formally integrated into DSM-5 in 2013 (Stunkard and Penick 1979). Overall, these historical milestones show that eating disorders are among the oldest documented mental health conditions.

1.3 Dysfunctional eating attitudes and behaviors catalyzed by pandemic confinement

In 2019, the Global Burden of Disease estimated an incidence of 176.2 cases of anorexia nervosa or bulimia nervosa per 100000 people, corresponding to approximately 13.6 million individuals (Amiri and Hosseini 2025, Santomauro et al. 2021). However, this categorical approach obscures a substantial proportion of individuals who experience food-related distress without meeting eating disorders diagnostic criteria (American Psychiatric Association 2023, Tournayre et al. 2024). The COVID-19 pandemic made this issue starkly visible, as dysfunctional eating attitudes and behaviors (DEAB) emerged as one of its major mental health consequences, constituting one of the five major mental health impacts of the COVID-19 pandemic (Cooper et al. 2022, Fernández-Aranda et al. 2020, Rodgers et al. 2020). Indeed, scientific literature published after pandemic confinement is unequivocal: vulnerable populations became more vulnerable, and individuals already sensitive to body image or food-related issues experienced heightened difficulties (Almandoz et al. 2020, Tester et al. 2020, Vavassori and Donzelli 2024). Pre-existing challenges related to body image and eating became increasingly complex (Linardon et al. 2022, Maunder and McNicholas 2021, Monga and Bhat 2024, Ponder et al. 2024). Pandemic confinement triggered a chain reaction of DEAB. DEAB unifies two distinct yet interconnected groups: individuals presenting disordered eating and those meeting criteria for eating disorders (Monthuy-Blanc et al. 2025).

Early in the pandemic, food hoarding, motivated by fear of shortages, evoked wartime behaviors. Constant access to stored foods at home, combined with "forced" sedentariness due to distancing measures, contributed to population-wide weight gain. This weight gain prompted alarmist discourse on social media through hashtags such as #Quarantine15, #COVID15, and #Covibesity (Khan and Smith 2020). Simultaneously, social media idealized paradoxically thin yet muscular body types, two physiologically distinct body compositions (Saiphoo and Vahedi 2019). Increasing time on social media placed individuals under double pressure: avoid gaining weight while also pursuing leanness (Ji et al. 2024, Scarmozzino and Visioli 2020, Vall-Roqué et al. 2021). Whether weight gain was actual or merely perceived (even among muscular individuals), this anxiety-laden context led to excessive or restrictive behaviors (Thompson et al. 2023), including compulsive exercise (Di Renzo et al. 2020, Galali 2021), or dietary restriction motivated either by intentional weight loss or unfounded fears of viral contamination (Canada Health 2023). Some people, however, benefited from preparing meals at home (Husain and Ashkanani 2020a), confronting their concerns through balanced food-related occupations. Others, including individuals with obesity, experienced decreased physical activity yet improved consumption of "healthy" foods such as fruits and vegetables (Husain and Ashkanani 2020b).

From the onset of the pandemic, researchers attempted to alert decision-makers to the impact of COVID-19 on DEAB, documenting population-level patterns such as: intentional dietary restriction (27.6%), binge eating without prior eating disorder diagnosis (34.6% to 81% depending on the country), voluntary meal skipping (52.8%), snacking between meals (80.9%), loss of control over eating (47.2%)

(Phillipou 2020, Ramalho et al. 2021). In conclusion, the COVID-19 pandemic shed light on the importance of considering the burden of DEAB, even in the absence of a formal eating disorder diagnosis.

1.4 Continuum of eating attitudes and behaviors: An inclusive model

Drawing from a dimensional approach to health education, which prioritizes human characteristics over clinical diagnoses (Forbush et al. 2024), the model of DEAB induced by bodily perceptions focuses on individuals who present such dysfunctional patterns (Monthuy-Blanc et al. 2023a). Within this perspective, the aim of this dimensional conceptualization is to characterize the *type* and *severity* of eating-related distress, as well as its consequences on daily functioning, rather than relying on a binary distinction between the presence or absence of an eating disorder, a form of labeling that can be stigmatizing and exclusionary (Goyal et al. 2012, Hay and Touyz 2018). Emphasis is therefore placed on *functionality* and its impact on the person's overall quality of life (Bohn et al. 2008, Jenkins et al. 2011, St-Pierre et al. 2023). As presented in Figure 1, this model conceptualizes eating behavior as driven by bodily perceptions and describes a continuum of functional to dysfunctional states, which may be transient or enduring expressions of these perceptions (Bonanséa et al. 2016, Bourbeau et al. 2025, Monthuy-Blanc et al. 2023a). A functional state corresponds to a physical, intuitive, and interoceptive eating pattern, in which the individual perceives, responds to, and ultimately satisfies internal bodily cues related to eating, such as hunger, thirst, freshness/fullness, satiety, and discomfort. A dysfunctional state, by contrast, is characterized by restrictive, binge-type, or negatively emotional eating patterns, which may contribute to or constitute a formal eating disorder. Along this continuum are found multiple profiles emerging from both the general and clinical populations, including intuitive, restrictive, binge-type, perceptual, and emotional profiles (Monthuy-Blanc et al. 2022, 2023b, Tylka et al. 2024, Van Strien et al. 1986, Westenhoefer 1991).

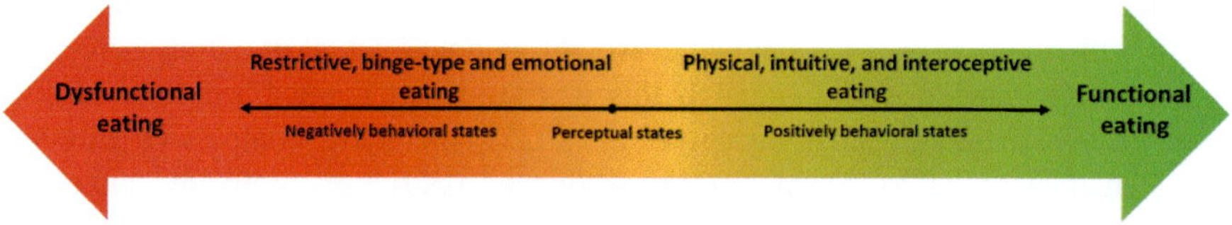

Figure 1. Continuum of eating attitudes and behaviors adapted from Monthuy-Blanc et al. (2023, 2025).

1.5 DEAB as expressions of negative bodily perceptions

Why body perceptions constitute the breaking point of the continuum of eating attitudes and behaviors? Historically, the position articulated by Hilde Bruch during the 1965 symposium, framing eating disorders as perceptual disorders, marked a critical turning point in the conceptualization of eating disorders (Meyer and Feldman 1965). Body perceptions, and more precisely body perception disturbances, common to anorexia nervosa, bulimia nervosa, and binge-eating disorder, remain a core aspect of how these conditions are understood. These disturbances constitute a "family of negative body-related perceptions," including (Cash 2012, Fox and Corbin 1989, McCabe et al. 2006, Shavelson et al. 1976, Slade 1985, Sarwer et al. 2005):

- Depreciated physical self-perceptions, extremely low or extremely high appearance-related self-appraisals;
- Body distortion, a discrepancy between actual and perceived body size, sometimes linked to broader conditions such as body dysmorphic disorder or gender dysphoria;
- Body dissatisfaction a discrepancy between perceived and desired or idealized body and a negative cognitive and emotional evaluation of one's own physical appearance;
- Body disembodiment, understood as immersion in a body-as-object perspective and a lack of connection with the lived body (i.e., the body-as-a-subject).

The nature and underlying mechanisms of body-perception disturbances remain subjects of ongoing scientific inquiry (Glashouwer et al. 2019). One line of evidence suggests that the overestimation of body size may arise from atypical functioning in neural systems implicated in body-related information processing (Suchan et al. 2015). An alternative account is provided by the allocentric lock hypothesis (see Chapters 3 and 7), which posits that individuals with eating disorders may become constrained within a stable, negative, allocentric body representation, one that fails to be updated by incoming egocentric perceptual signals (Riva and Dakanalis 2018, Riva and Gaudio 2017). Beyond this neural account, other researchers argue that perceptual body-image disturbances are not primarily driven by inaccurate size or weight awareness, but by cognitive–affective factors such as body dissatisfaction and the internalization of thin ideals (Cornelissen and Tovée 2021, Corno et al. 2018, Mölbert et al. 2017). Notably, attitudinal body-image disturbances have been shown to predict eating disorder symptoms and psychological distress more strongly than perceptual disturbances, both in clinical and non-clinical populations (Allen et al. 2008, Cash and Deagle 1997, Thompson et al. 1990). Body dissatisfaction, in particular, is widely recognized as one of the most potent predictors of the onset, maintenance, and relapse of DEAB (Bourbeau et al. 2025, McLean and Paxton 2019, Stice and Shaw 2002, Stice et al. 2011).

Recently, two major processes of perceptual exposure catalyzed by the pandemic context, had a major impact on body perceptions. First, exposure via social media to alarmist messages about weight gain (for example, "SkinnyTok") and to the internalization of a "muscular thinness" ideal (that is, adherence to a body shape that is simultaneously slender and sculpted). This reality reflects the dual exposure to social media pressures promoting weight control and "muscular thinness," and frequent exposure to one's own image through videoconferencing, deeply embedded in our daily TV show–like routines (Lucibello et al. 2021, Pearl 2020). These sociocultural forces shape a beauty ideal, lean, elongated, firm, and sculpted, that contradicts metabolic realities (Hoffmann and Warschburger 2019). This unattainable ideal becomes fertile ground for the "glorification" of eating disorders, posing significant risks for individuals vulnerable to food-related concerns (Levine and Smolak 2018). Second, in addition to the overuse of social media, exposure via videoconferencing to one's own image, now omnipresent in everyday life (Hudon et al. 2025). For nearly two years, daily life was reduced to the computer screen, leading to "compulsive and obsessive" self-viewing. With public health measures limiting in-person contact, remote life created an unprecedented situation centered around video-based interactions: seeing oneself while learning, working, receiving care, communicating, ultimately, while living. This constant self-viewing in everyday situations, a phenomenon known as autoscopic overexposure, led some individuals to develop disturbances in bodily perceptions, which in turn may precipitate DEAB (Monthuy-Blanc et al. 2025). This phenomenon is known as the "Zoom effect" or "Zoom dysmorphia", a concept derived from Snapchat and Instagram dysmorphia, which describes the tendency to apply filters to erase perceived bodily imperfections (Pino 2022, Pikoos et al. 2021, Ramphul 2022). Zoom dysmorphia refers to heightened preoccupation with, distortion of, and dissatisfaction toward one's physical appearance, triggered by continually seeing oneself on screen during remote interactions. Even today, the persistence of these attitudes and behaviors, remains one of the most significant psychological legacies of the pandemic context (Hezel et al. 2023, Lowenthal et al. 2020).

In resonance with Bruch's perceptual disorders, this new perceptual reality reinforces the central role of body perceptual disturbances in the predisposition, emergence, and maintenance of eating disorders (Ahuja and Banerjee 2021, Devoe et al. 2022, Gao et al. 2022, Haghshomar et al. 2022, Miniati et al. 2021, Monteleone et al. 2021, Sideli et al. 2021). Moreover, body perceptions, positive or negative, widens the gap between the two ends of the continuum of eating attitudes and behaviors: on one end, functional profiles associated with eating-related well-being, and on the other, dysfunctional profiles associated with eating-related distress (Bourbeau et al. 2025). The most affected groups often include girls and women (particularly those who are ethnicized or pregnant), students, athletes, clinical populations, and individuals belonging to LGBTQ+ communities (Crossland et al. 2023, Goltz et al. 2013, Gorrell et al. 2021, Mikhail et al. 2023, Mason et al. 2018). The relative invisibility of these issues in everyday life calls for health education and health programs that are explicitly grounded in people's lived realities.

2. Content of the book

The complexity of DEAB inspired this collective volume. Fifteen well-established research teams from seven countries (Belgium, Canada, France, Germany, Italy, Spain, and Switzerland; listed alphabetically) offer complementary approaches to understanding, assessing, and intervening on DEAB through the lens of bodily and body image–related perceptions. Across the chapters, DEAB and related phenomena are conceptualized using a range of terms and constructs, including:

- DEAB (Chapters 2, 3, 4, 5, 8, 9, 10, 11, 12, 13, 14), eating disorders (Chapters 1, 2, 3, 4, 7, 9, 12, 14), disordered eating and subclinical disordered eating symptoms (Chapters 2, 12, 14), emotional eating (Chapter 7), binge eating (Chapters 2, 3, 4, 7, 14), restrictive eating (Chapters 6, 10) and obesity as a clinical and sociocultural condition related to eating and body perceptions (Chapters 3, 7, 14).

- Bodily perceptions (Chapters 2, 4, 10, 14) and body perception disturbances (Chapters 4, 13, 14) are addressed through diverse but converging concepts, including: body as a lived, social, and cultural object (Chapter 10), body image (all Chapters, excepted Chapter 12), body image perceptions (Chapters 3, 4, 9, 14), embodiment (Chapters 3, 7, 8, 9, 14), interoceptive issues (such as deficit in interoceptive awareness, Chapters 3, 7, 8, 13, 14), self-perception, particularly physical self-perceptions (Chapters 1, 6, 9), body acceptance (Chapter 2), perceptual distortion (Chapter 3), body dissatisfaction (all Chapters, excepted Chapter 12).

Fourteen chapters structure this volume around two complementary thematic sections: "From Theoretical and Empirical Support ..." and "... To Practical Applications in Sociocultural Contexts." The first section consolidates theoretical and empirical foundations concerning DEAB and bodily perceptions, drawing on the most recent evidence. It addresses contemporary topics such as : the impact of social media on body image and eating behaviors (Chapter 1), the role of self-compassion as a protective factor (Chapter 2), contributions of virtual reality to the assessment and intervention of DEAB-related symptoms and perceptual body disturbances (Chapter 3), attentional bias mechanisms related to food and body cues (Chapter 4), and specific vulnerabilities and strengths among so-called priority populations, including LGBTQ+ communities (Chapter 5), athletes (Chapter 6), and individuals living with obesity (Chapter 7). The second section highlights the practical implications of this body of knowledge by presenting prevention and intervention initiatives rooted in distinct sociocultural contexts. These include: a Swiss prevention program targeting DEAB in community settings (Chapter 8); a Belgian clinical guide addressing DEAB within healthcare services (Chapter 9); a Canadian occupation-based intervention plan for DEAB (Chapter 10); a French support program for close caregivers (Chapter 11); a Canadian patient-partner intervention model in DEAB (Chapter 12); a German contribution emphasizing the integration of sex and gender diversity into DEAB assessment and care (Chapter 13); and a French intervention focusing on bodily embodiment among autistic individuals presenting DEAB (Chapter 14). Collectively, this volume underscores the central role of bodily perceptions in the understanding, assessment, and intervention of DEAB, while showcasing the richness of intercultural and international collaborations.

References

Ahuja, K.K. and D. Banerjee. 2021. A psychosocial exploration of body dissatisfaction: A narrative review with a focus on India during COVID-19. Frot. Glob. Women's Health. 2: 669013.

Allen, K.L., S.M. Byrne, N.J. McLean and E.A. Davis. 2008. Overconcern with weight and shape is not the same as body dissatisfaction: evidence from a prospective study of pre-adolescent boys and girls. Body Image 5: 261–270.

Almandoz, J.P., L. Xie, J.N. Schellinger, M.S. Mathew, C. Gazda, A. Ofori et al. 2020. Impact of COVID-19 stay-at-home orders on weight-related behaviours among patients with obesity. Clin. Obes. 10: e12386.

American Psychiatric Association. 2023. DSM-5-TR Manuel diagnostique et statistique des troubles mentaux, texte révisé. Elsevier Masson.

Amiri, S. and S.M. Hosseini. 2025. Trends, prevalence, incidence, and disability-adjusted life years of anorexia nervosa and bulimia nervosa in Iran: Global Burden of Disease Study. Eat. Weight Disord. 30: 59.

Bhattacharya, A., M. Cooper, C. McAdams, R. Peebles and C.A. Timko. 2022. Cultural shifts in the symptoms of Anorexia Nervosa: The case of Orthorexia Nervosa. Appetite 170: 105869.

Bohn, K., H.A. Doll, Z. Cooper, M. O'Connor, R.L. Palmer and C.G. Fairburn. 2008. The measurement of impairment due to eating disorder psychopathology. Behav. Res. Ther. 46: 1105–1110.

Bonanséa, M., J. Monthuy-Blanc, A. Aimé, P. Therme and C. Maïano. 2016. Attitudes et comportements alimentaires inappropriés et caractéristiques psychosociales des sportifs: comparaison entre deux niveaux de pratique sportive. Rev. Qué. Psychol. 37: 39–60.

Bourbeau, F., S. Bouchard, G. Corno and J. Monthuy-Blanc. 2025. The role of body image perception on a continuum from dysfunctional to healthy eating attitudes and behaviors among people seeking treatment. J. Clin. Med. 14: 597.

Bruch, H. 1961. Transformation of oral impulses in eating disorders: a conceptual approach. Psychiatric Quarterly.

Bruch, H. 1962. Perceptual and conceptual disturbances in anorexia nervosa. Psychosom. Med. 24: 187–194.

Bruch, H. 1973. Eating Disorders: Obesity, Anorexia Nervosa, and the Person Within. Basic Books.

Bruch, H. 1978. The Golden Cage: The Enigma of Anorexia Nervosa. Harvard University Press.

Canada Health. 2023. Coronavirus disease (COVID-19) and food safety.

Cash, T.F. and E.A. Deagle. 1997. The nature and extent of body-image disturbances in anorexia nervosa and bulimia nervosa: A meta-analysis. Int. J. Eat. Disord. 22: 107–125.

Cash, T.F. 2012. Cognitive-behavioral perspectives on body image. pp. 334–342. *In*: Cash, T.F. (ed.). Encyclopedia of Body Image and Human Appearance. Elsevier Academic Press, Cambridge, USA.

Cooper, M., E.E. Reilly, J.A. Siegel, K. Coniglio, S. Sadeh-Sharvit, E.M. Pisetsky et al. 2022. Eating disorders during the COVID-19 pandemic and quarantine: an overview of risks and recommendations for treatment and early intervention. Eat. Disord. 30: 54–76.

Cornelissen, P.L. and M.J. Tovée. 2021. Targeting body image in eating disorders. Curr. Opin. Psychol. 41: 71–77.

Corno, G., S. Serino, P. Cipresso, R.M. Baños and G. Riva. 2018. Assessing the relationship between attitudinal and perceptual component of body image disturbance using virtual reality. Cyberpsychol. Behav. Soc. Netw. 21: 679–686.

Crossland, A.E., L. Munns, E. Kirk and C.E.J. Preston. 2023. Comparing body image dissatisfaction between pregnant women and non-pregnant women: a systematic review and meta-analysis. BMC Pregnancy Childbirth 23: 709.

Devoe, J.D., A. Han, A. Anderson, D.K. Katzman, S.B. Patten, A. Soumbasis et al. 2022. The impact of the COVID-19 pandemic on eating disorders: a systematic review. Int. J. Eat. Disord. 56: 5–25.

Di Renzo, L., P. Gualtieri, F. Pivari, L. Soldati, A. Attinà, G. Cinelli et al. 2020. Eating habits and lifestyle changes during COVID-19 lockdown: an Italian survey. J. Transl. Med. 18: 1–15.

Fairburn, C.G. and P.J. Harrison. 2003. Eating disorders. The Lancet 361: 407–416.

Fernández-Aranda, F., M. Casas, L. Claes, D.C. Bryan, A. Favaro, R. Granero et al. 2020. COVID-19 and implications for eating disorders. Eur. Eat. Disord. Rev. 28: 239.

Forbush, K.T., Y. Chen, P.Y. Chen, B.K. Bohrer, K.E. Hagan, D.A. Chapa et al. 2024. Integrating "lumpers" versus "splitters" perspectives: toward a hierarchical dimensional taxonomy of eating disorders from clinician ratings. Clin. Psychol. Sci. 12: 625–643.

Fox, K.R. and C.B. Corbin. 1989. The physical self-perception profile: development and preliminary validation. J. Sport Exerc. Psychol. 11: 408–430.

Galali, Y. 2021. The impact of COVID-19 confinement on the eating habits and lifestyle changes: a cross sectional study. Food Sci. Nutr. 9: 2105–2113.

Gao, Y., N. Bagheri and L. Furuya-Kanamori. 2022. Has the COVID-19 pandemic lockdown worsened eating disorders symptoms among patients with eating disorders? A systematic review. J. Public Health. 30: 2743–2752.

Glashouwer, K.A., R.M.L. van der Veer, F. Adipatria, P.J. de Jong and S. Vocks. 2019. The role of body image disturbance in the onset, maintenance, and relapse of anorexia nervosa: a systematic review. Clin. Psychol. Rev. 74: 101771.

Goltz, F.R., L.M. Stenzel and C.D. Schneider. 2013. Disordered eating behaviors and body image in male athletes. Rev. Bras. Psiquiatri. 35: 237–242.

Gordon, R.A. 2001. Eating disorders East and West: a culture-bound syndrome unbound. pp. 1–16. *In*: Nasser, M., M.A. Katzman and R.A. Gordon (eds.). Eating Disorders and Cultures in Transition. Brunner-Routledge.

Gorrell, S., J.M. Nagata, K.B. Hill, J.L. Carlson, A.F. Shain, J. Wilson et al. 2021. Eating behavior and reasons for exercise among competitive collegiate male athletes. Eat. Weight Disord. 26: 75–83.

Goyal, S., Y.P.S. Balhara and S.K. Khandelwal. 2012. Revisiting classification of eating disorders-toward diagnostic and statistical manual of mental disorders-5 and international statistical classification of diseases and related health problems-11. Indian J. Psychol. Med. 34: 290–296.

Guitton, F.A. 2011. Anorexie mentale: Les vrais coupables. Europe éditions.

Haghshomar, M., P. Shobeiri, S. Brand, S.L. Rossell, A. Akhavan Malayeri and N. Rezaei. 2022. Changes of symptoms of eating disorders (ED) and their related psychological health issues during the COVID-19 pandemic: a systematic review and meta-analysis. J. Eat. Disord. 10: 1–18.

Hay, P. and S. Touyz. 2018. Classification challenges in the field of eating disorders: can severe and enduring anorexia nervosa be better defined? J. Eat. Disord. 6: 41.

Hezel, D.M., A.M. Rapp, S. Glasgow, G. Cridland and H.B. Simpson. 2023. Year of zoom in a year of doom: lessons learned delivering ERP remotely during the COVID-19 pandemic. Cogn. Behav. Pract. 30: 263–272.

Hoffmann, S. and P. Warschburger. 2019. Prospective relations among internalization of beauty ideals, body image concerns, and body change behaviors: considering thinness and muscularity. Body Image 28: 159–167.

Hudon, A., K. Perry, A.S. Plate, A. Doucet, L. Ducharme and O. Djona et al. 2025. Navigating the maze of social media disinformation on psychiatric illness and charting paths to reliable information for mental health professionals: observational study of TikTok videos. J. Med. Internet Res. 27: e64225.

Husain, M.I. and F. Ashkanani. 2020a. Does COVID-19 change dietary habits and lifestyle behaviours in Kuwait: a community-based cross-sectional study. Environ. Health Prev. Med. 25: 61.

Husain, M.I. and F. Ashkanani. 2020b. Impact of COVID-19 pandemic on dietary habits and physical activity in the general population. J. Nutri. Health Food Eng. 10: 112–118.

Jenkins, P.E., R.R. Hoste, C. Meyer and J.M. Blissett. 2011. Eating disorders and quality of life: A review of the literature. Clin. Psychol. Rev. 31: 113–121.

Ji, X., T. Zhan and T. Zhu. 2024. Impact of COVID-19 on negative body image: Evidence based on social media data. Soc. Sci. Med. 340: 116461.

Jie, Q., Y. Wu, L. Fanxiao, Z. Yikang, H. Jin, H. Zhang et al. 2022. An update on the prevalence of eating disorders in the general population: a systematic review and meta-analysis. Eat. Weight Disord. 27: 415–428.

Khan, M.A. and J.E.M. Smith. 2020. "Covibesity," a new pandemic. Obes. Med. 19: 100282.

Knapp, P.H. 1985. Current theoretical concepts in psychosomatic medicine. pp. 1113–1121. *In*: Kaplan, H.I. and B.J. Sadock (eds.). Comprehensive Textbook of Psychiatry (4th ed.). Baltimore: Williams & Wilkins.

Levine, M.P. and L. Smolak. 2018. Prevention of negative body image, disordered eating, and eating disorders: an update. pp. 1–14. *In*: Wonderlich, S., J. Mitchell and M. de Zwaan (eds.). Annual Review of Eating Disorders. CRC Press, London.

Linardon, J., M. Messer, R.F. Rodgers and T.M. Fuller. 2022. A systematic scoping review of research on COVID-19 impacts on eating disorders: A critical appraisal of the evidence and recommendations for the field. Int. J. Eat. Disord. 55: 3–38.

Lowenthal, P., J. Borup, R. West and L. Archambault. 2020. Thinking beyond Zoom: Using asynchronous video to maintain connection and engagement during the COVID-19 pandemic. JTATE 28: 383–391.

Lucibello, K.M., M.F. Vani, A. Koulanova, M.L. DeJonge, G. Ashdown-Franks and C.M. Sabiston. 2021. #quarantine15: a content analysis of Instagram posts during COVID-19. Body Image 38: 148–156.
Mason, T.B., R.J. Lewis and K.E. Heron. 2018. Disordered eating and body image concerns among sexual minority women: A systematic review and testable model. Psychol. Sex. Orientat. Gend. Divers. 5: 397.
Maunder, K. and F. McNicholas. 2021. Exploring carer burden amongst those caring for a child or adolescent with an eating disorder during COVID-19. J. Eat. Disord. 9: 1–8.
McCabe, M.P., L.A. Ricciardelli, G. Sitaram and K. Mikhail. 2006. Accuracy of body size estimation: Role of biopsychosocial variables. Body Image 3: 163–171.
McLean, S.A. and S.J. Paxton. 2019. Body image in the context of eating disorders. Psychiatr. Clin. North. Am. 42: 145–156.
Meyer, J.E. and H. Feldman. 1965. Anorexia Nervosa. Proceeding of a Symposium Göttinger, 24–25 April 1965. G. Thieme Verlag, Stuttgart.
Mikhail, M.E. 2023. Unheard voices: The impact of the COVID-19 pandemic on disordered eating in people with marginalized identities: Commentary on Deveci et al. (2022), Linardon et al. (2022) and Schneider et al. (2022). Int. J. Eat. Disord. 56: 68–71.
Miniati, M., F. Marzetti, L. Palagini, D. Marazziti, G. Orrù, C. Conversano et al. 2021. Eating disorders spectrum during the COVID pandemic: a systematic review. Front. Psychol. 12: 663376.
Mölbert, S.C., A. Thaler, S. Streuber, M.J. Black, H.O. Karnath, S. Zipfel et al. 2017. Investigating body image disturbance in anorexia nervosa using novel biometric figure rating scales: a pilot study. Eur. Eat. Disord. Rev. 607–612.
Monga, V. and R.M. Bhat. 2024. Eating behaviour and stress due to the psychological impact of COVID-19 among bariatric surgery patients resulting in weight regain: A narrative review. J. Clin. Diagn. Res. 18: 1–5.
Monteleone, A.M., G. Cascino, E. Barone, M. Carfagno and P. Monteleone. 2021. COVID-19 pandemic and eating disorders: What can we learn about psychopathology and treatment? A systematic review. Curr. Psychiatry Rep. 23: 1–15.
Monthuy-Blanc, J., G. Corno, M.-J. St-Pierre, S. Bouchard, F. Bourbeau, L. Mostefa-Kara et al. 2022. Body perceptions, occupations, eating attitudes, and behaviors emerged during the pandemic: An exploratory cluster analysis of eaters profiles. Front. Psychol. 13: 949373.
Monthuy-Blanc, J., G. Corno and S.A. Chakbe. 2023a. Exploring the impact of the COVID-19 pandemic on perceptual disturbances and dysfunctional eating attitudes and behaviours: A review of the literature. Front. Psychol. 14: 1139261.
Monthuy-Blanc, J., U. Faghihi, M.N. Ghazvini Fardshad, G. Corno, S. Iceta, M.-J. St-Pierre et al. 2023b. When eating intuitively is not always a positive response: Using machine learning to better unravel eaters profiles. J. Clin. Med. 12: 5172.
Monthuy-Blanc, J., E. Therrien and J. Harnois. 2025. Santé, boire et manger. L'alimentation en transdisciplinarité selon les perceptions. JFD éditions, QC.
Onnis, L. 2009. Lorsque la psyché est le reflet du corps Une nouvelle alliance entre les neurosciences et la psychothérapie. Cahiers Critiques de Thérapie Familiale et de Pratiques de Réseaux 43: 65–91.
Pearce, J. 2004. Richard Morton: origins of anorexia nervosa. Eur Neurol. 52: 191–192.
Pearl, R.L. 2020. Weight stigma and the "Quarantine-15". Obesity 28: 1180–1181.
Phillipou, A., D. Meyer, E. Neill, E.J. Tan, W.L. Toh, T.E. Van Rheenen et al. 2020. Eating and exercise behaviors in eating disorders and the general population during the COVID-19 pandemic in Australia: Initial results from the COLLATE project. Int. J. Eat. Disord. 53: 1158–1165.
Pikoos, T.D., S. Buzwell, G. Sharp and S.L. Rossell. 2021. The Zoom effect: exploring the impact of video calling on appearance dissatisfaction and interest in aesthetic treatment during the COVID-19 pandemic. Aesthet. Surg. J. 41: NP2066–NP2075.
Pino, O. 2022. Is Zoom dysmorphia a new disorder? Acta Biomed. 92: e2021303.
Ponder, M.L., B.M. Jenkins and W. Sun. 2024. The impact of stigma on sexual and gender minority communities during the COVID-19 pandemic. Howard J. Commun. 36: 209–229.
Raimbault, G. and C. Eliacheff. 2001. Les indomptables. Odile Jacob.
Ramalho, S.M., A. Trovisqueira, M. de Lourdes, S. Gonçalves, I. Ribeiro, A.R. Vaz et al. 2021. The impact of COVID-19 lockdown on disordered eating behaviors: the mediation role of psychological distress. Eat. Weight Disord. 27: 179–188.

Ramphul, K. 2022. "Zoom dysmorphia": the rise of a new issue amidst the pandemic. Acta Biomed. 92: e2021348.
Riva, G. and A. Dakanalis. 2018. Altered processing and integration of multisensory bodily representations and signals in eating disorders: A possible path toward the understanding of their underlying causes. Front. Hum. Neurosci. 12: 49.
Riva, G. and S. Gaudio. 2018. Locked to a wrong body: Eating disorders as the outcome of a primary disturbance in multisensory body integration. Conscious Cogn. 59: 57–59.
Rodgers, R.F., C. Lombardo, S. Cerolini, D.L. Franko, M. Omori, M. Fuller-Tyszkiewicz et al. 2020. The impact of the COVID-19 pandemic on eating disorder risk and symptoms. Int. J. Eat. Disord. 53: 1166–1170.
Russell, G. 1979. Bulimia nervosa: an ominous variant of anorexia nervosa. Psychol. Med. 9: 429–448.
Saiphoo, A.N. and Z. Vahedi. 2019. A meta-analytic review of the relationship between social media use and body image disturbance. Comput. Hum. Behav. 101: 259–275.
Santomauro, D.F., S. Melen, D. Mitchison, T. Vos, H. Whiteford and A.J. Ferrari. 2021. The hidden burden of eating disorders: an extension of estimates from the Global Burden of Disease Study 2019. Lancet Psychiatry 8: 320–328.
Sarwer, D.B., J.K. Thompson and T.F. Cash. 2005. Body image and obesity in adulthood. Psychiatr. Clin. North. Am. 28: 69–87.
Scarmozzino, F. and F. Visioli. 2020. COVID-19 and the subsequent lockdown modified dietary habits of almost half the population in an Italian sample. Foods 9: 675.
Shavelson, R.J., J.J. Hubner and G.C. Stanton. 1976. Self-concept: Validation of construct interpretations. Rev. Educ. Res. 46: 407–441.
Sideli, L., G. Lo Coco, R.C. Bonfanti, B. Borsarini, L. Fortunato, C. Sechi et al. 2021. Effects of COVID-19 lockdown on eating disorders and obesity: A systematic review and meta-analysis. Eur. Eat. Disord. Rev. 29: 826–841.
Slade, P. 1985. A review of body-image studies in anorexia nervosa and bulimia nervosa. J. Psychiatr. Res. 19: 255–265.
Stice, E. and H.E. Shaw. 2002. Role of body dissatisfaction in the onset and maintenance of eating pathology: a synthesis of research findings. J. Psychosom. Res. 53: 985–993.
Stice, E., C.N. Marti and S. Durant. 2011. Risk factors for onset of eating disorders: evidence of multiple risk pathways from an 8-year prospective study. Behav. Res. Ther. 49: 622–627.
St-Pierre, M.-J., P.-Y. Therriault, U. Faghihi and J. Monthuy-Blanc. 2023. Eating disorders: When food "eats" time. Appetite 185: 106509.
Stunkard, A.J. and S.B. Penick. 1979. Behavior modification in the treatment of obesity: The problem of maintaining weight loss. Arch. Gen. Psychiatry 36: 801–806.
Suchan, B., S. Vocks and M. Waldorf. 2015. Alterations in activity, volume, and connectivity of body-processing brain areas in anorexia nervosa. Eur. Psychol. 20: 27–33.
Tester, J.M., L.G. Rosas and C.W. Leung. 2020. Food insecurity and pediatric obesity: a double whammy in the era of COVID-19. Curr. Obes. Rep. 9: 442–450.
Thompson, J.K., L.A. Penner and M.N. Altabe. 1990. Procedures, problems, and progress in the assessment of body images. pp. 21–48. *In*: Cash, T.F. and T. Pruzinsky (eds.). Body Images: Development, Deviance, and Change. The Guilford Press, New York, USA.
Thompson, K.A., E.L. Hedlund, Q. Sun, C.M. Peat, R.W. Goode, J.D. Termorshuizen et al. 2023. Course and predictors of eating disorder symptoms, anxiety symptoms, and pandemic-related eating disorder concerns among adults with eating disorders during the first year of the COVID-19 pandemic. Int. J. Eat. Disord. 56: 151–168.
Tournayre, L., M.A.A. Balbinotti and J. Monthuy-Blanc. 2024. Some hope for a dimensional assessment? A critical review of psychometric validated (semi-)structured interview to assess eating disorders. Eur. Eat. Disord. Rev. 32: 1138–1156.
Tylka, T.L., C. Maíno, M. Fuller-Tyszkiewicz, J. Linardon, C.B. Burnette, J. Todd et al. 2024. The Intuitive Eating Scale-3: Development and psychometric evaluation. Appetite 199: 107407.
Vall-Roqué, H., A. Andrés and C. Saldaña. 2021. The impact of COVID-19 lockdown on social network sites use, body image disturbances and self-esteem among adolescent and young women. Prog. Neuro-Psychopharmacol. Biol. Psychiatry 110: 110293.

Van Son, G.E., D. van Hoeken, E.F. van Furth, G.A. Donker and H.W. Hoek. 2010. Course and outcome of eating disorders in a primary care-based cohort. Int. J. Eat. Disord. 43: 130–138.

Van Strien, T., J.E.R. Frijters, G.P.A. Bergers and P.B. Defares. 1986. The Dutch Eating Behavior Questionnaire (DEBQ) for assessment of restrained, emotional, and external eating behavior. Int. J. Eat. Disord. 5: 295–315.

Vavassori, M. and G. Donzelli. 2024. Impact of COVID-19 restrictive measures during lockdown period on eating disorders: An umbrella review. Nutrition 124: 112463.

Westenhoefer, J. 1991. Dietary restraint and disinhibition: Is restraint a homogeneous construct? Appetite 16: 45–55.

Contents

Preface iii

Part I: From Theoretical and Empirical Support...

1. **Social Media and Body Image** 3
Daniela Villani, Gaia Cuccì and *Anna Flavia Di Natale*

2. **The Role of Self-Compassion in Body Image** 16
Diana Burychka, Marta Miragall and *Rosa Mª Baños*

3. **Applications of Virtual Reality in the Assessment and Treatment of Eating Disorders** 30
Giulia Corno, Johana Monthuy-Blanc and *Stéphane Bouchard*

4. **Attentional Bias and Body Perceptions in Dysfunctional Eating Attitudes and Behaviors** 44
José Gutiérrez-Maldonado and *Marta Ferrer-Garcia*

5. **Dysfunctional Eating Attitudes and Behaviors, and Body Dysmorphia Among LGBTQ+ People** 58
Gabriel Desjardins, Frederick Aardema and *Robert-Paul Juster*

6. **Negative Physical Self-perception in Athletes with Dysfunctional Eating Attitudes and Behaviors** 73
Stéphanie Mériaux-Scoffier

7. **Beyond the Mirror: Exploring Body Image in Individuals with Obesity** 87
Giuseppe Riva, Fabio Frisone and *Giulia Brizzi*

Part II: ... To Practical Applications in Sociocultural Contexts

8. **Prevention of Dysfunctional Eating Attitudes and Behaviors Focusing on Body Image** 103
Isabelle Carrard and *Sophie Bucher Della Torre*

9. **Body Experience in Eating Disorders: Clinical Guidelines** 116
Michel Probst

10. Dysfunctional Eating Attitudes and Behaviours, Meaningful Occupations and Perceptual Disturbances: A Multidimensional Perspective **132**
Marie-Josée St-Pierre, Anick Sauvageau and *Émie Therrien*

11. Challenges and Perspectives for Informal Caregivers in Dysfunctional Eating Attitudes and Behaviors: French Insights **148**
Elisabetta Scanferla and *Romain Rey*

12. Patient Partner in DEAB Intervention: Experiential Knowledge of the Body **162**
Liette St-Pierre

13. Bodies in Context: How Gender and Sexuality Shape Body Perception Disturbances and Dysfunctional Eating Attitudes and Behaviors **175**
Georg Halbeisen and *Georgios Paslakis*

14. Body Image and Embodied Cognition in Eating Disorders: Clinical and Therapeutic Perspectives **188**
Amandine Turcq and *Pierre Dechelotte*

Conclusion **202**

Index **209**

Part I
From Theoretical and Empirical Support…

Chapter 1

Social Media and Body Image

Daniela Villani,[1,*] *Gaia Cucci*[2] and *Anna Flavia Di Natale*[1]

INTRODUCTION

In recent years, social media has transformed the way individuals perceive and present themselves, particularly in terms of physical appearance. Visual platforms such as Instagram have become powerful arenas for self-expression, yet they also promote idealized standards of beauty that can significantly impact users' body image. This chapter explores the psychological mechanisms underlying social media use, especially selfie-related practices, and their influence on body satisfaction and self-objectification. By drawing from sociocultural and social comparison theories, we examine how online behaviors such as photo editing, posting, and social comparison contribute to photo-investment and body image concerns, and how individual differences such as gender and age shape these experiences.

1. Social media and body image

Social media platforms have become one of the primary ways that people leverage the internet to build connection and community, and social network activities can be considered today an integral part of daily life. In addition to various opportunities in terms of entertainment, access to information, relationships and others, the literature has increasingly focused on the negative consequences of social media interaction on well-being and mental health of the general population, reporting harmful effects such as body image ideals, anxiety, depression, and suicide risk for some individuals and groups based on their characteristics and other vulnerabilities (Wang et al. 2022).

[1] Research Centre in Communication Psychology, Department of Psychology, Università Cattolica del Sacro Cuore, Largo Gemelli 1, Milan, Italy.

[2] CRIdee, Department of Psychology, Università Cattolica del Sacro Cuore, Milan, Italy.

Emails: gaia.cucci@unicatt.it, annaflavia.dinatale@unicatt.it

* Corresponding author: daniela.villani@unicatt.it

DOI: 10.1201/9781032718125-2

1.1 Social media and risks on body image

Risks associated with social media use have been identified in both adults and youths (Rasmussen et al. 2020). In response, the Surgeon General's public health advisory on social media issued in May 2023 highlighted the need to implement preventive interventions. In particular, highly visual social media such as Instagram and Snapchat, which are primarily photo-based (Marengo et al. 2018) seems to enhance different processes compared to low visual social media, such as Twitter, and to some extent Facebook, that are primarily text-based. First, high visual social media have become powerful means through which people convey and present a certain self-image and may encourage more frequent engagement in appearance-related behaviors. In fact, through Social Networking Sites (SNS) people can manipulate and edit their appearance (Mingoia et al. 2019) and present idealized versions of themselves through selfie-posting (Boursier and Manna 2018). Second, SNS also lead to greater feelings of intimacy than text-based platforms, as they present social experience more similar to real life and identification processes (Pittman and Reich 2016). Thus, some people aspire to fit in with internalized beauty-ideals and adopt a series of behaviors aimed to reach likes and social approval, including digitally modifying one's physical characteristics in photographs. Among Visual SNS, Instagram has increasingly drawn scholarly attention over the years (i.e., Lee and Borah 2020), due to its widespread popularity and large user base. As of April 2024, approximately 32% of users worldwide were aged between 18 and 24 years, while 30.6% were aged between 25 and 34 years (Statista Research Department 2024). Instagram has gathered attention from body-image researchers due to its focus on aesthetic content and the frequent use of photo-editing tools within its smartphone camera app (Fardouly and Vartanian 2015). Consequently, Instagram has become a popular platform for posting "selfies," or self-portraits typically captured at arm's length with a smartphone and shared online. Research has consistently shown that appearance-focused activities on social media are stronger predictors of body image disturbance than general social media use, as evidenced by reviews and meta-analyses (Fardouly and Vartanian 2015, Saiphoo and Vahedi 2019). This raises a critical question: what specific mechanisms enacted by social media heighten individuals' focus on their own body image and the appearance of others, thereby contributing to body image concerns?

1.2 Sociocultural theory, an understanding approach of social media

Sociocultural theory posits that body dissatisfaction results from exposure to Westernized body image 'ideals' where bodies are displayed as objects, along with the internalization of the belief that rewards are gained when one meets said body image ideals (Tiggerman 2011). The internalization of these body ideals lends itself to using similar others as a comparison point to ascertain if one is measuring up (e.g., Social Comparison Theory, Festinger 1954). Repeated exposure to these media ideals also contributes to self-objectification, where one feels the need to constantly monitor/surveil one's appearance as compared to those ideals (Fredrickson and Roberts 1997). Social comparison theory (Festinger 1954) explains the process by which individuals understand themselves in relation to others. In the absence of an objective standard for self-evaluation, people look to those who are similar to them to assess their social position and performance. These comparisons can occur in one of three directions: upward comparisons (the individual perceives themselves as doing worse in a particular domain than a target individual); lateral comparisons (the individual perceives themselves as performing at a comparable level to a target individual); and downward comparisons (the individual perceives themselves as doing better than a target individual). Downward and lateral comparisons generally lead to positive psychological outcomes (e.g., inspiration for behavior change or reassurance that the individual is doing well), while upward comparisons, though sometimes inspiring, more often lead to negative outcomes (e.g., feelings of discouragement and derogation of self and others).

In the context of social media, upward social comparisons are likely to occur due to exposure to images that are often heavily edited and/or filtered. Upward-directed physical appearance comparisons (Fardouly et al. 2015) and unfavorable comparisons to others have been associated with body image disturbance, body dissatisfaction and problematic eating behaviors (Myers and Crowther 2009, Casale et al. 2021). Appearance comparison on Instagram is thought to heighten body dissatisfaction by encouraging the internalization of societal standards of physical attractiveness, leading to greater awareness of personal flaws. This focus on others is linked to higher levels of body surveillance and increased self-objectification behaviors on social media. Additionally, constant comparison with idealized images may contribute to greater perfectionism regarding physical appearance (Simon et al. 2022), prompting individuals to adopt a self-presentational style aimed at defensively hiding perceived imperfections. This can lead to increased shame and dissatisfaction with one's body (Casale et al. 2024).

2. Selfie and selfie practices

Particular importance has been assumed in recent years by the phenomenon of selfies. The introduction of the term selfie has had a boost thanks to the introduction of front cameras on smartphones in 2010. The first hashtag #selfie appeared in 2011 in relation to a photo posted on Instagram (Sung et al. 2016) and became progressively successful.

The Oxford Dictionary first included the term *selfie* in 2013, but the definition currently endorsed by the scientific community is the one proposed by Lim (2016) who describes selfie as "*a self-expressive photograph featuring the photographer (...) that is consciously created, modified and shared with others to varying degrees, conditional on the dynamic interaction between the personal and situational factors present and facilitated by technology*" (p.1775). This definition recognized an active role for the individual who has control over the type of image he/she wants to create and share. Selfie, indeed, can be considered as a form of self-presentation online and it is also a tool to obtain information (i.e., likes, comments) about how much a person fits with the beauty standards of the relevant social context. In this sense, a person may present him/herself as maximally attractive to gain more approval. Selfies are indeed a tool for self-presentation and self-promotion (e.g., Boursier and Manna

2018, Mills et al. 2018) which, through the reinforcement of positive feedback, may influence self-esteem and self-confidence when the expectations related to social acceptance are met.

The literature on the theme of selfie suggested that people may engage in several selfie practices (e.g., Chang et al. 2019, McLean et al. 2015, 2019). The first one is selfie-taking which consists of taking a picture of oneself with or without the intention to share it on SNS. It, indeed, differs from selfie-posting (also known as selfie-sharing) that is a form of online self-presentation where the person actually posts the selfie on SNS. Posting and sharing selfies online may include a sort of "backstage" process of selfie preparation in order to show the best representation of oneself and or to reach an ideal online self-presentation. This process is defined as selfie-editing, and it may include the use of filters or the modification of certain aspects of the photo such as lights or color saturation. Concerning the process of selfie modification, another practice is the one selfie-manipulation which involves altering the appearance of photo elements, such as people's features using specific programs or apps. Finally, selfie browsing (or selfie viewing) implies that a person views or is exposed to others' selfies (both of celebrities and people from the personal social context) on SNS. Despite this is a more passive practice, since it does not imply an active role of the person, it is strongly associated with processes of social comparison.

Overall, selfie appears to be a complex phenomenon which cannot be reduced to just "taking a photo of oneself" but includes specific control and manipulation strategies as well as specific psychosocial processes (i.e., social-comparison) that influence body image and body satisfaction, as will be explored further in the following paragraph.

3. Photo investment

The growing focus on selfies and its relationship with physical appearance underscores a heightened attention to the body in the digital age and has led to the definition of a new construct related to self-photos: Photo Investment (PI). PI has been defined as the concern individuals have regarding the quality and portrayal of their photos, as well as the effort they invest in selecting, editing, and sharing these images on SNSs. It also involves individual concerns about how the photo will be evaluated by others considering the number of "likes" (McLean et al. 2015). PI is considered a multidimensional construct, encompassing cognitive (e.g., strategic thinking about timing of photo posts, planning or anticipatory thoughts about potential reactions to photos), emotional (e.g., feelings related one's photos, such as anxiety about how a photo will be evaluated or satisfaction/dissatisfaction with one's appearance in images) and behavioral (e.g., time and mental energy spent choosing which photos to share or editing photos) components that interact and influence each other in complex ways. For example, cognitive evaluations of photo quality might trigger emotional responses like anxiety, which in turn could lead to behavioral actions such as increased editing. Similarly, the positive emotions elicited by receiving positive feedback on a photo might reinforce cognitive beliefs about the importance of photo quality, leading to more investment in photo-related behaviors.

The concept of PI has been further investigated by Nesi and colleagues (2021), who identified two specific components of PI: Selfie Appearance Investment, which involves the effort individuals put into enhancing their physical appearance in selfies, such as through photo editing and posing, as well as concerns about how they look in these photos; and Peer Feedback Concern, which captures the social and feedback-seeking aspects of sharing photos online, including worries about the number of comments or likes a photo receives, asking friends to like or comment on photos, and the importance placed on peer reactions to shared photos.

Although research on PI is still in its early stages, along with studies on related behaviors such as photo editing and other selfie practices, it has identified several psychological correlates, highlighting the broader impact of PI and selfie practices on mental health and well-being. For example, photo editing has been linked to lower *self-esteem*, indicating that individuals who invest heavily in their online images may be more prone to negative self-evaluations and perceptions of their own value (Chen et al. 2019). Higher levels of PI have been consistently linked to increased symptoms of *depression* and *anxiety* (Lamp et al. 2019, McLean et al. 2015), suggesting that excessive concern with one's online photographic self-presentation may contribute to broader mental health issues. Additionally, certain personality traits, such as lower conscientiousness and higher narcissism, have been associated with selfie-posting and selfie-editing (Kim and Chock 2017).

One key aspect, which will be explored in the next paragraph, is the impact of PI and related practices on body image. The way individuals engage in photo editing and selfie-related behaviors not only affects their mental health but also plays a significant role in shaping their perceptions of their physical appearance and body satisfaction.

3.1 Gender differences

Gender plays a crucial role in selfie practices and PI, with differences emerging between females and males. Studies on the topic have been conducted mainly in western-culture countries (i.e., North America, Australia and Europe) and Asian-culture countries (e.g., Singapore, China...). However, to the best of our knowledge, no cross-cultural studies have been conducted to date. In general, literature showed that females have higher engagement in selfie-practices than their male counterparts (e.g., Boursier and Manna 2018, McLean et al. 2015, 2019, Mingoia et al. 2019). Research, indeed, consistently showed that females are more likely than males to take, post, and edit selfies (Dhir et al. 2016). Females also place greater importance on appearing attractive in social media photos and are more invested in receiving positive peer feedback (Nesi and Prinstein 2019), they also tend to report higher PI than males (Mingoia et al. 2019, Lonergan et al. 2020) and are more concerned about not meeting the internalized beauty ideals (Mingoia et al. 2019). This heightened investment in appearance is linked to higher levels of body surveillance, body shame, and self-objectification among females, aligning with objectification theory that highlights societal pressures on girls and women to prioritize their physical appearance (Salomon and Brown 2019).

However, research is increasingly showing that SNSs can emphasize the importance of physical appearance across all genders, with males also experiencing body-related concerns and self-objectification (Barlett et al. 2008, Boursier and Gioia 2002, Boursier et al. 2020, Gioia et al. 2020, Manago et al. 2015, Ridgeway and Tylka 2005, Strelan and Hargrweaves 2005). Studies further reveal that also males engage in selfie-editing, however, they usually focus their attention on achieving a lean, muscular, and physically fit body. Mingoia and colleagues (2019), for example, found associations between selfie-editing and the internalization of the muscular ideal among adolescent boys. Selfie-editing in boys is more similar to females since it resulted to be associated with appearance comparisons, body dissatisfaction, and disordered eating behaviors (Lonergan et al. 2020, Mingoia et al. 2019), further highlighting the broader impact of appearance-related pressures in males.

3.2 Age differences

Age also plays a critical role in selfie practices and PI, with different age groups being characterized by distinct psychological processes and patterns of social media use. Research has primarily focused on adolescents and emerging adults, highlighting key differences in how these groups engage with social media and the impact on body image and well-being.

Adolescence is a developmental stage marked by rapid and sudden physical changes, requiring adolescents to continually adjust their body image to keep up with these changes, leading to heightened concerns about their own appearance. Research has shown that SNSs intensify these concerns by engaging in key psychological processes such as social comparison, feedback-seeking, and self-presentation (Nesi et al. 2018). Through constant exposure to peer content and idealized images, adolescents are driven to compare themselves with others, actively seek validation through likes and comments, and carefully curate their online appearance to align with societal beauty standards, as in the case of selfie. These mechanisms collectively heighten the pressure to conform and enhance self-presentation, ultimately contributing to increased body dissatisfaction and PI (McLean et al. 2015, Rousseau 2021). As a result, adolescents are likely to invest time and effort into selecting, editing, and posting self-photos on SNS in order to post a photo representing an ideal self.

Similarly, research shows that also emerging adults frequently engage in photo-related activities such as selfie-taking, editing and posting (Mingoia et al. 2019) and thus suggesting that during this stage of life people still invest time and effort in their online self-presentation. Indeed, despite the end of biological development, emerging adults experience unique psychological and social challenges as they navigate identity formation, intimacy, and self-presentation (Arnett 2003). This makes them especially sensitive to external evaluations and the opinions of others (Lonergan et al. 2019), heightening the importance they place on how they appear to others and resulting in photo-editing behaviors where individuals selectively edit their images to present an enhanced version of themselves (Mustafa and Akram 2022).

4. Photo-based social media behaviors and body image

In the past years, research has explored the implications of selfie practices for body image. The majority of studies (e.g., McLean et al. 2015, Lonergan et al. 2019, Modica 2020, Tiggemann et al. 2020) indicates that these kinds of behavior were generally associated with greater body dissatisfaction for both males and females. Interesting results also emerged from two studies conducted in Singapore among female adolescents (Chang et al. 2019, Chua et al. 2016) who considered selfie editing as a necessary practice to achieve ideal self-presentation to impress peers and to manage insecurity and low self-esteem. Consistently, viewing selfies posted by peers on SNS could result in lower body confidence or desires to change appearance after comparing their own appearance, thus confirming the central role of peers' feedback and social acceptance. These findings are in line with those carried out in USA and Australia in which greater exposure to appearance-related photo and engagement in selfie-editing was associated with lower body confidence (e.g., Meier and Gray 2014, McLean et al. 2015).

Furthermore, another contribution that could be interesting to mention, is the one of Mills and colleagues (2018), who conducted an experimental study with a sample of young women to explore whether taking and posting selfies, with and without the option of photo-retouching the selfie, would influence mood and body image. Findings showed that those who took and posted selfies, even with the possibility to modify them, reported higher feelings of anxiety, less self-confidence and perceived themselves as less physically attractive, compared to those who did not post a photo, highlighting important implications of social media for female psychological well-being.

Some other authors focused their attention in particular on body esteem, that is typically divided into three subscales: appearance, which reflects general feelings and satisfaction with one's physical appearance; attribution, which captures the extent to which individuals believe their appearance influences social evaluations and self-worth; and weight, which assesses how individuals feel about their body size and weight relative to societal or personal ideals (Mendelson et al. 2001). In particular, Wang (2019) explored the relationship between body esteem and selfie-editing, showing that individuals with lower satisfaction of their appearance and higher attribution of their self-worth to their appearance are more likely to engage in frequent photo-editing as a way to enhance their online self-presentation and seek external validation. Similarly, Chang and colleagues (2019) and Pham and colleagues (2022) found a negative correlation between photo-editing frequency and body esteem, further highlighting the detrimental impact of editing behaviors on body image and reinforcing the idea that frequent editing can contribute to lower self-perception.

In line with these literature evidence, photo-based social media behaviors, such as frequent photo manipulation and posting, resulted also to be closely linked to self-objectification, as individuals may come to view themselves primarily through the lens of how they appear to others (Caso et al. 2020, Veldhuis et al. 2020) and body shame (Gioia et al. 2024, Salomon and Brown 2019), where individuals feel inadequate or embarrassed about their appearance when they perceive themselves as failing to meet societal or peer standards of beauty.

Despite few studies have specifically examined the construct of PI in relation to body image, the findings consistently showed associations with body concerns, social comparison regarding physical appearance, and body dissatisfaction (McLean et al. 2015, Cohen et al. 2018, Lonergan et al. 2019, Mingoia et al. 2019, Rousseau 2021). These findings suggest that individuals who invest significant time and emotional energy into curating and editing their photos are more likely to report dissatisfaction with their bodies.

Another interesting aspect with respect to the topic of social media and body image that is worthy of attention, despite still understudied in literature, is the associations between selfie practices and attitudes and behaviors towards cosmetic surgery. Nowadays, cosmetic surgery interventions are increasing worldwide, also among adolescents. The International Society of Aesthetic Plastic Surgery (2023) in the annual report registered an increase of 11.2% in procedures performed by plastic surgeons in 2022 compared to 2021, with face and head procedures as the most popular ones. Therefore, it is important to deepen the understanding of the phenomenon and the associated factors. Selfies might play an important role in the increase of cosmetic surgery (especially in terms of facial cosmetic surgery). For example, individuals may resort to selfie taking and selfie editing and modification to reach an ideal self-representation and then look for cosmetic surgery interventions to replicate the selfie and appear like their photos.

Literature on the theme is still meagre, however some interesting findings emerged. Firstly, authors agreed upon the idea that selfie practices are associated with body dissatisfaction, which in turn represents a strong predictor for both a more positive attitude towards cosmetic surgery and the actual consideration of cosmetic surgery (e.g., Di Gesto et al. 2022). In particular, when considering selfie practices, it seems that facial-dissatisfaction is a key factor that mediates the relationship between selfie editing and cosmetic surgery consideration (e.g., Lyu et al. 2023). Moreover, the use of filters in the selfies was related to higher desire to undergo facial cosmetic procedures (e.g., Aldosari 2020, Varman et al. 2021). Finally, for adolescents, peers played a pivotal role since the engagement in selfie practices may set a process of upward social comparison, which in turn increase their acceptance of cosmetic surgery (Lyu et al. 2023).

Finally, shifting the focus toward more maladaptive and less normative outcomes, studies investigated the associations between photo-based social media behaviors and eating disorders. This is because in the context of social media, selfie practices together with monitoring strategies related to social feedback may reflect some behaviors that are typical of an individual with an eating disorder. For example, body-surveillance can be translated into an extensive and excessive process of selfie selection before posting it (Lonergan et al. 2020). In particular, several studies (e.g., McLean et al. 2015, Cohen et al. 2018, Lonergan et al. 2020, Niu et al. 2020, Rousseau 2021) showed that higher engagement in selfie practices and photo-based behaviors were associated with overvaluation of shape and weight, dietary restraint, internalization of the thin ideal, restrained eating and eating disorders (i.e., anorexia and bulimia nervosa). These results confirmed that those who are more engaged and invested in selfie practices may develop higher body-related and eating concerns, thus suggesting the importance to develop specific interventions.

5. Preventing body dissatisfaction and other negative effects of media exposure

In recent years, researchers also focused their attention on the identification of key protective factors that can help individuals avoid the negative effects on body image of social media usage. Concurrently, authors explored and developed a range of strategies to support and promote healthier attitudes toward the body. Given the pervasive role of social media in shaping perceptions of beauty and self-worth, these protective factors are essential in mitigating the harmful effects of constant exposure to idealized, and often unrealistic, body standards. Several protective factors have been identified, such as: *emotion regulation*, that helps individuals manage the emotional distress that often accompanies exposure to idealized body images online (Rodgers and Rousseau 2022, Zerhouni et al. 2022); *self-efficacy* that provides individuals with the resilience to counter societal pressures and reduce the impact of appearance-related comparisons (Zerhouni et al. 2022); *mindfulness*, that protects against the internalization of unrealistic beauty standards often seen on social media by disengaging individuals from automatic negative thoughts and judgments about their appearance (Pidgeon and Appleby 2014).

Coherently with these factors, more recently researchers in the field of social media and body image started to focus more on the role of self-compassion. Self-compassion involves treating oneself with kindness, understanding, and non-judgmental acceptance, particularly in moments of perceived inadequacy or failure and encourages individuals to recognize that suffering, imperfection, and personal struggles are part of the shared human experience (Neff 2003). Self-compassion has shown to be a key protective factor against the negative impacts of social media on body image as it reduces self-criticism and the pressure to meet unattainable beauty standards often propagated by social media platforms (Siegel et al. 2020). Self-compassion interventions, such as brief meditation practices or writing exercises, have been shown to effectively reduce body dissatisfaction and body shame, particularly in women. These interventions help shift the focus from appearance-based self-worth to a more holistic appreciation of oneself (Albertson et al. 2015). Studies have demonstrated that even short-term interventions, such as a 3-week self-compassion meditation program, can significantly improve body image and self-acceptance. Participants in such programs reported lasting increases in body appreciation and decreases in body dissatisfaction and other negative outcomes, as well as reduced engagement in harmful comparisons on social media (Davies et al. 2024, Davies et al. 2023, Gobin et al. 2022, Maohn and Hevey 2023, Turk et al. 2022).

Furthermore, a crucial role is played by social media literacy (Paxton et al. 2022) whose key aspect is teaching individuals to recognize the extent of digital manipulation involved in media content, such as photo editing and filters. This awareness reduces the internalization of the thin ideal by revealing that many media images are highly stylized and unattainable in real life (McLean et al. 2015). As a matter of fact, studies indeed showed that interventions highlighting the artificial nature of media images can protect individuals, and in particular adolescents, from engaging in harmful social comparisons, which are linked to increased body dissatisfaction. As a result, media literacy interventions were increasingly recognized as an effective tool to prevent body dissatisfaction and mitigate the harmful effects of media exposure, particularly regarding the portrayal of idealized body images (McLean et al. 2016, Paxton et al. 2022). These interventions, indeed, focus on developing critical thinking skills that enable individuals to analyze and deconstruct media messages, fostering a deeper understanding of the unrealistic beauty standards often promoted on social media platforms (McLean et al. 2016). By empowering individuals to critically evaluate media, these interventions not only reduce the risk of body dissatisfaction but also decrease the likelihood of engaging in disordered eating (Bennet et al. 2023).

These strategies for mitigating the negative effects of social media on body image and promoting a more compassionate, balanced self-perception are promising, and it is recommended that future interventions incorporate them.

Conclusion

Overall, the chapter underscores how photo-based social media engagement can exacerbate body dissatisfaction, especially through appearance-focused activities like selfie-editing and photo investment. These behaviors not only influence self-perception but also correlate with broader psychological outcomes such as anxiety, depression, and disordered eating. However, protective strategies, including self-compassion and media literacy, can mitigate these effects and foster a healthier relationship with one's body. Understanding these dynamics is essential for developing effective interventions aimed at promoting positive body image in the digital age.

References

Albertson, E.R., K.D. Neff and K.E. Dill-Shackleford. 2015. Self-compassion and body dissatisfaction in women: A randomized controlled trial of a brief meditation intervention. Mindfulness 6: 444–454.

Aldosari, B. 2020. Do filters and pose in selfies have an effect on cosmetic procedures. Saudi J. Otorhinolaryngol. Head Neck Surg. 22: 21–23.

Bennett, B.L., P. Pokhrel and J.D. Latner. 2023. Delivering a media literacy intervention for body dissatisfaction using an app-based intervention: A feasibility and pilot trial. Eat. Behav. 50: 101770.

Boursier, V. and V. Manna. 2018. Selfie expectancies among adolescents: Construction and validation of an instrument to assess expectancies toward selfies among boys and girls. Front. Psychol. 9: 1–14.

Casale, S., G. Gemelli, C. Calosi, B. Giangrasso and G. Fioravanti. 2019. Multiple exposure to appearance-focused real accounts on Instagram: Effects on body image among both genders. Curr. Psychol. 40: 2877–2886.

Casale, S., C. Pettini, G. Fioravanti, M. Padovani and S. Ghinassi. 2024. The link between Problematic Instagram Use and body-image investment dimensions: the mediating role of social comparison on Instagram and the need to conceal body flaws. Clin. Neuropsychiatry 21: 79.

Caso, D., G. Schettino, R. Fabbricatore and M. Conner. 2020. "Change my selfie": Relationships between self-objectification and selfie-behavior in young Italian women. J. Appl. Soc. Psychol. 50: 538–549.

Chang, L., P. Li, R.S.M. Loh and T.H.H. Chua. 2019. A study of Singapore adolescent girls' selfie practices, peer appearance comparisons, and body esteem on Instagram. Body Image 29: 90–99.

Chen, J., M. Ishii, K.L. Bater, H. Darrach, D. Liao, P.P. Huynh et al. 2019. Association between the use of social media and photograph editing applications, self-esteem, and cosmetic surgery acceptance. JAMA Facial Plast. Surg. 21: 361–367.

Chua, T.H.H. and L. Chang. 2016. Follow me and like my beautiful selfies: Singapore teenage girls' engagement in self-presentation and peer comparison on social media. Comput. Hum. Behav. 55: 190–197.

Cohen, R., T. Newton-John and A. Slater. 2018. 'Selfie'-objectification: The role of selfies in self-objectification and disordered eating in young women. Comput. Hum. Behav. 79: 68–74.

Davies, B., M. Turner and J. Udell. 2023. Are humorous or distractor images more effective than self-compassion messages for combatting the negative body image consequences of social media? An experimental test of possible micro-intervention stimuli. Body Image 46: 356–371.

Davies, B., M. Turner and J. Udell. 2024. It helps to be funny or compassionate: An exploration of user experiences and evaluation of social media micro-intervention designs for protecting body image. Comput. Hum. Behav. 150: 107999.

Di Gesto, C., A. Nerini, G.R. Policardo and C. Matera. 2022. Predictors of acceptance of cosmetic surgery: Instagram images-based activities, appearance comparison and body dissatisfaction among women. Aesthetic Plast. Surg.: 1–11.

Fardouly, J. and L.R. Vartanian. 2015. Negative comparisons about one's appearance mediate the relationship between Facebook usage and body image concerns. Body Image 12: 82–88.

Fredrickson, B.L. and T.A. Roberts. 1997. Objectification theory: Toward understanding women's lived experiences and mental health risks. Psychol. Women Q. 21: 173–206.

Gioia, F., S.A. McLean, V. Rega and V. Boursier. 2024. What about young adults' photo manipulation activity? The predictive role of body shame and the mediating effect of body esteem. Curr. Psychol. 43: 10418–10433.

Gobin, K.C., S.E. McComb and J.S. Mills. 2022. Testing a self-compassion micro-intervention before appearance-based social media use: Implications for body image. Body Image 40: 200–206.

Office of the Assistant Secretary for Health (OASH). 2023. Surgeon General Issues New Advisory About Effects Social Media Use Has on Youth Mental Health. [Internet]. [cited 2024 September 6]. Available from: https://www.hhs.gov/about/news/2023/05/23/surgeon-general-issues-new-advisory-about-effects-social-media-use-has-youth-mental-health.html.

International Society of Aesthetic Plastic Surgery. 2022. Global survey 2022. https://www.isaps.org/discover/about-isaps/global-statistics/global-survey-2022-full-report-and-press-releases/.

Kim, J.W. and T.M. Chock. 2017. Personality traits and psychological motivations predicting selfie posting behaviors on social networking sites. Telemat. Inform. 34: 560–571.

Lamp, S.J., A. Cugle, A.L. Silverman, M.T. Thomas, M. Liss and M.J. Erchull. 2019. Picture perfect: The relationship between selfie behaviors, self-objectification, and depressive symptoms. Sex Roles 81: 704–712.

Lim, W.M. 2016. Understanding the selfie phenomenon: current insights and future research directions. Eur. J. Mark. 50: 1773–1788.

Lyu, Z., Y. Wang, C. Chen and P. Zheng. 2023. Selfie behavior and cosmetic surgery consideration in adolescents: the mediating roles of physical appearance comparisons and facial appearance concern. Psychol. Health Med. 28: 2273–2285.

Lonergan, A.R., K. Bussey, J. Fardouly, S. Griffiths, S.B. Murray, P. Hay et al. 2020. Protect me from my selfie: Examining the association between photo-based social media behaviors and self-reported eating disorders in adolescence. Int. J. Eat. Disord. 53: 755–766.

Lonergan, A.R., K. Bussey, J. Mond, O. Brown, S. Griffiths, S.B. Murray et al. 2019. Me, my selfie, and I: The relationship between editing and posting selfies and body dissatisfaction in men and women. Body Image 28: 39–43.

Mahon, C. and D. Hevey. 2023. Pilot trial of a self-compassion intervention to address adolescents' social media-related body image concerns. Clin. Child Psychol. Psychiatry 28: 307–322.

Marengo, D., C. Longobardi, M.A. Fabris and M. Settanni. 2018. Highly-visual social media and internalizing symptoms in adolescence: The mediating role of body image concerns. Comput. Hum. Behav. 82: 63–69.

McLean, S.A., S.J. Paxton, E.H. Wertheim and J. Masters. 2015. Photoshopping the selfie: Self photo editing and photo investment are associated with body dissatisfaction in adolescent girls. Int. J. Eat. Disord. 48: 1132–1140.

McLean, S.A., S.J. Paxton and E.H. Wertheim. 2016. The role of media literacy in body dissatisfaction and disordered eating: A systematic review. Body Image 19: 9–23.

McLean, S.A., H.K. Jarman and R.F. Rodgers. 2019. How do "selfies" impact adolescents' well-being and body confidence? A narrative review. Psychol. Res. Behav. Manag.: 513–521.

Meier, E.P. and J. Gray. 2014. Facebook photo activity associated with body image disturbance in adolescent girls. Cyberpsychol. Behav. Soc. Netw. 17: 199–206.

Mendelson, B.K., M.J. Mendelson and D.R. White. 2001. Body Esteem Scale for adolescents and adults. J. Pers. Assess. 76: 90–106.

Mills, J.S., S. Musto, L. Williams and M. Tiggemann. 2018. "Selfie" harm: Effects on mood and body image in young women. Body Image 27: 86–92.

Mingoia, J., A.D. Hutchinson, D.H. Gleaves and C. Wilson. 2019. The relationship between posting and photo manipulation activities on social networking sites and internalization of a tanned ideal among Australian adolescents and young adults. Soc. Media Soc. 5: 1–10.

Modica, C.A. 2020. The associations between Instagram use, selfie activities, appearance comparison, and body dissatisfaction in adult men. Cyberpsychol. Behav. Soc. Netw. 23: 90–99.

Mustafa, S. and M. Akram. 2022. Self-consciousness, self-objectification, and social anxiety as predictors of photo editing behavior among emerging adults. Hum. Behav. Emerg. Technol. 2022: 6609752.

Myers, T.A. and J.H. Crowther. 2009. Social comparison as a predictor of body dissatisfaction: A meta-analytic review. J. Abnorm. Psychol. 118: 683–698.

Niu, G., L. Sun, Q. Liu, H. Chai, X. Sun and Z. Zhou. 2020. Selfie-posting and young adult women's restrained eating: The role of commentary on appearance and self-objectification. Sex Roles 82: 232–240.

Oxford Dictionaries. 2013. Oxford Dictionaries Word of the Year 2013. Oxford Dictionaries. Available at: http://blog.oxforddictionaries.com/press-releases/oxford-dictionaries-wordof-the-year-2013/.

Paxton, S.J., S.A. McLean and R.F. Rodgers. 2022. "My critical filter buffers your app filter": Social media literacy as a protective factor for body image. Body Image 40: 158–164.

Pham, H.C., L. Nguyen, T.A. Vu and P. Tran. 2022. Body image esteem and photo manipulation among social media users. Acta Inform. Pragensia 1: 62–79.

Pidgeon, A.M. and L. Appleby. 2014. Investigating the role of dispositional mindfulness as a protective factor for body image dissatisfaction among women. Curr. Res. Psychol. 52: 96.

Pittman, M. and B. Reich. 2016. Social media and loneliness: Why an Instagram picture may be worth more than a thousand Twitter words. Comput. Hum. Behav. 62: 155–167.

Rasmussen, E.E., N. Punyanunt-Carter, J.R. LaFreniere, M.S. Norman and T.G. Kimball. 2020. The serially mediated relationship between emerging adults' social media use and mental well-being. Comput. Hum. Behav. 102: 206–213.

Rodgers, R.F. and A. Rousseau. 2022. Social media and body image: Modulating effects of social identities and user characteristics. Body Image 41: 284–291.

Rousseau, A. 2021. Adolescents' selfie-activities and idealized online self-presentation: An application of the sociocultural model. Body Image 36: 16–26.

Saiphoo, A.N. and Z. Vahedi. 2019. A meta-analytic review of the relationship between social media use and body image disturbance. Comput. Hum. Behav. 101: 259–275.

Salomon, I. and C.S. Brown. 2019. The selfie generation: Examining the relationship between social media use and early adolescent body image. J. Early Adolesc. 39: 539–560.

Siegel, J.A., K.L. Huellemann, C.C. Hillier and L. Campbell. 2020. The protective role of self-compassion for women's positive body image: An open replication and extension. Body Image 32: 136–144.

Simon, P.D., S.M.O. Cu, K.E.M. De Jesus, N.T.S. Go, K.T.F. Lim and C.L.C. Say. 2022. Worried about being imperfect? The mediating effect of physical appearance perfectionism between Instagram addiction and body esteem. Pers. Individ. Dif. 186: 111346.

Statista Research Department. 2024, May 2. Distribution of Instagram users worldwide as of April 2024, by age group. Retrieved September 9, 2024. Available from; https://www.statista.com/statistics/325587/instagram-global-age-group/.

Sung, Y., J.A. Lee, E. Kim and S.M. Choi. 2016. Why we post selfies: Understanding motivations for posting pictures of oneself. Pers. Individ. Dif. 97: 260–265.

Tiggemann, M., I. Anderberg and Z. Brown. 2020. Uploading your best self: Selfie editing and body dissatisfaction. Body Image 33: 175–182.

Turk, F., S. Kellett and G. Waller. 2022. Comparing self-compassion versus body exposure for adult women with moderate to severe body dissatisfaction: A feasibility and pilot trial. Clin. Psychol. Psychother. 29: 1475–1480.

Varman, R.M., N. Van Spronsen, M. Ivos and J. Demke. 2021. Social media filter use and interest to pursue cosmetic facial plastic procedures. Am. J. Cosmet. Surg. 38: 181–186.

Veldhuis, J., J.M. Alleva, A.J. Bij de Vaate, M. Keijer and E.A. Konijn. 2020. Me, my selfie, and I: The relations between selfie behaviors, body image, self-objectification, and self-esteem in young women. Psychol. Pop. Media 9: 3.

Wang, Y., J. Yang, J. Wang, L. Yin and L. Lei. 2020. Body talk on social networking sites and body dissatisfaction among young women: A moderated mediation model of peer appearance pressure and self-compassion. Curr. Psychol. 1–11.

Wang, Y., X. Xie, J. Fardouly, L.R. Vartanian and L. Lei. 2021. The longitudinal and reciprocal relationships between selfie-related behaviors and self-objectification and appearance concerns among adolescents. New Media Soc. 23: 56–77.

Zerhouni, O., V. Flaudias, M. Barré and R.F. Rodgers. 2022. The effects of exposure to social media images of thin and average size women on body satisfaction among young women: Emotion regulation and self-efficacy as modulating factors. Body Image 43: 292–300.

Chapter 2

The Role of Self-Compassion in Body Image

Diana Burychka,[1,2,3,*] *Marta Miragall*[1,2,3] and *Rosa Mª Baños*[1,2,3]

INTRODUCTION

Body perception disturbance (BPD), including body dissatisfaction or perceptual distortions, plays a crucial role in both the onset and maintenance of eating disorders (EDs) (Glashouwer et al. 2019). Extensive evidence shows that these concerns can lead individuals, particularly women, to engage in body surveillance and unhealthy eating behaviors in pursuit of the thin ideal (Fredrickson and Roberts 1997, McKinley and Hyde 1996). Given the adverse consequences associated with BPD, fostering resilience against the Western beauty standards can improve the effectiveness of the prevention and early intervention programs of EDs (Levine and Smolak 2016). Among the established protective factors, self-compassion has gained increased attention for helping to cope with negative body image (Braun et al. 2016) and to foster positive body image (Seekis et al. 2017).

In the following chapter, the protective role of self-compassion on body perceptions (BP) will be reviewed. To do so, the chapter will analyze: (1) the definition and theoretical foundations of the self-compassion construct; (2) the association between self-compassion and both negative and positive body image; (3) the effect of compassion-focused interventions on BP; and (4) the future research directions, identifying existing gaps and areas for further exploration.

[1] Department of Personality, Evaluation and Psychological Treatment, University of Valencia, Avenida Blasco Ibáñez, 21. 46010, Valencia, Spain.
[2] Polibienestar Research Institute, University of Valencia. Calle del Serpis, 29. 46022, València, Spain.
[3] CIBERObn Physiopathology of Obesity and Nutrition, Instituto de Salud Carlos III, Madrid, Spain.
Emails: marta.miragall@uv.es, rosa.banos@uv.es
* Corresponding author: diana.burychka@uv.es

DOI: 10.1201/9781032718125-3

1. Definition of self-compassion

Self-compassion—defined as a kind and non-judgmental attitude towards oneself as well as the acceptance of one's flaws or failures (Neff 2003a)—has been found to significantly contribute to the reduction of stress, anxiety and depression (Neff and Germer 2013) and to promote adaptive psychological functioning such as self-soothing behaviors and adaptive emotional regulation (Inwood and Ferrari 2018). Self-compassion may also help to buffer individual's responses during situations that may challenge self-assessment (Neff 2003a).

Meta-analyses carried out across diverse age groups consistently show an inverse relationship between self-compassion and various mental health concerns (e.g., suicidal thoughts and behaviors or anxiety), with effect sizes ranging from moderate to large (e.g., Ferrari et al. 2019). Research points out that men, compared to women, generally report higher self-compassion levels (Yarnell et al. 2015). Among women, the lower self-compassion levels are often accompanied by higher levels of self-criticism and a tendency to overidentify with negative emotions (Neff 2003b).

Regarding dysfunctional eating attitudes and behaviors (DEAB), self-compassion has also emerged as a promising protective factor across clinical and non-clinical populations (e.g., Braun et al. 2016). By fostering feelings of being cared for, connected to others and emotionally at ease, a self compassionate attitude helps to decrease body-related distress particularly when confronted with BP threats (Gilbert 2009).

2. Theoretical models of self-compassion

Two leading theories of self-compassion are discussed in literature.

2.1 Self-compassion model

Rooted in Buddhist psychology, Neff's self-compassion framework (2003a) emphasizes treating oneself with the same kindness and understanding that one would offer a friend in distress identifying three main components:

- **Self-kindness** (vs. self-judgment) in moments of failure or imperfection, instead of being self-critical, self-compassion encourages individuals to be kind and understanding towards themselves. Self-kindness can contribute to healthy coping mechanisms (e.g., balanced eating patterns) when faced with body-related distress.
- **Common humanity** (vs. isolation) involves recognizing that suffering and imperfection are part of the shared human experience. For individuals struggling with BP concerns, understanding this may help to decrease feelings of isolation and shame by interpreting the body-related concerns as part of a universal human experience.
- **Mindfulness** (vs. over-identification) refers to observing one's painful thoughts and emotions without becoming overwhelmed or over-identified with them. This

component helps to keep a healthy approach to eating behaviors and physical appearance by decreasing the intensity of negative body-related thoughts and, as a result, fostering healthier psychological functioning (e.g., adaptive emotional regulation).

This perspective on self-compassion has been found to protect against maladaptive psychological traits, such as emotional distress, while fostering a more adaptive way to managing eating behaviors and body-related concerns (Neff 2003a).

2.2 Social mentality theory and compassionate mind model

As an alternative approach to Neff's model (2003a), Gilbert's framework for understanding self-compassion is grounded in evolutionary psychology, incorporating insights from evolutionary biology, neurobiology and attachment theory. The Social Mentality Theory—developed to explain the evolutionary basis of emotions like compassion and their role in management of social interaction or roles—and the Compassionate Mind Model—a practical model to promote compassion in therapeutic contexts—(Gilbert 2010) highlight the importance of recognizing suffering and nurturing a motivation to alleviate it. Both models integrate three primary emotion-regulation systems—threat, drive, and safeness—that explain individual's responses to stressors:

- **The threat-protection system** is activated in response to perceived internal or external threats triggering defensive responses such as fight-or-flight. In the field of body image, this system becomes active when individuals engage in appearance comparison or receive negative comments from others that lead to feelings of inadequacy.
- **The drive system** generates positive emotions that motivate goal-oriented behaviors and resource-seeking to reach personal aspirations. In the field of body image, this can manifest as an attempt to reach certain appearance ideals (e.g., thin ideal).
- **The safeness-soothing system** plays a central role in calming/deactivating the threat response by fostering emotional balance through compassion. This system is associated with feelings of ease, attachment and social connection to mitigate the isolating effects of body-related shame.

This model facilitates adaptive emotional regulation by fostering balance among these three systems. Practicing self-compassion helps to deactivate the threat response, reduce the feelings of shame and cultivate social connectedness (Gilbert 2009).

Moreover, the Compassion-Focused Therapy model (Gilbert 2009) has incorporated the construct of "fear of compassion" as a barrier to compassion that arises from evolutionary survival mechanisms. Considering the attachment theory, individuals with insecure attachment styles may find emotional closeness distressing as it may trigger memories of negative relationships from the past and reactivate their fears of intimacy (Gilbert et al. 2011). As a result, these beliefs that one is unworthy of kindness, the concerns about being perceived as weak, and the fear of vulnerability can prevent individuals from being able to accept self-compassionate attitudes (Gilbert 2010). Thus, addressing fears of compassion early in treatment and promoting self-compassion is key to developing effective interventions for BPD and disordered eating (Kirby et al. 2024).

3. Body compassion: A specific approach to self-compassion in body image

The concept of body compassion has gained attention in recent years. Combining the constructs of body image and self-compassion, this construct is defined as the attitude of specifically focusing compassion on one's body. This concept emphasizes the importance of treating the body with kindness and understanding, particularly in response to perceived flaws or societal pressures regarding one's appearance (Altman et al. 2020). Although relatively new, emerging evidence highlights the potential role of body compassion in promoting healthier BP. For instance, Oliveira et al. (2018) reported that body compassion moderated the impact of general shame on body-related shame as well as on disordered eating. Further supporting these findings, studies such as by de Carvalho Barreto et al. (2020) indicated that body compassion mediated the relationship between self-compassion and disordered eating behaviors. Additionally, research has identified an inverse association between body compassion and binge eating symptoms among Portuguese women (Barata-Santos et al. 2019), physique anxiety (Abdollahi et al. 2023) or body image shame and appearance anxiety (Khanjani et al. 2025) in Irani women. Finally, Burychka et al. (2024) highlighted body compassion's protective effects on body dissatisfaction and disordered eating. However, although these findings are promising, longitudinal studies are needed to better establish the distinct clinical value of body compassion beyond general self-compassion.

3.1 The role of self-compassion in body image

Over the past decade, research has extensively focused on the potential of self-compassion-based interventions to decrease the risk factors for DEAB (e.g., body dissatisfaction) as well as to foster positive body image dimensions (e.g., body appreciation) (Linardon et al. 2024). Theoretical frameworks suggest that self-compassion can act as a direct predictor, mediator or moderator among the body-image related constructs. Nonetheless, according to Tylka et al. (2015), it is highly probable that self-compassion influences body image through multiple concurrent pathways. To further clarify these relationships, a deeper understanding of the mechanisms underlying self-compassion's effects on negative and positive body image is essential.

The following section reviews key findings on specific dimensions of negative and positive body image that are significantly associated with self-compassion.

3.2 The role of self-compassion in reducing negative body image

Self-compassion can effectively mitigate established risk factors for disordered eating and negative body image while also having a preventive role in the development of ED-related issues (Braun et al. 2016).

Drive for thinness and thin-ideal internalization. Sociocultural theory affirms that societal appearance ideals, such as the thin ideal for women and a muscular ideal for men, are disseminated through a variety of sources (e.g., media, family, and peers), being a significant risk factor for body dissatisfaction and disordered eating (Thompson et al. 1999). Research indicates that self-compassion acts as a buffer against societal pressures on the drive for thinness (Ferreira et al. 2013, Tylka et al. 2015) or the muscular body ideal (Maher et al. 2021). Regarding the societal pressures, evidence indicates that self-compassion can reduce the effects of critical family comments on body concerns among undergraduate women (Daye et al. 2014). Thøgersen-Ntoumani et al. (2017) also found that self-compassion was associated with lower drive for thinness and social physique anxiety, emphasizing its protective role in young women even in the presence of upward social comparisons. Similarly, Ferreira et al. (2013) found that self-compassion was also associated with a lower drive for thinness in women diagnosed with EDs.

Body and weight concerns. Higher self-compassion levels have been associated with less weight and shape concerns, helping individuals to value themselves for their intrinsic worth rather than appearances and, thus, helping them to resist internalizing harmful standards. For example, self-compassion has been associated with less body concerns in undergraduate women and to mediate the relationship between body concerns and depressive symptoms (Wasylkiw et al. 2012). Self-compassion also buffers the relationship between body mass index and weight concerns, specifically among young women with higher body mass index (Kelly et al. 2014). This suggests that self-compassion may allow individuals to approach their bodies with acceptance and decreased self-criticism (Wasylkiw et al. 2012).

Body surveillance and body shame. Theories such as objectified body consciousness (McKinley and Hyde 1996) and objectification theory (Fredrickson and Roberts 1997) posit that individuals, especially women, are socialized to perceive their bodies as objects to be evaluated based on appearance. This self-objectification—defined as a state where individuals internalize an external observer's perspective—leads individuals to continuously monitor their appearance (i.e., body surveillance) in pursuit of appearance ideals. The surveillance of one's body in order to reach the thin ideal not only is a risk factor for the development of an ED but it also contributes to body-related shame (Fredrickson and Roberts 1997, McKinley and Hyde 1996). Body shame—defined as negative feelings directed at one's body that are shaped by both external (others' perceptions) and internal (self-critical) judgments (Gilbert 2011) is one of the main factors that contribute to EDs (Nechita et al. 2021). Research has found that higher self-compassion is negatively associated with body surveillance and body shame (Braun et al. 2016). In their systematic review, Braun et al. (2016) established that self-compassion acts as a buffer against the harmful

BP-related threats by promoting kindness and understanding toward oneself, which can help individuals resist negative self-evaluation. Furthermore, by fostering mindful acceptance of distressing emotions, self-compassion allows individuals to confront and to adaptively process these emotions (Ferreira et al. 2013). Self-compassionate protective processes can disrupt the cycle of negative self-evaluation (Goss and Allan 2010), protecting against body-related shame.

Disordered eating. Self-compassion has also gathered evidence as a protective factor against disordered eating behaviors in both non-clinical and clinical populations (Braun et al. 2016). Individuals with higher levels of self-compassion report fewer symptoms of disordered eating such as binge eating and dietary restrictions. For instance, experimental research has indicated that self-compassionate practices reduce eating-related distress and promote mindful eating (Adams and Leary 2007). A systematic review by Sarda et al. (2025) further indicated that self-compassion could buffer or interrupt the impact of social media on self-objectifications and BPD. Furthermore, in populations receiving treatment for EDs, individuals with higher self-compassion levels experienced better treatment outcomes (Kelly et al. 2014). Regarding the buffering effect of compassion on risk factors, self-compassion may act as both a moderator and a mediator in the pathways leading to lower BPD and DEAB. Self-compassion can decrease the strength of the association between external pressures to achieve thinness and appearance comparisons (e.g., Lonergan et al. 2019). Moreover, self-compassion mediates the relationship between risk factors (i.e., shame and perfectionism) and BPD (e.g., drive for thinness) or DEAB (Braun et al. 2016) in both clinical and non-clinical populations of women (Ferreira et al. 2013).

3.3 The role of self-compassion in fostering positive body image

Positive body image, which involves a loving and respectful attitude toward one's body, appreciating its uniqueness and functionality, and emphasizing one's body's assets rather than dwelling on its imperfections (Webb et al. 2015), is supported by self-compassion's core principles (Neff 2003a). A self-compassionate attitude can foster a development of a balanced and accepting view of the own body, contributing to individual's well-being (Turk and Waller 2020).

Body appreciation. Body appreciation is defined as the acceptance, respect and gratitude individuals have for their bodies with independence of the ideals promoted by society (Avalos et al. 2005). Self-compassion has been shown to positively influence body appreciation by fostering a shift away from critical self-evaluation towards a more supportive and understanding mindset (Homan and Tylka 2015). Sullivan et al. (2024) found that self-compassionate texts and body-positive contents improved body appreciation in undergraduates. This shift from the appearance-based comparison allows individuals to appreciate their bodies for their inherent worth and to resist societal standards of beauty (Andrew et al. 2016).

Body image flexibility. Body image flexibility involves accepting negative body-related thoughts and emotions without avoiding or modifying them (Sandoz et al. 2013). Self-compassion supports body image flexibility by promoting non-judgmental awareness and reducing self-criticism regarding body-related experiences (e.g., Daye et al. 2014). Kelly et al. (2014) showed that self-compassion moderated the impact of body mass index on body image flexibility resulting in lesser weight-related concerns. Linardon et al. (2024) also provided evidence supporting the efficacy of self-compassion training in boosting body image flexibility and reducing internalized self-criticism.

Adaptive eating behaviors. Adaptive eating behaviors—defined by mindful and intuitive eating practices that respond to internal hunger and satiety cues—are also positively associated with self-compassion (Kelly and Stephen 2016). Similarly, a tree week self-compassion-based intuitive eating intervention led to an increase in body appreciation, self-compassion and intuitive eating, with gains maintained at one month (Liu et al. 2025). Through these processes, individuals learn to engage in eating behaviors that reflect their bodily needs instead of responding to emotional or societal pressures by engaging in maladaptive eating behaviors. The mindfulness component of self-compassion has been shown to improve adaptive or intuitive eating, enhancing body satisfaction and reducing the likelihood of disordered eating (Kelly and Stephen 2016). These findings suggest that fostering a kinder relationship with oneself may support healthier eating patterns guided by internal cues.

4. Self-compassion-focused interventions

Self-compassion interventions show from moderate to large effects on the increase in self-compassion scores, supporting self-compassion as a flexible construct that can be cultivated (Ferrari et al. 2019). In the literature, two primary evidence-supported interventions related to self-compassion—Mindful Self-Compassion (Neff and Germer 2013) and Compassion-Focused Therapy (Gilbert 2009)—have been adapted for their study in the field of body perceptions and DEAB. On the one hand, the Mindful Self-Compassion, an 8-week program, designed to promote mindfulness and compassion in daily life based on Buddhist approach. Primarily elaborated for non-clinical populations, Mindful Self-Compassion program teaches individuals to respond to their flaws and failures with kindness and to manage emotional distress by cultivating a compassionate inner voice. The program covers topics like core values, emotional resilience and body acceptance through activities such as meditation, mindful eating or silent retreats. Research has shown that Mindful Self-Compassion can significantly enhance self-compassion, life satisfaction, and emotional well-being, while also reducing anxiety, stress, and depressive symptoms (Neff and Germer 2013). On the other hand, the Compassion-Focused Therapy extends the foundational principles of Compassionate Mind Model and integrates practices from attachment theory, affective neuroscience and cognitive-behavioral therapy. The Compassion-Focused Therapy is particularly effective for individuals struggling with self-criticism, shame and negative self-perceptions that are common among individuals with disordered eating. According to Gilbert's affect regulation systems (2009), individuals with high levels of shame and self-criticism often have limited access to the affiliative-soothing system and are led by the highly activated threat system. Through compassionate imagery, breathing exercises, and self-soothing practices, Compassion-Focused Therapy may promote the development of a self-compassionate identity, and, as a result, decrease the impact of psychological distress. In the field of EDs, the specific format of Compassion-Focused Therapy for EDs has been designed to address onset and maintenance factors in EDs while teaching practical skills to address disordered thoughts, feelings and behaviors. Compassion-Focused Therapy for EDs aims to regulate eating patterns and help to restore weight by fostering self-soothing and self-compassionate responses. Learning new self-compassionate ways of managing body-related threats (e.g., social criticism due to weight gain) can be particularly effective for individuals with internalized shame and self-blame as well as disordered eating, leading to reduced DEAB and an improvement in individual's relationship with food and their body (Goss and Allan 2010).

The practices derived from the Mindful Self-Compassion and Compassion-Focused Therapy for EDs have been further tested to examine their role in relation to several positive and negative body image dimensions. In order to do so, the aforementioned self-compassion interventions have been widely adapted to a variety of formats, modalities and durations. Current evidence from recent meta-analyses and reviews (e.g., Ferrari et al. 2019, Turk and Waller 2020) supports the effectiveness of these self-compassion interventions in improving body perceptions. The following section discusses different adaptations of self-compassion interventions and their impact on body perceptions and related psychological outcomes.

4.1 Self-guided interventions

Audio-based meditations for cultivating self-compassion. Self-compassion guided audio meditations, such as compassionate body scan, affectionate breathing and loving-kindness practices, help individuals develop more kind and accepting attitude toward their bodies. Several studies have explored this approach by adapting Neff and Germer's (2013) Mindful Self-Compassion meditations into daily podcasts. Albertson et al. (2015) found that a three-week self-compassion meditation intervention led to significant improvements in body appreciation and reductions in body dissatisfaction, body shame, and appearance-based self-worth, and these benefits were maintained for three months. Papini et al. (2022) extended these findings to pregnant and postpartum women, finding significant reductions in body shame and body dissatisfaction and an increase in body appreciation. Toole and Craighead (2016) tested a shorter one-week version of the intervention among undergraduate women. Participants began with an in-lab session for baseline measures and the first meditation, afterwards they received daily links to the three guided practices. They found increases in body appreciation and decreases in body surveillance; however, body shame and dissatisfaction were not significantly affected. Nevertheless, in another brief audio self-compassion intervention designed to promote compassion (vs. nature-focused guided imagery group) (de Wet et al. 2020), young women in both conditions experienced improvements in self-compassion and body appreciation.

Although being a promising approach, these findings highlight the need for further research to improve the effect of these audio interventions on BP outcomes.

Writing-based meditations for cultivating self-compassion. Writing-based self-compassion exercises, such as self-compassionate diaries or compassionate letters, help individuals shift from negative self-perceptions to a more kind and understanding view of their bodies. For example, Moffitt et al. (2018) found that self-compassionate writing (i.e., expressing compassion toward body shape, weight, and appearance) improved affective states, especially in those women with high body dissatisfaction. Similarly, Gobin et al. (2022) reported reduced body dissatisfaction after women completed a brief three-minute writing task following exposure to thin-ideal media. In line with these findings, Li et al. (2025) showed that self-compassion writing (vs. Mindful breathing) effectively protected body image after appearance-focused social media exposure, improving state body image, particularly among wound women with high self-objectification. Gracias and Stutts (2024) further highlighted the effectiveness of compassionate writing (both self-compassion and compassion directed on others) on decreasing body dissatisfaction and fat phobia among women. Furthermore, Nightingale and Cassin (2023) study confirmed that self-compassion writing may also have benefits in women with higher body mass index and weight bias internalization. Barbeau et al. (2021) found that the self-compassion writing condition (vs. self-esteem condition) significantly reduced the emphasis on weight and appearance as a source of self-worth. Additionally, writing exercises focused on self-compassion and self-esteem have been shown to improve body image in men, including sexual minority groups (Grey et al. 2022). In the case of positive body image, short exercises of writing have shown to enhance body appreciation (Seekis et al. 2017) and adaptive eating behaviors (Kelly and Stephen 2016). For women with anorexia nervosa, self-compassion writing has also shown to help in reducing body-related shame and fear of self-compassion (Kelly and Waring 2018).

Digital self-compassion interventions. Digital interventions are commonly self-guided structured lessons or modules supported by websites or smartphone applications. A recent meta-analysis conducted by Conboy et al. (2024) showed that digital body image interventions were found to be effective in improving global body satisfaction and reducing cognitive body dissatisfaction in non-clinical adult women. These interventions showed small to medium effect sizes suggesting that digital interventions can be a viable tool for addressing body dissatisfaction that are unable to access conventional treatment. Intervention type (e.g., psychoeducation, cognitive dissonance, media literacy, body and self-compassion) was not found to be a statistically significant moderator, which may suggest that a range of intervention types can produce similar reductions in body dissatisfaction. Compassion-focused digital interventions have proven to be effective in improving BP. For instance, a 10-week intervention for women increased self-compassion and reduced self-judgment, perfectionism and shame, with effects maintained at a one-month follow-up (Nadeau et al. 2021). Additionally, other studies have shown that these interventions can increase appearance esteem in adolescents (Rodgers et al. 2018).

Recently, these interventions have been found to be particularly in addressing BP threats related to social media. Ong and Sündermann (2022) assessed a self-guided mHealth app focused on body image and self-compassion over a nine-day period in young adult university students. The program included activities aimed at enhancing media literacy, minimizing appearance-based comparisons, and fostering greater self-compassion. Female participants reported notable reductions in body dissatisfaction, along with improvements in body appreciation and self-compassion. Moreover, Davies et al. (2024) showed that appearance-related self-compassion messages, as part of social media micro-interventions, were the most effective at enhancing body satisfaction. Nevertheless, despite their potential, improving engagement strategies and delivery methods is necessary to enhance their effectiveness (Toole and Craighead 2016).

Group-based self-compassion interventions. Group-based self-compassion interventions have shown promise in addressing BP issues and disordered eating. The Bodies in Motion program (Voelker et al. 2019) for female athletes combines self-compassion and cognitive dissonance to promote healthier responses to appearance pressures and sports-related body expectations. Participants, guided to challenge unrealistic body ideals and to cultivate a kind, nonjudgmental self-view, reported significant reductions in thin-ideal internalization. Self-compassion online group programs, such as the SMART program, a five-week social media resilience training for adolescents, have also improved body appreciation and reduced self-criticism in this sample, with effects maintained at a three-month follow-up (Mahon and Hevey 2023). Lastly, a recent pilot trial showed that a brief self-compassion intervention can lead to reduced body shame and body surveillance in women with internalized weight bias (Haley et al. 2025), highlighting the potential value of group approaches for populations affected by weight stigma.

Additionally, programs targeting DEAB have proven effective. The BEfree program for binge eating disorder (Pinto-Gouveia et al. 2017)—which combines psychoeducation, mindfulness and self-compassion to help participants manage emotional triggers and reduce binge eating behaviors in twelve sessions—showed significant reductions in binge eating symptoms and psychological distress. Its digital adaptation, eBEfree app, recently extended these benefits, showing significant decreases in binge eating symptoms, self-criticism and BMI, with effects maintained at 26-weeks follow-up (Serna et al. 2025). Similarly, Duarte et al. (2017) implemented a low-intensity four-week online group program that improved binge eating symptoms, self-criticism, and body image flexibility in women diagnosed with binge eating. Recent evidence also highlights benefits on positive mental health in women with anorexia nervosa: in a two-week diary study, higher self-compassion was associated with greater positive affect and social safeness (Katan et al. 2025).

5. Future directions

The field of self-compassion research in BP has grown significantly over recent decades, yet important theoretical and methodological considerations remain to fully elucidate the role of self-compassion in BP. Future research should aim to diversify participant demographics, extending beyond the WEIRD samples that are predominantly young, White, cisgender and female (Egbert et al. 2024), to include men, transgender individuals and individuals across various racial, socio-economic and age groups as a way to generalize the findings. Furthermore, longitudinal research designs are essential to clarify the sustained impact of self-compassion on body image (Turk et al. 2021).

Moreover, specific positive body image dimensions –such as body appreciation or body functionality—should also be examined independently to determine which aspects are most closely influenced by self-compassion practice. Additionally, future studies should also explore the mechanisms underlying self-compassion's effectiveness in body image interventions. This includes exploring resistance to self-compassion as a potential therapeutic barrier and addressing fears associated with self-compassionate practice, as these may play a role in the BP-related intervention outcomes (Geller et al. 2019).

Conclusion

In conclusion, research indicates that individuals with higher levels of self-compassion are more likely to respond to perceived body flaws with kindness and warmth, recognizing the unattainable nature of societal standards while maintaining a mindful awareness of their emotions and thoughts. Rather than feeling isolated in their body distress or avoiding negative emotions, self-compassion enables a more supportive and adaptive response. Addressing these areas in future research and practice will contribute to the development of self-compassion-based interventions that will effectively promote positive body image, improving BPD and prevent DEAB.

Acknowledgements

This work was supported by the project BODY-R-VALUED, funded by the Ministry of Science, Innovation, and Universities, with reference number PID2023-148700OB-I00, as well as CIBEROBN, an initiative of ISCIII (ISCIII CB06 03/0052).

References

Abdollahi, A., K.D.V. Prasad, N.S.G. Abdelrasheed, S.H. Alshahrani, S.J. Shoja, G.R.L. Al-Awsi et al. 2023. An investigation of relationships between body compassion, social physique anxiety and physical appearance perfectionism in young people from Iran. J. Eat. Disord. 11: 90.

Adams, C.E. and M.R. Leary. 2007. Promoting self-compassionate attitudes toward eating among restrictive and guilty eaters. J. Soc. Clin. Psychol. 26: 1120–1144.

Albertson, E.R., K.D. Neff and K.E. Dill-Shackleford. 2015. Self-compassion and body dissatisfaction in women: A randomized controlled trial of a brief meditation intervention. Mindfulness 6: 444–454.

Altman, J.K., K. Linfield, P.G. Salmon and A.O. Beacham. 2020. The body compassion scale: Development and initial validation. J. Health Psychol. 25: 439–449.

Andrew, R., M. Tiggemann and L. Clark. 2016. Predicting body appreciation in young women: An integrated model of positive body image. Body Image 18: 34–42.

Avalos, L., T.L. Tylka and N. Wood-Barcalow. 2005. The body appreciation scale: Development and psychometric evaluation. Body Image 2: 285–297.

Barata-Santos, M., J. Marta-Simões and C. Ferreira. 2019. Body compassion safeguards against the impact of major life events on binge eating. Appetite 134: 34–39.

Barbeau, K., C. Guertin, K. Boileau and L. Pelletier. 2022. The effects of self-compassion and self-esteem writing interventions on women's valuation of weight management goals, body appreciation, and eating behaviors. Psychol. Women Q. 46: 82–98.

Braun, T.D., C.L. Park and A. Gorin. 2016. Self-compassion, body image, and disordered eating: A review of the literature. Body Image 17: 117–131.

Burychka, D., M. Miragall and R.M. Baños. 2024. The role of body compassion in the risk of eating disorders: mediational effects of body appreciation and body shame. Psicothema 36: 36–45.

Conboy, L., J. Mingoia, A.D. Hutchinson, B.A. Reisinger and D.H. Gleaves. 2024. Digital body image interventions for adult women: A meta-analytic review. Body Image 51: 101776.

Davies, B., M. Turner and J. Udell. 2024. It helps to be funny or compassionate: An exploration of user experiences and evaluation of social media micro-intervention designs for protecting body image. Comput. Hum. Behav. 150: 107999.

Daye, C.A., J.B. Webb and N. Jafari. 2014. Exploring self-compassion as a refuge against recalling the body-related shaming of caregiver eating messages on dimensions of objectified body consciousness in college women. Body Image 11: 547–556.

de Carvalho Barreto, M., C. Ferreira, J. Marta-Simões and A.L. Mendes. 2020. Exploring the paths between self-compassionate attributes and actions, body compassion and disordered eating. Eat. Weight Disord. 25: 291–297.

de Wet, A.J., B.R. Lane and K.E. Mulgrew. 2020. A randomised controlled trial examining the effects of self-compassion meditations on women's body image. Body Image 35: 22–29.

Duarte, C., J. Pinto-Gouveia and R.J. Stubbs. 2017. Compassionate Attention and Regulation of Eating Behaviour: A pilot study of a brief low-intensity intervention for binge eating. Clin. Psychol. Psychother. 24: O1437–O1447.

Duarte, C., J. Pinto-Gouveia, C. Ferreira and D. Batista. 2015. Body image as a source of shame: A new measure for the assessment of the multifaceted nature of body image shame. Clin. Psychol. Psychother. 22: 656–666.

Egbert, A.H., R.A. Hunt, K.L. Williams, N.L. Burke and K.J. Mathis. 2022. Reporting racial and ethnic diversity in eating disorder research over the past 20 years. Int. J. Eat. Disord. 55(4): 455–462.

Ferrari, M., C. Hunt, A. Harrysunker, M.J. Abbott, A.P. Beath and D.A. Einstein. 2019. Self-compassion interventions and psychosocial outcomes: A meta-analysis of RCTs. Mindfulness 10: 1455–1473.

Ferreira, C., J. Pinto-Gouveia and C. Duarte. 2013. Self-compassion in the face of shame and body image dissatisfaction: Implications for eating disorders. Eat. Behav. 14: 207–210.

Fredrickson, B.L. and T.A. Roberts. 1997. Toward understanding women's lived experiences and mental health risks. Psychol. Women Q. 21: 173–206.

Gilbert, P. 2009. The Compassionate Mind: A New Approach to Life's Challenges. Constable, London.

Gilbert, P. 2010. An introduction to compassion-focused therapy in cognitive behavior therapy. Int. J. Cogn. Ther. 3: 97–112.

Gilbert, P., K. McEwan, M. Matos and A. Rivis. 2011. Fears of compassion: Development of three self-report measures. Psychol. Psychother. Theory Res. Pract. 84: 239–255.

Glashouwer, K.A., R.M. van der Veer, F. Adipatria et al. 2019. The role of body image disturbance in the onset, maintenance, and relapse of anorexia nervosa: A systematic review. Clin. Psychol. Rev. 74: 101771.

Gobin, K.C., S.E. McComb and J.S. Mills. 2022. Testing a self-compassion micro-intervention before appearance-based social media use: Implications for body image. Body Image 40: 200–206.

Goss, K. and S. Allan. 2010. Compassion focused therapy for eating disorders. Int. J. Cogn. Ther. 3: 141–158.

Gracias, K.R. and L.A. Stutts. 2024. The impact of compassion writing interventions on body dissatisfaction, self-compassion, and fat phobia. Mindfulness 15: 1793–1802.

Grey, W., E.A. Harris and S. Griffiths. 2022. A randomized controlled trial of a brief self-compassion intervention designed to improve the body image of sexual minority men. Body Image 42: 385–400.

Haley, E.N., C.L. Dolbier, L.C. Campbell, R.A. Carels and J.M. Braciszewski. 2025. Brief self compassion intervention for women of higher weight and internalised weight bias: a randomized pilot study. Int. J. Behav. Med. 32: 293–307.

Homan, K.J. and T.L. Tylka. 2015. Self-compassion moderates body comparison and appearance self-worth's inverse relationships with body appreciation. Body Image 15: 1–7.

Inwood, E. and M. Ferrari. 2018. Mechanisms of change in the relationship between self-compassion, emotion regulation, and mental health: A systematic review. Appl. Psychol. Health Well Being 10: 215–235.

Katan, A., A.C. Kelly and J. Geller. 2025. Self compassion promotes positive mental health in women with anorexia nervosa: a two week daily diary study. Eat. Disord. 33: 198–213.

Kelly, A.C. and E. Stephen. 2016. A daily diary study of self-compassion, body image, and eating behavior in female college students. Body Image 17: 152–160.

Kelly, A.C. and S.V. Waring. 2018. A feasibility study of a 2-week self-compassionate letter-writing intervention for nontreatment seeking individuals with typical and atypical anorexia nervosa. Int. J. Eat. Disord. 51: 1005–1009.

Kelly, A.C., K. Vimalakanthan and K.E. Miller. 2014. Self-compassion moderates the relationship between body mass index and both eating disorder pathology and body image flexibility. Body Image 11: 446–453.

Khanjani, S., A.A. Foroughi, A.A. Parvizifard, M. Soleymani Moghadam, M. Rajabi, P. Mojtahedzadeh et al. 2025. Evaluation of psychometric properties of the Persian version of the Body Compassion Scale: validation with clinical and nonclinical samples. J. Res. Med. Sci. 30: 12.

Kirby, J.N., A. Hoang and C.R. Crimston. 2024. A brief compassion-focused therapy intervention can increase moral expansiveness: A randomized controlled trial. Mindfulness 15: 282–294.

Levine, M.P. and L. Smolak. 2016. The role of protective factors in the prevention of negative body image and disordered eating. Eat. Disord. 24: 39–46.

Li, E., W. Cheng, H. Yuan and X. Gao. 2025. Protecting young women's body image from appearance based social media exposure: a comparative study of self compassion writing and mindful breathing interventions. J. Psychosom. Res. 192: 112121.

Linardon, J., R. Moffitt, C. Anderson and T.L. Tylka. 2024. Testing for longitudinal bidirectional associations between self-compassion, self-criticism, and positive body image components. Body Image 49: 101722.

Liu, Y., J. Zhou, Y. Wang and X. Zeng. 2025. Self compassion cultivates intuitive eating: A randomized controlled trial of a new intervention among Chinese adults. Curr. Psychol. 44: 1675–1685.

Lonergan, A.R., K. Bussey, J. Mond, O. Brown, S. Griffiths, S.B. Murray et al. 2019. Me, my selfie, and I: The relationship between editing and posting selfies and body dissatisfaction in men and women. Body Image 28: 39–43.

Maher, A.L., B.R. Lane and K.E. Mulgrew. 2021. Self-compassion and body dissatisfaction in men: Extension of the tripartite influence model. Psychol. Men Masculinities 22: 345.

Mahon, C. and D. Hevey. 2023. Pilot trial of a self-compassion intervention to address adolescents' social media-related body image concerns. Clin. Child Psychol. Psychiatry 28: 307–322.

McKinley, N.M. and J.S. Hyde. 1996. The objectified body consciousness scale: Development and validation. Psychol. Women Q. 20: 181–215.

Moffitt, R.L., D.L. Neumann and S.P. Williamson. 2018. Comparing the efficacy of a brief self-esteem and self-compassion intervention for state body dissatisfaction and self-improvement motivation. Body Image 27: 67–76.

Nadeau, M.M., N.A. Caporale-Berkowitz and A.B. Rochlen. 2021. Improving women's self-compassion through an online program: A randomized controlled trial. J. Couns. Dev. 99: 47–59.

Nechita, D.M., S. Bud and D. David. 2021. Shame and eating disorders symptoms: A meta-analysis. Int. J. Eat. Disord. 54: 1899–1945.

Neff, K. 2003a. Self-compassion: An alternative conceptualization of a healthy attitude toward oneself. Self Identity 2: 85–101.

Neff, K. 2003b. The development and validation of a scale to measure self-compassion. Self Identity 2: 223–250. https://doi.org/10.1080/15298860309027.

Neff, K.D. and C.K. Germer. 2013. A pilot study and randomized controlled trial of the mindful self-compassion program. J. Clin. Psychol. 69: 28–44.

Nightingale, B.A. and S.E. Cassin. 2023. Self-compassion may have benefits for body image among women with a higher body mass index and internalized weight bias. Healthcare 11: 970.

Oliveira, S., I.A. Trindade and C. Ferreira. 2018. The buffer effect of body compassion on the association between shame and body and eating difficulties. Appetite 125: 118–123.
Ong, W.Y. and O. Sündermann, 2022. Efficacy of the mental health app "Intellect" to improve body image and self-compassion in young adults: A randomized controlled trial with a 4-week follow-up. JMIR Mhealth Uhealth 10(11): e41800.
Papini, N.M., T.B. Mason, S.D. Herrmann and N.V. Lopez. 2022. Self-compassion and body image in pregnancy and postpartum: A randomized pilot trial of a brief self-compassion meditation intervention. Body Image 43: 264–274.
Pinto-Gouveia, J., S.A. Carvalho, L. Palmeira, P. Castilho, C. Duarte, C. Ferreira et al. 2017. BEfree: A new psychological program for binge eating that integrates psychoeducation, mindfulness, and compassion. Clin. Psychol. Psychother. 24: 1090–1098.
Rodgers, R.F., E. Donovan, T. Cousineau, K. Yates, K. McGowan, E. Cook et al. 2018. BodiMojo: efficacy of a mobile-based intervention in improving body image and self-compassion among adolescents. J. Youth Adolesc. 47: 1363–1372.
Sandoz, E.K., K.G. Wilson, R.M. Merwin and K.K. Kellum. 2013. Assessment of body image flexibility: The Body Image-Acceptance and Action Questionnaire. J. Contextual Behav. Sci. 2: 39–48.
Sarda, E., C. El-Jor, R. Shankland, Q. Hallez, D. Patiram, C. Nguyen et al. 2025. Social media use and roles of self-objectification, self-compassion and body image concerns: a systematic review. J. Eat. Disord. 13: 192.
Seekis, V., G.L. Bradley and A. Duffy. 2017. The effectiveness of self-compassion and self-esteem writing tasks in reducing body image concerns. Body Image 23: 206–213.
Senra, H., C. Duarte, S.A. Carvalho, L. Simões, C. Ferreira, L. Palmeira et al. 2025. eBEfree: Combining psychoeducation, mindfulness, and self-compassion in an app-based psychological intervention to manage binge-eating symptoms: A randomized controlled trial. Int. J. Eat. Disord. 58: 293–307.
Sullivan, E.J., J.P. Trammell and J.A. Harriger. 2024. Two sides of the self-love coin: Self-compassion text-only posts and body positive photo-based content both positively affect body image. Body Image 49: 101686.
Thøgersen-Ntoumani, C., L. Dodos, N. Chatzisarantis and N. Ntoumanis. 2017. A diary study of self-compassion, upward social comparisons, and body image-related outcomes. Appl. Psychol. Health Well-Being 9: 242–258.
Thompson, J.K., M.D. Coovert and S.M. Stormer. 1999. Body image, social comparison, and eating disturbance: A covariance structure modeling investigation. Int. J. Eat. Disord. 26: 43–51.
Toole, A.M. and L.W. Craighead. 2016. Brief self-compassion meditation training for body image distress in young adult women. Body Image 19: 104–112.
Turk, F. and G. Waller. 2020. Is self-compassion relevant to the pathology and treatment of eating and body image concerns? A systematic review and meta-analysis. Clin. Psychol. Rev. 79: 101856.
Turk, F., S. Kellett and G. Waller. 2021. Determining the potential links of self-compassion with eating pathology and body image among women and men: A cross-sectional mediational study. Body Image 37: 28–37.
Tylka, T.L., H.L. Russell and A.A. Neal. 2015. Self-compassion as a moderator of thinness-related pressures' associations with thin-ideal internalization and disordered eating. Eating Behaviors 17: 23–26.
Voelker, D.K., T.A. Petrie, Q. Huang and A. Chandran. 2019. Bodies in Motion: An empirical evaluation of a program to support positive body image in female collegiate athletes. Body Image 28: 149–158.
Wasylkiw, L., A.L. MacKinnon and A.M. MacLellan. 2012. Exploring the link between self-compassion and body image in university women. Body Image 9: 236–245.
Yarnell, L.M., R.E. Stafford, K.D. Neff, E.D. Reilly, M.C. Knox and M. Mullarkey. 2015. Meta-analysis of gender differences in self-compassion. Self Identity 14: 499–520.

Chapter 3

Applications of Virtual Reality in the Assessment and Treatment of Eating Disorders

Giulia Corno,[1,2,3,*] *Johana Monthuy-Blanc*[3,4,5] and *Stéphane Bouchard*[1,2,3]

INTRODUCTION

Eating disorders (EDs) represent the severe end of the continuum of dysfunctional eating attitudes and behaviors and are psychiatric disorders characterised by disturbances in behaviours and cognitions associated with eating, eating-related behaviours, weight and body shape (Grilo 2024). It could be argued that EDs are conditions that have only emerged in recent times, coinciding with the rise in the importance of body image as a defining aspect of the individual identity. Nevertheless, the reality of the situation is in fact quite distinct. The origins of EDs are longstanding. To illustrate this point, the first documented cases of self-starvation in Western countries, known as "holy anorexia" or *anorexia mirabilis*, are known

[1] Department of Psychoeducation and Psychology, Université du Québec en Outaouais, 283, boulevard Alexandre-Taché, J8X 3X7, Gatineau, QC, Canada.

[2] Centre Intégré de Santé et des Services Sociaux de l'Outaouais, 909, boulevard de la Vérendrye Ouest, J8P 7H2, Gatineau, QC, Canada.

[3] Montreal Mental Health University Institute Research Center, 7401, rue Hochelaga, H1N 3MG, Montréal, QC, Canada.

[4] Department of Education Sciences, Université du Québec à Trois-Rivières, 3351, boulevard des Forges, G9A 5H7, Trois-Rivières, QC, Canada.

[5] Department of Psychiatry and Addiction Medicine, Université de Montréal, Pavillon Roger-Gaudry 2900, boulevard Édouard-Montpetit, bureau S-750 Montréal (Québec) H3T 1J4.

Emails: johana.monthuy-blanc@uqtr.ca, stephane.bouchard@uqo.ca

* Corresponding author: giulia.corno@uqo.ca

DOI: 10.1201/9781032718125-4

to have occurred during the Middle Ages (Harris 2014). In this particular instance, the practice of self-starvation was imbued with a religious significance, prioritising spiritual purification over the pursuit of thinness (Dell'Osso et al. 2016). The first modern definition of an ED can be traced back to the late 1800s, when anorexia nervosa (AN) was defined by Gull (1874, 1997). Today, the DSM-5-TR section of feeding and eating disorders comprises six main diagnoses: AN, bulimia nervosa (BN), binge-eating disorder (BED), pica, rumination and avoidant/restrictive food intake disorder (American Psychiatric Association 2022). Additionally, the DSM-5-TR includes other specified feeding or eating disorder and unspecified feeding or eating.

Psychological treatments for EDs have been developed among the years. Cognitive behavioural therapy (CBT) has been a prominent approach, with the enhanced transdiagnostic version of CBT (CBT-E; Fairburn et al. 2003, Fairburn 2008), being a particularly significant contribution to the field. Nevertheless, psychological treatments for EDs still encounter some limitations, with only 50% of those therapies resulting in complete recovery (Södersten et al. 2017). Consequently, innovations in this field remain imperative for the enhancement of treatment outcomes. This chapter proposes an overview of the utilization of virtual reality (VR) in the treatment of EDs and the assessment of the body image disturbances frequently encountered in these disorders.

1. Virtual reality in mental health

VR is a computer-based technology that enables the recreation of real or imagined environments and simulates the user's presence within them. This is achieved through real-time interaction with the virtual environment using tools such as hand controllers, motion tracking systems, and sensory feedback devices. VR engages multiple sensory modalities, sight, touch, proprioception, smell, and hearing, thereby enhancing the immersive experience (Clus et al. 2018, Di Natale et al. 2024). A key psychological concept for VR-based technologies is the feeling of presence (Riva et al. 2021). The feeling of presence, in other words the feeling of actually being in a virtual environment, allows the individual to live experiences in the virtual environment, that are comparable to experiences in the physical reality (Berthiaume et al. 2021). This has meaningful therapeutic implications, as it will be illustrated in the following paragraph.

VR has been employed by researchers in mental health since the late 1980. Indeed, the concept of VR was formally articulated in 1989, marking the beginning of its broader integration into research and mental health applications (Maples-Keller et al. 2017). VR offers numerous advantages for researchers and clinicians in the field of mental health. First, it allows for the creation of personalized scenarios and stimuli that can be tailored to address individual triggers or symptoms (Arrom-Llabrés et al. 2025). Second, VR makes it possible to simulate, within a safe, confidential, and controlled setting, situations that may be difficult or impossible to recreate in real life and are often reliant on the client's imagination (Arrom-Llabrés et al. 2025, Clus et al. 2018). Moreover, VR-based exposure, also called *in virtuo* exposure, is generally perceived as safer than *in vivo* exposure, which can increase patients' willingness to engage more rapidly in therapeutic exercises, particularly exposure-based interventions (Arrom-Llabrés et al. 2025). Compared to imagery-based exposure, *in virtuo* exposure offers a significantly higher level of immersion by engaging multiple sensory modalities, thus enhancing emotional engagement (Ferrer-García and Gutiérrez-Maldonado 2012). Another advantage is the clinician's/researcher's ability to adjust the intensity or complexity of scenarios in real time, according to the patient's needs and progress. Additionally, therapists can monitor, in real time, the specific stimuli presented to the patient, thereby facilitating the identification of triggers associated with particular emotional responses (Ferrer-García and Gutiérrez-Maldonado 2012). Furthermore, VR facilitates the collection of real-time psychophysiological data, such as eye tracking, heart rate, or skin conductance, that are difficult to obtain using traditional methods. Finally, VR may enhance client engagement in therapy by reducing dropout rates related to distance, monotony, or fatigue, while also offering the opportunity for at-home practice.

Initially made popular for the treatment of phobias, the use of VR has expanded to other mental health disorders such as other anxiety disorders, depressive disorders, trauma- and stressor-related disorders, obsessive-compulsive and related disorders, substance-related and addictive disorders, neurodevelopmental disorders, and EDs (e.g., Bell et al. 2024). The first VR-based studies in the field of EDs were conducted in the late 1990s and early 2000s by the research team led by Giuseppe Riva in Milan (Italy), and the group headed by Conxa Perpiñá et al. in Castellón and Valencia (Spain) (Perpiñá et al. 2000, Riva 1998). Their pioneering projects focused on the development of VR-based tools aimed at assessing and treating body image disturbances in individuals with EDs. Benefits of using VR-based interventions in the context of EDs can include allowing automation and standardization of psychoeducational interventions, providing immersive and real-life based opportunities to practice emotion regulation skills, modifying attentional bias (please refer to Chapter 4 of this book), improving self-awareness of body image disturbances, modifying implicit and explicit body image perceptions, or strengthening exposure-based therapy (Brown et al. 2020).

In the following sections. We will examine how VR has been utilized in the treatment of EDs. We will then explore its use in the assessment of body image disturbances in this population.

2. VR for the treatment of EDs

In this section, we examine VR-based interventions targeting specific features of EDs, such as fear of food, fear of gaining weight, urge to be physically active, and body image disturbances. Specifically, we provide an overview of VR-based applications including cue exposure-based therapy, experiential cognitive therapy (which is described in more details in Chapter 7), body image exposure, exposure-based interventions targeting the acute urge to be physically active, and interventions aimed to change categorical boundaries for what an individual judges to be a thin versus a fat body. It is important to note that VR-based attention bias training has also been employed in the treatment of EDs. However, this approach will not be discussed here, as it is the focus of Chapter 4.

2.1 VR-based cue exposure intervention

Cue exposure-based therapy is a subcategory of exposure interventions, primarily applied to eating and substance-related disorders (Brown et al. 2020). Cue exposure intervention is grounded in the conditioning model of binge eating (Jansen 1998). It aims to break the association between specific cues (i.e., the conditioned stimuli that signal food intake, such us sight, smell, taste or a certain environment such as a kitchen or a restaurant) and the dysfunctional binge eating response (conditioned response). This is achieved through systematic, gradual exposure to these cues while preventing the eating behavior (Nameth et al. 2021). Based on the inhibitory learning model, the individual forms new associations between the conditioned stimuli and the conditioned response, inhibiting the dysfunctional association between food-related cues and binge eating (Nameth et al. 2021).

Several studies have reported the efficacy of cue exposure intervention in reducing food cravings, anxiety, episodes of binge eating and associated purging behaviors (Ferrer-Garcia et al. 2019). Traditionally, cue exposure intervention is done *in vivo*. However, it requires to bring sufficient quantities and types of binge foods to therapy sessions, and it can be limited to a reduced number of settings (Ferrer-Garcia et al. 2019). When done outside the laboratory or the therapist' office, this type of exercise limits confidentiality and control on the situation. It requires also some costs for the clients in terms of purchased food and time taken to travel to specific settings. VR-based cue exposure intervention allow to overcome these limits. Studies have demonstrated that virtual foods are able to generate the same emotional response of real food in individuals with EDs, and they are able to elicit stronger emotional reactions than the ones generated by pictures of food (Gorini et al. 2010). Before starting the VR-based cue exposure sessions, individuals are asked to rate a series of virtual food and food-related everyday life scenarios (e.g., restaurants, kitchens, supermarkets) in terms of their level of food craving. A personalised exposure hierarchy of virtual stimuli and situations is then organised for each individual. They are then progressively exposed to different combinations of food stimuli and situations according to their personalised exposure hierarchy. During VR-based exposure sessions, individuals are asked to interact with the environment and virtual foods, for instance by holding and manipulating foods, bringing the food closer to their face, and engaging different sensory modalities (Nameth et al. 2021). VR-based cue exposure intervention also offer greater confidentiality and safety, as well as being more cost-effective, since it can be carried out in the therapist's office or remotely from home, instead of going to restaurants and public places.

The use of VR-based cue exposure intervention for EDs has empirical support (e.g., Ferrer-Garcia et al. 2017, 2019, Nameth et al. 2021). For instance, patients with BN and BED who continued to experience symptoms after receiving standard CBT demonstrated a significantly greater reduction in binge eating, as well as higher rates of abstinence from binge eating and purging, following randomization to six sessions of VR-based cue exposure intervention compared to six additional sessions of CBT (Ferrer-Garcia et al. 2017). A 6-month follow-up of the same study indicated that the reduction in binge, purge, and overeating episodes was more pronounced after VR-based cue exposure intervention (Ferrer-Garcia et al. 2019). More recently, an uncontrolled pilot study has explored the feasibility and acceptability of implementing VR-based cue exposure intervention in real-world settings (Nameth et al. 2021). Results showed high acceptability from both adults with a history of BED or BN and therapists, as well as an early indication of effectiveness in terms of decrease of binge eating episodes (Nameth et al. 2021).

2.2 Experiential cognitive therapy

Experiential Cognitive Therapy combines nutritional and physical activity group intervention with a VR-based body image rescripting protocol. This protocol is based on the Allocentric Lock Theory, and it is aimed at "unlocking" the body memory by enhancing the contribution of novel egocentric somatosensory information related to the negative allocentric memory (e.g., Riva and Dakanalis 2018, Riva and Gaudio 2018). The VR-based protocol is further described in Chapter 7. Indeed, Experiential Cognitive Therapy has been used among individuals living with obesity, BED and BN (Manzoni et al. 2016, Riva et al. 2003). Studies involving BN and BED patients demonstrated the effectiveness of this treatment in decreasing concerns with weight, fear of gaining weight, and reducing purging and binge eating as well as increasing body satisfaction (Riva et al. 2003).

2.3 VR-based body exposure intervention

Another exposure-based procedure, body exposure, has been integrated into treatments for EDs, especially for AN, to address fear of gaining weight and body image disturbances through habituation (Key et al. 2002, Porras-Garcia et al. 2021, Vock et al. 2008). Traditionally, body exposure is conducted through mirror exposure. This typically involves the patient observing in a mirror their body or specific body parts for a designated period, either in a neutral, non-judgmental manner (Hilbert et al. 2002), a positive and descriptive manner (cognitive dissonance-based mirror exposure intervention) (Luetchcke et al. 2011), or in a more open and expressive way, where the individual shares their thoughts and emotions regarding their body (Moreno-Domínguez et al. 2012).

VR technology can be utilized to create three-dimensional bodies that replicate the individual's body shape, skin tone, height, hair and clothing (Gutiérrez-Maldonado et al. 2016, 2018). Moreover, VR technology enables individuals to experience what is known as "full body illusion" or "body swapping", where they perceive a virtual body as their own real body by integrating various types of sensory information, and effectively feeling as though they own the virtual body (e.g., Piryankova et al. 2014, Serino et al. 2016). This kind of illusion is achieved by visuomotor and/or visuo-tactile stimulations (e.g., Malighetti et al. 2020, Serino et al. 2019). In other words, the illusion of owning the virtual body is achieved by granting synchronous movements between the real and the virtual body, and/or by performing synchronous visuo-tactile stimulations on the real body of the participant while the virtual body is stimulated at the same time and place.

Furthermore, VR technology enables the development of software that allows to modify an individual's virtual body shape, by gradually increasing or decreasing the overall size or specific body parts (Corno et al. 2022). This can be particularly beneficial for individuals with a fear of gaining weight, as VR-based body exposure allows them to be progressively exposed to, and embody, virtual bodies with increasing body mass index (BMI). In this regard, for instance, a randomized controlled clinical study, provided evidence of efficacy of VR-based body exposure in reducing fear of weight gain and body image disturbances in a sample of adults and adolescents with AN (Porras-Garcia et al. 2021). Specifically, during exposure sessions, participants were exposed to virtual bodies starting with their actual BMI and gradually progressing to virtual bodies with higher BMIs, until reaching a healthy BMI (Porras-Garcia et al. 2021). Another more recent non-controlled study with a sample of women with AN confirmed that repeated exposure to virtual bodies with increasing BMI improved fear of weight gain (Behrens et al. 2023).

Regarding body image disturbances, studies have shown that embodying a virtual body corresponding to a healthy BMI could subsequently lead to a diminished misestimation of body parts among women with AN (Keizer et al. 2016, Serino et al. 2019). In a pilot study, Malighetti et al. (2020) proposed combining VR-based body exposure with autobiographical recollection to treat body image disturbances in seven young women with AN. The intervention consisted of four sessions in which patients embodied virtual bodies of different sizes. Starting in session 1 and 2 with a virtual body corresponding to the patient's BMI (underweight), this progressed to a virtual body corresponding to a BMI of 17.5 kg/m^2 in session 3, and finally to a virtual body corresponding to a healthy BMI (18.5 kg/m^2) in session 4. During the VR-based exposure intervention, participants were asked to recall negative life events while embodying underweight virtual bodies, and positive life events while embodying the healthy-weight virtual body. The rationale behind combining VR-based body exposure and autobiographical recall was to associate negative feelings related to negative life events with underweight virtual bodies and positive feelings related to positive memories with a healthy virtual body. The results of this pilot study showed that, following the intervention, patients exhibited a decreased level of body dissatisfaction, body image concerns, and body shame (Malighetti et al. 2020).

2.4 VR-based exposure for the acute urge to be physically active

Acute urge to engage in physical activity, is often reported by EDs patients (Amin et al. 2023, Casper et al. 2020, Graap et al. 2018). It is characterised by multiple behavioural/motor (e.g., elevated drive for activity, increased motor restlessness), emotional (e.g., increased sense of agitation, anxiety), and cognitive (e.g., compulsive and intrusive thoughts about physical activity, concerns about activity) components (Boltri et al. 2025, Paslaskis et al. 2107). Even though it is often reported by EDs patients, especially by individuals suffering from AN and BN (Amin et al. 2023, Casper et al. 2020, Graap et al. 2018), disordered-specific treatments do not explicitly target this symptom (Boltri et al. 2025, Casper et al. 2020, Graap et al. 2018, Paslakis et al. 2017). In a first proof-of-concept pilot study, Paslakis and colleagues (2017) developed a VR-based exposure paradigm that was hypothesized to help reducing the urge of being physically active through habituation, in a sample of AN and BN patients. The 3D virtual environment consisted in a 360°-based video which participants watched through VR googles. The VR-based experience consisted in watching a jogger's running from an egocentric (i.e., first-person) perspective. Participants were able to move their head and further explore the virtual surroundings. They were instructed to devote themselves to the running experience and to self-report the urge of engage in physical activity through a questionnaire. The results of this pilot study indicated a significant decrease of the urge to engage in physical activity from baseline to postexposure (Paslakis et al. 2017). More recently, a case series study, explored the feasibility of a VR-based running exposure protocol to target the urge to be physically active in AN patients, as part of a multidisciplinary treatment approach (Boltri et al. 2025). Indeed, three women with severe AN were enrolled in an inpatient rehabilitation treatment program which included inpatient activities (e.g., enteral nutrition, monitored meals), nutritional support, movement therapy and psychological support. The VR-based running exposure protocol consisted of four weekly VR-based exposure sessions. During each session, women were asked to passively watch a 360° first-person video that reproduced a jogging session in a rural landscape. Participants could move their head, but no other physical movement was required or performed. Acute urge to move decreased for all the three participants after each VR session. Additional promising changes were reported in other clinically relevant variables such as drive for thinness, body image dissatisfaction, interoceptive deficits, and emotional regulation (Boltri et al. 2025). Furthermore, patients expressed the desire for the integration of this VR-based protocol into outpatient programs (Boltri et al. 2025).

2.5 Interventions targeting categorical boundaries

Moving beyond the treatment of EDs symptoms, a recent body image-based intervention paradigm focused on changing the categorical boundary for what an individual judges to be a thin versus a fat body. Based on the paradigm used in studies aiming at shifting the categorical boundary in the recognition of emotions in faces, Gledhill et al. (2017) modified this training to adapt it to categorization of bodies. Their aim was to change the categorical boundary, in other words the subjective point in the BMI continuum at which bodies change from being categorized as thin to being categorises as fat, towards higher BMI. This training, originally performed with a standard computer and two-dimensional bodies, was replicated in VR using three-dimensional bodies by Irvine et al. (2020). The authors invited women with high, but yet sub-clinical, body image concerns, to participate to one between three conditions: one intervention group characterized by limited stimulus presentation time, one condition with no time limits and a control condition. In all the conditions, women were asked to categorise a series of 15 three-dimensional female bodies with BMI ranging from 15.45 kg/m^2 to 33.70 kg/m^2. In the two intervention groups, participants received inflationary feedback to change their categorisation towards higher BMIs. The results of the study of Irvine et al. (2020) showed that both interventions were able to shift the categorical boundaries of participants, with participants assigned to the unlimited presentation times showing a larger training effect. The categorical training did not have effect only on the subjective categorical boundary of participants. Indeed, participants of both intervention groups reported statistically significant reduction about concerns related to their body, weight, and eating, with clinically meaningful changes only in the group with the unlimited presentation times.

3. VR for the assessment of body image disturbances

3.1 Body image and body image disturbances

Body image is a complex phenomenon which encompasses attitudes (cognitions, behaviours, and emotions) and perceptions related to one's body image (e.g., Cash and Smolak 2011). Two main disturbances in body image have been identified: body dissatisfaction and body distortion. Body dissatisfaction, defined as the negative subjective evaluation of one's body, is so common among women in Western societies that it is deemed as "normative discontent" (e.g., Fiske et al. 2014, Stice and Shaw 2002). Body dissatisfaction is also a well-recognized predictor and maintenance factor for EDs (e.g., Neumark-Sztainer et al. 2006). Body distortion is defined as a disturbance in estimating (i.e., underestimating or overestimating) one's body size. It is commonly identified in individuals with AN and BN, who tend to overestimate their body size (e.g., Fisher et al. 2020, Lewer et al. 2016, 2017). Regarding individuals with BED, studies report no significant differences from non-clinical samples, thereby suggesting relatively realistic estimates (e.g., Lewer et al. 2016, 2017). Different methods have been used to assess body dissatisfaction and distortion. In the following paragraph, the traditional assessment methods and their limitations will be presented.

3.2 Traditional assessment methods of body image disturbances and their limitations

The assessment of body dissatisfaction can be conducted through the utilisation of visual-perceptual methods or by means of self-reported questionnaires. Visual-perceptual methods traditionally imply the use of paper-based figure-rating scales (e.g., the Stunkard Figure Rating Scale by Stunkard et al. 1983). They consist in a series of two-dimensional figure drawings ranging from underweight to obesity, presented in an allocentric (i.e., third person) perspective (e.g., Sob et al. 2021). Individuals are asked to select from the range of bodies presented, those that better represent their perceived and ideal body size. The discrepancy between perceived and ideal body size provides a measure of body dissatisfaction (Corno et al. 2024, Ferrer-García and Gutiérrez-Maldonado 2012). Body dissatisfaction measured by self-reported questionnaires is conceptually different than body dissatisfaction assessed by visual-perceptual methods (Corno et al. 2024, Mölbert et al. 2017). Questionnaires-based measures evaluate a broad concept of body dissatisfaction, including global feelings about the body, concerns related to specific body parts or appearance-related fears. On the other hand, visual-perceptual methods allow to capture weight-related body concerns and ideals (Corno et al. 2024, Mölbert et al. 2017). Regarding body distortion, assessment is typically conducted through visual-perceptual methods, where individuals are asked to indicate their perceived body size. The difference, mainly calculated in terms of BMI, between the real body size and the perceived body size is regarded as a measure of body distortion (Corno et al. 2024, Ferrer-García and Gutiérrez-Maldonado 2012, Monthuy-Blanc et al. 2020, 2022).

Traditional paper-based visual-perceptual methods present some limitations. First, they are limited to the assessment of allocentric body image perceptions, neglecting the egocentric (i.e., first person) perspective. Second, drawings used in conventional figure-rating scales can be unrealistic and poorly proportionated, and the stepwise changes in body weight are often inconsistent from one figure to the next (e.g., Corno et al. 2024, Mölbert et al. 2017). Third, their two-dimensional format renders them flat and lacking depth (Corno et al. 2024). Together, these limitations may reduce the ability of traditional paper-based figure rating scales to accurately capture individuals' body image perceptions (Corno et al. 2024, Monthuy-Blanc et al. 2020, 2022). As it will be discussed in the following paragraphs, VR-based technologies have been used to overcome the limitations of visual-perceptual methods.

3.3 VR-based assessment methods of body image disturbances

As it was discussed at the beginning of this chapter, the research group of Riva and Perpiña were the first to develop VR-based assessment tools for body image and body image disturbances. The software developed by Riva and colleagues at the end of the late 1990, the BIVRS (i.e., Body Image Virtual Reality Scale), was the first non-immersive virtual environment that introduced a third dimension to a continuum of nine female and male virtual bodies of increasing dimensions (Riva 1998). A few years later, Perpiña et al. (2000) developed a VR software featuring a three-dimensional virtual human whose body-part dimensions could be enlarged or reduced via a slider. This tool enabled assessment of multiple facets of body image perceptions, including perceived, ideal and normative body size.

Today, VR enables the creation of high definition, near photorealistic three-dimensional bodies that can be experienced from both allocentric and egocentric perspectives, in immersive virtual environments. Two VR assessment paradigms are common. In modulation tasks, individuals adjust the entire virtual body, or certain body parts, to match their perceived or ideal body size (Corno et al. 2018). In continuum tasks, which mirror traditional paper-based figure rating scales, individuals can choose from a lineup of virtual bodies (Fisher et al. 2020, Mölbert et al. 2017, Monthuy-Blanc et al. 2020, 2022).

Emerging work in the VR field has developed novel VR-based body image assessment tools, contributing to the understanding of body image disturbances in EDs. For instance, Mölbert et al. (2018) investigated body image perceptions and body distortion in women with AN and community controls using biometric allocentric virtual bodies that varied ±20% of each participant's weight. The authors found that both groups underestimated their body size, with women with AN choosing a thinner ideal body than controls. Fisher et al. (2020) compared a traditional paper-based figure rating scale with a VR-based assessment method in adolescent girls with AN. The VR tool presented standardized, non-biometric female virtual bodies spanning BMI 10–30 kg/m^2, which could be viewable in 360°. Perceived and ideal body selections were consistent across the two methods: participants overestimated their body size, and body dissatisfaction and body distortion did not different between tools. Head-tracking analyses further indicated greater engagement with underweight bodies and the least engagement with bodies representing obesity.

Despite technological advances, relatively few studies have used VR to examine body image perceptions and disturbances from both allocentric and egocentric perspectives (e.g., Bourbeau et al. 2025, Corno et al. 2018, Monthuy-Blanc et al. 2020, 2022). Why it could be interesting to further investigate differences in body image perceptions and disturbances depending on visuospatial reference frames of the body? Conceptually, it has been proposed that individuals may view the body as an object (non-embodied) from an allocentric standpoint and as a subject (embodied) from an egocentric one (Bourbeau et al. 2025, Monthuy-Blanc et al. 2022). Furthermore, the Allocentric Lock Theory proposes that egocentric and allocentric perspectives differentially shape body experience: the egocentric perspective is grounded in somatoperceptions (i.e., real-time sensory input about the body), while the allocentric perspective is linked to somatorepresentations (i.e., abstract beliefs, attitudes and knowledge about one's body) (e.g., Riva et al. 2014). Further research is needed to clarify whether and how these perspectives differ and what roles they play in body-image assessment in community and EDs populations.

Conclusion

In conclusion, research on the use VR as an assessment and intervention tool in EDs has been progressively developed during the last 30 years. Specifically, research on the use of VR as an intervention tool to target specific EDs symptoms has been more developed than research on the use of VR to understand and assess body image disturbances in individuals with EDs. In the imminent future, the potential exists for the implementation of novel technologies (e.g., artificial intelligence) with a view of further enhancing the possibilities offered by VR.

Acknowledgments

This chapter was supported by postdoctoral grants by the Foundation of the Montreal Mental Health University Institute affiliated to the Montreal Mental Health University Institute Research Center, the CIHR Fellowship (Health Research Training A - Post-PhD), a research funding from the Fondation Santé Gatineau (FSG PR-590183), and a research funding from Social Sciences and Humanities Research Council (430-2024-00013) awarded to GC; the settlement fund of the Foundation of the Montreal Mental Health University Institute affiliated to the Montreal Mental Health University Institute Research Center (2021–2025), the Foundations of RBC Royal Bank and the Takeda Canada (2021–2024) awarded to JMB.

References

American Psychiatric Association. 2022. Diagnostic and Statistical Manual of Mental Disorders (5th ed., text rev.). American Psychiatric Association, Washington, DC.

Amin, L., G. Halbeisen, K. Braks, T.J. Huber and G. Paslakis. 2023. The State Urge to be Physically Active-Questionnaire (SUPA-Q): Development and validation of a state measure of activity urges in patients with eating disorders. Brain Behav. 13: e3220.

Arrom-Llabrés, M., M.T. Mendoza-Medialdea and J. Gutiérrez-Maldonado. 2025. Innovative approaches to eating disorders treatment: a systematic review on the effectiveness of virtual reality. Appli. Sci. 15: 3334.

Behrens, S.C., J. Tesch, P.J.B. Sun, S. Starke, M.J. Black, H. Schneider et al. 2023. Virtual reality exposure to a healthy weight body is a promising adjunct treatment for Anorexia Nervosa. Psychother. Psychosom. 92: 170–179.

Bell, I.H., R. Pot-Kolder, A. Rizzo, M. Rus-Calafell, V. Cardi, M. Cella et al. 2024. Advances in the use of virtual reality to treat mental health conditions. Nat. Rev. Psychol. 3: 552–567.

Berthiaume, M., G. Corno, K. Nolet and S. Bouchard. 2018. A novel integrated information processing model of presence. Presence 27: 378–399.

Boltri, M., G. Brizzi, F. Brusa, C. Gabutti, G. Cera, A. Scalia et al. 2025. Virtual reality-based running exposure to target the acute urge to be physically active in Anorexia Nervosa: A case series. Neuropsychobiology 1–13.

Bourbeau, F., S. Bouchard, G. Corno and J. Monthuy-Blanc. 2025. The role of body image perception on a continuum from dysfunctional to healthy eating attitudes and behaviors among people seeking treatment. J. Clin. Med. 14: 597.

Brown, T., E. Nauman Vogel, S. Adler, C. Bohon, K. Bullock, K. Nameth et al. 2020. Bringing virtual reality from clinical trials to clinical practice for the treatment of eating disorders: an example using virtual reality cue exposure therapy. Journal Med. Internet Res. 22: e16386.

Cash, T.F. and L. Smolak. 2011. Body Image. A Handbook of Science, Practice, and Prevention (2nd ed.). The Guildford Press

Casper, R.C., U. Voderholzer, S. Naab and S. Schlegl. 2020. Increased urge for movement, physical and mental restlessness, fundamental symptoms of restricting anorexia nervosa? Brain Behav. 10: e01556.

Clus, D., M.E. Larsen, C. Lemey and S. Berrouiguet. 2018. The use of virtual reality in patients with eating disorders: systematic review. J. Med. Internet Res. 20: e157.

Corno, G., S. Serino, P. Cipresso, R.M. Baños and G. Riva. 2018. Assessing the relationship between attitudinal and perceptual component of body image disturbance using virtual reality. Cyberpsychol. Behav. Soc. Netw. 21: 679–686.

Corno, G., M. Berthiaume, A. Paquette and S. Bouchard. 2022. La réalité virtuelle : un outil validé et polyvalent pour l'étude de l'image corporelle. pp. 211–224. *In*: Maïano, C., J. Dion and A. Aimé (eds.). L'image corporelle sous toutes ses formes. Presses de l'Université du Québec.

Corno, G., A. Paquette, D. Burychka, M. Miragall, M.C. Rivard, R.M. Baños et al. 2024. Development of a visual-perceptual method to assess body image: A cross-cultural validation in Canadian and Spanish women. Eur. Eat. Disord. Rev. 32: 771–783.

Dell'Osso, L., M. Abelli, B. Carpita, S. Pini, G. Castellini, C. Carmassi et al. 2016. Historical evolution of the concept of anorexia nervosa and relationships with orthorexia nervosa, autism, and obsessive-compulsive spectrum. Neuropsychiatr. Dis. Treat. 12: 1651–1660.

Di Natale, A.F., S.F.M. Pizzoli, G. Brizzi, D. Di Lernia, F. Frisone, A. Gaggioli et al. 2024. Harnessing immersive virtual reality: a comprehensive scoping review of its applications in assessing, understanding, and treating eating disorders. Curr. Psychiatry Rep. 26: 470–486.

Fairburn C.G., Z. Cooper and R. Shafran 2003. Cognitive behaviour therapy for eating disorders: a "transdiagnostic" theory and treatment. Behav. Res. Ther. 41: 509–28.

Fairburn, C.G. 2008. Cognitive Behavior Therapy and Eating Disorders. Guilford Press.

Ferrer-García, M. and J. Gutiérrez-Maldonado. 2012. The use of virtual reality in the study, assessment, and treatment of body image in eating disorders and nonclinical samples: a review of the literature. Body Image 9: 1–11.

Ferrer-García, M., J. Gutiérrez-Maldonado, J. Pla-Sanjuanelo, F. Vilalta-Abella, G. Riva, M. Clerici et al. 2017. A randomised controlled comparison of second-level treatment approaches for treatment-resistant adults with bulimia nervosa and binge eating disorder: Assessing the benefits of virtual reality cue exposure therapy. Eur. Eat. Disord. Rev. 25: 479–490.

Ferrer-Garcia, M., J. Pla-Sanjuanelo, A. Dakanalis, F. Vilalta-Abella, G. Riva, F. Fernandez-Aranda et al. 2019. A randomized trial of virtual reality-based cue exposure second-level therapy and cognitive behavior second-level therapy for bulimia nervosa and binge-eating disorder: Outcome at six-month followup. Cyberpsychol. Behav. Soc. Netw. 22: 60–68.

Fisher S., A. Abdullah, I. Charvin, D. Da Fonseca and F. Bat-Pitault. 2020. Comparison of body image evaluation by virtual reality and paper-based figure rating scales in adolescents with anorexia nervosa: retrospective study. Eat. Weight Disord. 25: 735–743.

Fiske, L., E.A. Fallon, B. Blissmer and C.A. Redding. 2014. Prevalence of body dissatisfaction among United States adults: Review and recommendations for future research. Eat. Behav. 15: 357–365.

Gledhill, L.J., K.K. Cornelissen, P.L. Cornelissen, I.S. Penton-Voak, M.R. Munafò and M.J. Tovée. 2017. An interactive training programme to treat body image disturbance. Br. J. Health Psychol. 22: 60–76.

Gorini, A., E. Griez, A. Petrova and G. Riva. 2010. Assessment of the emotional responses produced by exposure to real food, virtual food and photographs of food in patients affected by eating disorders. Ann. Gen. Psychiatry 9: 30.

Graap, H., Y. Erim and G. Paslakis. 2018. The effect of dronabinol in a male patient with anorexia nervosa suffering from severe acute urge to be physically active. Int. J. Eat. Disord. 51: 180–183.

Grilo, C.M. 2024. Treatment of eating disorders: current status, challenges, and future directions. Annu. Rev. Clin. Psychol. 20: 97–123.

Gull, W.W. 1874. Anorexia nervosa. Trans. Clin. Soc. Lond. 7: 22–28.

Gull, W.W. 1997. Anorexia nervosa (apepsia hysterica, anorexia hysterica). 1868. Obes. Res. 5: 498–502.

Gutiérrez-Maldonado, J., B.K. Wiederhold and G. Riva. 2016. Future directions: how virtual reality can further improve the assessment and treatment of eating disorders and obesity. Cyberpsychol. Behav. Soc. Netw. 19: 148–153.

Gutiérrez-Maldonado, J., M. Ferrer-García, A. Dakanalis and G. Riva. 2018. Virtual reality: applications to eating disorders. pp. 470–491. *In*: Agras, W.S. and A. Robinson (eds.). The Oxford Handbook of Eating Disorders. Oxford University Press, Oxford, UK.

Harris, J.C. 2014. Anorexia nervosa and anorexia mirabilis: Miss K. R--and St Catherine of Siena. JAMA Psychiatry 71: 1212–1213.

Hilbert, A., B. Tuschen-Caffier and C. Vögele. 2002. Effects of prolonged and repeated body image exposure in binge-eating disorder. J. Psychosom. Res. 52: 137–144.

Irvine, K.R., A.R. Irvine, N. Maalin, K. McCarty, K.K. Cornelissen, M.J. Tovée et al. 2020. Using immersive virtual reality to modify body image. Body Image 33: 232–243.

Jansen, A. 1998. A learning model of binge eating: Cue reactivity and cue exposure. Behav. Res. Ther. 36: 257–272.

Keizer, A., A. van Elburg, R. Helms and H.C. Dijkerman. 2016. A virtual reality full body illusion improves body image disturbance in Anorexia Nervosa. PLOS ONE 11: e0163921.

Key, A., C.L. George, D. Beattie, K. Stammers, H. Lacey and G. Waller. 2002. Body image treatment within an inpatient program for anorexia nervosa: The role of mirror exposure in the desensitization process. Int. J. Eat. Disord. 31: 185–190.

Lewer, M., N. Nasrawi, S. Schroeder and S. Vocks. 2016. Body image disturbance in binge eating disorder: a comparison of obese patients with and without binge eating disorder regarding the cognitive, behavioral and perceptual component of body image. Eat. Weight Disord. 21: 115–125.

Lewer, M., A. Bauer, A.S. Hartmann and S. Vocks. 2017. Different facets of body image disturbance in binge eating disorder: a review. Nutrients 9: 1294.

Luethcke, C.A., L. McDaniel and C.B. Becker. 2011. A comparison of mindfulness, nonjudgmental, and cognitive dissonance-based approaches to mirror exposure. Body Image 8: 251–258.

Malighetti, C., A. Chirico, S. Serino, S. Cavedoni, M. Matamala-Gomez, C. Stramba-Badiale et al. 2020. Manipulating body size distortions and negative body-related memories in patients with Anorexia Nervosa: A virtual reality-based pilot study. Annu. Rev. CyberTherapy Telemed. 18: 177–181.

Manzoni, G.M., G.L. Cesa, M. Bacchetta, G. Castelnuovo, S. Conti, A. Gaggioli et al. 2016. Virtual reality-enhanced cognitive-behavioral therapy for morbid obesity: a randomized controlled study with 1 year follow-up. Cyberpsychol. Behav. Soc. Netw. 19: 134–140.

Maples-Keller, J.L., B.E. Bunnell, S.J. Kim and B.O. Rothbaum. 2017. The use of virtual reality technology in the treatment of anxiety and other psychiatric disorders. Harv. Rev. Psychiatry 25: 103–113.

Mölbert, S.C., A. Thaler, S. Streuber, M.J. Black, H. Karnath, S. Zipfel et al. 2017. Investigating body image disturbance in anorexia nervosa using novel biometric figure rating scales: A pilot study. Eur. Eat. Disord. Rev. 25: 607–612.

Mölbert, S.C., A. Thaler, B.J. Mohler, S. Streuber, J. Romero, M.J. Black et al. 2018. Assessing body image in anorexia nervosa using biometric self-avatars in virtual reality: Attitudinal components rather than visual body size estimation are distorted. Psychol. Med. 48: 642–653.

Monthuy-Blanc, J., S. Bouchard, M. Ouellet, G. Corno, S. Iceta and M. Rousseau. 2020. eLoriCorps immersive body rating scale: Exploring the assessment of body image disturbances from allocentric and egocentric perspectives. J. Clin. Med. 9: 2926.

Monthuy-Blanc, J., G. Corno, M. Ouellet, F. Touré, F. Bourbeau, M. Rousseau et al. 2022. eLoriCorps immersive body rating scale and eLoriCorps mobile versions: Valid ation to assess body image disturbances from allocentric and egocentric perspectives in a nonclinical sample of adolescents. J. Clin. Med. 11: 1156.

Moreno-Domínguez, S., S. Rodríguez-Ruiz, M.C. Fernández-Santaella, A. Jansen and B. Tuschen-Caffier. 2012. Pure versus guided mirror exposure to reduce body dissatisfaction: A preliminary study with university women. Body Image 9: 285–288.

Nameth, K., T. Brown, K. Bullock, S. Adler, G. Riva, D. Safer et al. 2021. Translating virtual reality cue exposure therapy for binge eating into a real-world setting: an uncontrolled pilot study. J Clin. Med. 10: 1511.

Neumark-Sztainer, D., S. Paxton, P. Hannan, J. Haines and M. Story. 2006. Does body satisfaction matter? Five-Year longitudinal associations between body satisfaction and health behaviors in adolescent females and males. J. Adolesc. Health. 39: 244–244251.

Paslakis, G., V. Fauck, K. Röder, E. Rauh, M. Rauh and Y. Erim. 2017. Virtual reality jogging as a novel exposure paradigm for the acute urge to be physically active in patients with eating disorders: Implications for treatment. Int. J. Eat. Disord. 50: 1243–1246.

Perpiñá, C., C. Botella and R. Baños. 2000. Imagen Corporal en los Trastornos Alimentarios. Evaluación y Tratamiento Mediante Realidad Virtual. Promolibro, Valencia.

Piryankova, I.V., H.Y. Wong, S.A. Linkenauger, C. Stinson, M.R. Longo, H.H. Bülthoff et al. 2014. Owning an overweight or underweight body: distinguishing the physical, experienced and virtual body. PLoS ONE 9: e103428.

Porras-Garcia, B., M. Ferrer-Garcia, E. Serrano-Troncoso, M. Carulla-Roig, P. Soto-Usera, H. Miquel-Nabau et al. 2021. AN-VR-BE. A randomized controlled trial for reducing fear of gaining weight and other eating disorder symptoms in Anorexia Nervosa through virtual reality-based body exposure. J. Clin. Med. 10: 682.

Riva, G. 1998. Virtual reality in psychological assessment: The body image virtual reality scale. CyberPsychol. Behav. 1: 37–44

Riva, G., M. Bacchetta, G. Cesa, S. Conti and E. Molinari. 2003. Six-month follow-up of in-patient experiential cognitive therapy for binge eating disorders. Cyberpsychol Behav. 6: 251–258.

Riva, G., S. Gaudio and A. Dakanalis. 2014. I'm in a virtual body: A locked allocentric memory may impair the experience of the body in both obesity and anorexia nervosa. Eat. Weight Disord. 19: 133–134.

Riva, G. and A. Dakanalis. 2018. Altered processing and integration of multisensory bodily representations and signals in eating disorders: A possible path toward the understanding of their underlying causes. Front. Hum. Neurosc. 12: 49.

Riva, G. and S. Gaudio. 2018. Locked to a wrong body: Eating disorders as the outcome of a primary disturbance in multisensory body integration. Conscious. Cogn. 59: 57–59.

Riva, G., C. Malighetti and S. Serino. 2021. Virtual reality in the treatment of eating disorders. Clin. Psychol. Psychother. 28: 477–488.

Serino, S., E. Pedroli, A. Keizer, S. Triberti, A. Dakanalis, F. Pallavicini et al. 2016. Virtual reality body swapping: a tool for modifying the allocentric memory of the body. Cyberpsychol. Behav. Soc. Netw. 19: 127–133.

Serino, S., N. Polli and G. Riva. 2019. From avatars to body swapping: The use of virtual reality for assessing and treating body-size distortion in individuals with anorexia. J. Clin. Psychol. 75: 313–322.

Sob, C., L. Giacone, K. Staub, N. Bender, M. Siegrist, C. Hartmann et al. 2021. Drawings or 3D models: Do illustration methods matter when assessing perceived body size and body dissatisfaction? PLoS One 16: e0261645.

Södersten, P., C. Bergh, M. Leon, U. Brodin and M. Zandian. 2017. Cognitive behavior therapy for eating disorders versus normalization of eating behavior. Physiol. Behav. 174: 178–190.

Stice, E. and H.E. Shaw. 2002. Role of body dissatisfaction in the onset and maintenance of eating pathology: A synthesis of research findings. J. Psychosom. Res. 53: 985–993.

Stunkard, A.J., T. Sørensen and F. Schulsinger. 1983. Use of the Danish Adoption Register for the study of obesity and thinness. Res. Publ. Assoc. Res. Nerv. Ment. Dis. 60: 115–120.

Vocks, S., A. Wächter, M. Wucherer and J. Kosfelder. 2008. Look at yourself: Can body image therapy affect the cognitive and emotional response to seeing oneself in the mirror in eating disorders? Eur. Eat. Disord. Rev. 16: 147–154.

Chapter 4

Attentional Bias and Body Perceptions in Dysfunctional Eating Attitudes and Behaviors

*José Gutiérrez-Maldonado** and *Marta Ferrer-Garcia*

INTRODUCTION

This chapter offers a comprehensive examination of how attentional processes contribute to body perception disturbances and the development and maintenance of dysfunctional eating attitudes and behaviors (DEAB). Drawing from both experimental psychology and clinical practice, the chapter underscores the importance of bridging the gap between basic research and applied therapeutic interventions. It presents a compelling case for the integration of eye-tracking (ET) and virtual reality (VR) technologies as innovative tools to investigate and address attentional biases in individuals with body dissatisfaction and DEAB. The content is organized around three primary objectives. First, it delineates the theoretical and empirical foundations of attentional biases in the context of DEAB, detailing how these biases manifest differently in individuals depending on gender, body dissatisfaction, and clinical status. Second, it critically reviews methodological advancements in the assessment of attentional bias, highlighting the precision and ecological validity offered by ET and VR. Third, the chapter explores the emerging field of Attention Bias Modification Training, particularly its application within VR environments, presenting preliminary evidence for its potential to reduce body-related anxiety and

Department of Clinical Psychology and Psychobiology, Universitat de Barcelona, Passeig de la Vall d'Hebron 171, 08035 Barcelona (Spain).
Email: martaferrerg@ub.edu
* Corresponding author: jgutierrezm@ub.edu

DOI: 10.1201/9781032718125-5

improve therapeutic outcomes. Through this analysis, readers are expected to gain a nuanced understanding of the mechanisms by which attentional biases reinforce negative body perception and contribute to disordered eating behaviors. Additionally, the chapter aims to familiarize readers with state-of-the-art technologies that offer both diagnostic insight and therapeutic promise. Ultimately, it invites researchers and clinicians to consider how attentional bias interventions, especially those incorporating immersive and interactive elements, may enhance current approaches to DEAB treatment and prevention.

1. Attentional biases in relation to body perceptions and DEAB

Attentional bias refers to the tendency to selectively focus on certain types of information while ignoring others, often in a way that aligns with one's pre-existing concerns or fears. This phenomenon has been extensively studied in various psychological disorders, including anxiety and DEAB, where it manifests as an increased focus on disorder-related stimuli. In anxiety disorders, attentional bias modification has proven effective in some randomized controlled trials (Amir et al. 2009a, Amir et al. 2009b, Amir et al. 2011, Eldar et al. 2012, Hakamata et al. 2010), highlighting its therapeutic relevance. In recent years, technological advancements have enabled more precise and ecologically valid investigations into attentional biases. The integration of ET and VR technologies offers promising opportunities in this regard. ET provides objective, quantitative data on visual attention in highly controlled environments, while VR adds ecological validity by simulating real-world settings. Together, these tools allow researchers to assess attentional processes with both rigor and realism. Several studies have already employed this combination to examine attentional biases toward various body parts in individuals with differing levels of body dissatisfaction (Porras-Garcia et al. 2018, Porras-Garcia et al. 2019).

A growing body of research demonstrates that individuals with DEAB, particularly those with anorexia nervosa, exhibit distinct patterns of attentional bias toward body-related information. These individuals allocate more cognitive resources to weight- and shape-related body parts, such as the hips and thighs, often at the expense of more neutral stimuli or other body parts, such as the head and chest (Rodgers and DuBois 2016, Williamson et al. 2004). This hypervigilance is consistent with a broader dysfunctional focus on body perceptions and has been strongly linked to body dissatisfaction, a key risk factor for both the onset and maintenance of DEAB (Stice et al. 2017). Research shows that patients with DEAB disproportionately attend to body areas they perceive as unattractive, unlike individuals without DEAB, who tend to distribute their visual attention more evenly across their bodies (von Wietersheim et al. 2012, Freeman et al. 1991, Jansen et al. 2005, Kerr-Gaffney et al. 2018, Rodgers and DuBois 2016, Roefs et al. 2008, Tuschen-Caffier et al. 2015). This phenomenon is also evident in non-clinical populations. Women with high levels of body dissatisfaction tend to fixate more on self-identified unattractive body parts when viewing images of themselves (Bauer et al. 2017, Glashouwer et al. 2016, Janelle et al. 2009, Roefs et al. 2008). Interestingly, while most findings suggest a hypervigilant focus on negatively evaluated body parts, some studies have documented avoidance patterns instead, particularly when individuals view others' bodies rather than their own (e.g., Janelle et al. 2003). These conflicting attentional patterns, specifically, scrutiny and avoidance, are thought to fluctuate within individuals and may serve as short-term coping mechanisms that negatively reinforce the disorder over time by temporarily reducing anxiety about weight gain. This line of investigation has been enriched through studies employing ET and VR technologies. In one such series of experiments, participants with varying levels of body dissatisfaction (but no clinical diagnosis) interacted with virtual avatars of themselves, either at actual size or with digitally increased body mass indexes. Visual fixations on different body parts, categorized as weight-related (i.e., thighs, buttocks, hips, stomach, legs, and waist) or non-weight-related (i.e., head, shoulders, arms, décolletage, neck, and chest) using the Physical Appearance State and Trait Anxiety Scale (Reed et al. 1991), were recorded using ET. Results revealed that women, regardless of body dissatisfaction levels, focused significantly more on weight-related areas, whereas men directed their attention predominantly toward non-weight-related regions (Porras-Garcia et al. 2018, Porras-Garcia et al. 2019). These findings suggest that attentional bias toward weight-related body parts may be a gendered risk factor, more prevalent among women even in the absence of clinical symptoms.

Several theoretical models have been proposed to explain the role of attentional biases in DEAB, often drawing from both cognitive and behavioral frameworks. Cognitive models posit that attentional biases contribute to and maintain body dissatisfaction by selectively attending to information congruent with pre-existing, weight-related schemas. Information that challenges these schemas is either ignored or processed less thoroughly (Vitousek and Hollon 1990, Rodgers and DuBois 2016, Tuschen-Caffier et al. 2015, Williamson et al. 2004). Fairburn (1981) argued that sociocultural pressures lead individuals, particularly women, to overvalue weight and body shape, which in turn fosters selective attention to perceived physical flaws. Later, Fairburn et al. (1999) expanded on this view, suggesting that individuals with DEAB engage in repeated scrutiny of specific body parts as a means of validating distorted beliefs about body fat and weight, further entrenching disordered thinking. In contrast, behavioral models offer an alternative perspective, grounded in principles of conditioning. Drawing from research on anxiety disorders (Cisler and Koster 2010), these models suggest that attentional biases in DEAB develop as conditioned responses to stimuli interpreted as threatening, such as the visual perception of body fat. These biases manifest through safety behaviors and avoidance strategies that, while reducing immediate distress, reinforce maladaptive patterns in the long term. This is consistent with findings that many patients exhibit an initial orienting response followed by avoidance of distressing stimuli (Giel et al. 2011, Blechert et al. 2010, Phillipou et al. 2016). More precisely, the observed overlap between eating disorders and anxiety disorders in symptoms, comorbidity, and even genetic factors further supports the notion that shared mechanisms may underlie attentional biases in both disorders. Bridging the gap between basic and applied research remains a critical challenge in psychological science. However, advances in our understanding of attentional biases in eating disorders, particularly when informed by tools like ET and VR, open promising avenues for therapeutic innovation. While attentional bias modification has shown efficacy in treating anxiety disorders, its application to eating disorders remains underexplored. Nevertheless, given the theoretical and empirical parallels between these disorders, there is considerable potential for developing interventions that target attentional biases to improve outcomes for individuals struggling with eating disorders.

2. Assessing attentional biases using eye-tracking

Attentional bias in individuals with DEAB has been assessed using a variety of cognitive and behavioral tasks. Common methods include modified Stroop tasks, which reveal interference effects when participants are slower to name the color of disorder-relevant words, and dot-probe tasks, which indicate bias through faster responses to probes replacing emotionally salient stimuli. Visual search tasks assess how quickly individuals locate disorder-related targets among distractors, providing insight into attention allocation in complex scenes. Less frequently used techniques such as dichotic listening, lexical decision, and spatial cueing tasks examine auditory attention, word recognition, and spatial orienting, respectively, offering additional dimensions of cognitive processing related to attentional control. A comprehensive review of these methods can be found in Jiang and Vartanian (2018). Among these, ET is considered the most direct and informative method, as it provides continuous, real-time data on gaze behavior while participants view visual stimuli. This technique allows for a direct and objective assessment of attentional biases, whereas other cognitive tasks (e.g., Stroop, dot-probe, and lexical decision tasks) only infer these biases through response latencies. Moreover, ET facilitates the decomposition of visual behavior into voluntarily controlled and automatic responses, which enables more valid differentiation between automatic orienting responses (vigilance), voluntary attention (maintenance), and avoidance responses, as well as the temporal progression of these behaviors. For example, saccadic latency, the time it takes to initiate an eye movement toward a stimulus after its appearance, is commonly interpreted as an indicator of attentional vigilance. In contrast, first fixation duration and total fixation time are typically used to assess attentional maintenance, reflecting how long attention is held on a stimulus once it has been fixed.

Despite its potential, ET has been underutilized in the study of DEAB compared to its application in anxiety and mood disorders. Most studies using ET in DEAB research have focused on general visual behavior rather than differentiating between these specific attentional processes (e.g., vigilance, maintenance, avoidance). However, some studies have investigated these mechanisms in more detail. For instance, Gao et al. (2011, 2014) used first fixation latency and saccadic movements as indicators of vigilance, and the duration of the first fixation and total fixation time as indicators of attentional maintenance (Gao et al. 2011, 2014, Giel et al. 2011, Jiang and Vartanian 2012). Some studies have compared attention toward different body parts, while others have evaluated the competition between images of the self and others. For example, Blechert et al. (2010) found that patients with anorexia nervosa showed shorter saccadic latency when viewing images of themselves compared to images of others, suggesting heightened vigilance toward self-related stimuli. Similar to research on attentional biases in anxiety and depressive disorders, it is important to examine specific biased aspects of attentional processes in DEAB, rather than merely identifying the presence of an attentional bias. Attentional biases have important implications for treatment, as they can hinder habituation during exposure therapy due to unstable attentional patterns. For example, in mirror exposure therapy, a technique commonly used in the treatment of body perception disturbances in eating disorders, patients are asked to observe their own body in a mirror for a prolonged period. Individuals with DEAB often display attentional avoidance or hypervigilance toward specific body parts they perceive negatively. This prevents emotional processing and habituation to the distressing stimulus (i.e., their own body). Modifying these unstable patterns into more sustained attentional focus may be essential for habituation to occur during exposure. Therapists might use real-time feedback from eye-tracking devices or verbal prompts to encourage sustained attention. Over time, this can help reduce the emotional reactivity associated with body perception and support the effectiveness of exposure-based interventions.

The ecological validity of ET can be further enhanced by combining ET with VR technology, which allows for the assessment of visual attention while the participant is immersed in virtual simulations of real-life situations (Lutz et al. 2017). Additionally, VR addresses the issue that arises in studies where patients must evaluate their body perceptions using mirrors: patients may feel uncomfortable wearing tight-fitting or revealing clothing that allows full observation of their body, which can influence the results. With VR, participants do not need to change their clothing during the sessions, as the virtual body's characteristics are defined by the software and are independent of what the participant is wearing at the time.

3. Attentional bias modification in VR-based interventions for DEAB

Although extensive research has been conducted on attentional and cognitive biases in severe DEAB like eating disorders, very little work has been done to apply these findings to enhance the effectiveness of current treatments. Some of the few studies in this area include those by Cardi et al. (2015) and Turton et al. (2018) on reducing negative interpretational biases toward social stimuli in patients with anorexia nervosa, and by Boutelle et al. (2016) and Schmitz and Svaldi (2017) on patients with binge eating disorder. Research specifically on modifying attentional biases toward the body in patients with anorexia nervosa and other DEAB is still in its infancy. While mirror exposure is frequently used to complement cognitive-behavioral therapy, it is primarily aimed at extinguishing negative cognitive, emotional, and behavioral responses to one's body, rather than directly altering attentional processes (Renwick et al. 2013).

Given the current state of knowledge outlined in previous sections, it seems highly relevant to explore whether the efficacy of body exposure treatment could be improved by incorporating training to modify attentional biases in patients with DEAB. If this line of research confirms that modifying attentional biases can enhance the effects of body exposure therapy, for example, by reducing the anxiety and fear of weight gain that patient with anorexia nervosa experience, then a new therapeutic tool could be developed to improve current treatments and make them more adaptable to a broader range of patients. This goal aligns with the growing interest in "stratified medicine," which aims to tailor treatments to individual patient profiles (Lester and Eley 2013, Trusheim et al. 2007). To pursue this research, a limited number of studies have focused on using cutting-edge technology to develop systems capable of modifying body-related attentional biases through virtual simulations. Immersive VR systems, equipped with head-mounted displays and integrated ET devices, have been used alongside custom-designed virtual environments that guide patients' visual attention. These setups enable both the assessment and modification of attentional biases related to body perception.

3.1 VR-based applications for assessing body perception-related attentional bias

The integration of VR and ET technologies has introduced a novel and ecologically valid approach to assessing attentional biases related to body perceptions. Unlike traditional laboratory tasks, VR environments allow participants to engage with realistic, immersive simulations of their own bodies, while ET provides precise, real-time data on visual attention. This combination enables researchers to capture subtle attentional patterns that may be critical in understanding the cognitive mechanisms underlying body dissatisfaction and disordered eating behaviors. A notable example of this approach is the system developed by Porras-Garcia et al. (2019), which embedded ET devices into a head-mounted VR display to examine how gender and body dissatisfaction influence visual attention to different body areas. Participants were immersed in a virtual room with a full-length mirror and viewed personalized avatars from both first- and third-person perspectives. Through synchronized visuo-motor and visuo-tactile stimulation, the system induced a strong sense of embodiment (Mottelson et al. 2023), enhancing the realism of the experience and the relevance of the attentional data collected. Using predefined body areas based on the Physical Appearance State and Trait Anxiety Scale, the researchers measured gaze fixations on weight-related and non-weight-related body parts. The findings revealed gender-specific attentional patterns and suggested that individuals with higher body dissatisfaction may exhibit selective attention toward body areas they perceive as problematic. These results underscore the potential of VR and ET not only for assessment but also as a foundation for developing targeted interventions that address maladaptive attentional processes in individuals at risk for or experiencing DEAB.

Using the same methodology, Porras-Garcia et al. (2020) evaluated the usefulness of VR-based body exposure software for the assessment of fear of weight gain, body anxiety and body-related attentional bias in 30 female patients with anorexia nervosa and 43 non-clinical female college students (25 with low body dissatisfaction and 18 with high body dissatisfaction). All participants were embodied in an avatar that had their silhouette and body mass index by means of synchronous visuo-motor and visuo-tactile stimulation. Visuo-motor stimulation involved syncing the movements of the participant and their avatar. This was done by attaching motion sensors to the participant's hands, feet, and waist. Inside the virtual environment, participants saw themselves from a first-person view and could also look at their avatar in a mirror (third-person view). Visuo-tactile stimulation involved syncing touch and sight. When a researcher touched the participant's body (like their arms, legs, or stomach) with a controller, the participant could see their avatar being touched in the exact same place at the same time by a virtual controller. After inducing full body illusion over the avatar, participants rated how strongly they felt the avatar was their body, their level of body anxiety, and their concern about weight. Finally, the researchers measured how much attention participants paid to their virtual body using ET technology. Participants wore a VR headset that tracked their gaze while they looked at their avatar in the mirror for 30 seconds. To avoid biasing their behavior, participants were told this was part of recalibrating their avatar's position, and they were asked to stay still and avoid sudden head movements. Findings revealed that patients with anorexia nervosa reported significantly higher levels of fear of weight gain and body anxiety compared to women with low body dissatisfaction, with strong effect sizes. In fact, among the variables studied, fear of weight gain was the most effective at distinguishing anorexia nervosa patients from healthy participants and differentiating healthy participants with high body dissatisfaction from those with low body dissatisfaction. Additionally, results indicated that anorexia nervosa patients exhibited a body-related attentional bias, spending more time and looking more frequently at weight-related areas of their bodies, such as the thighs, stomach, and hips, compared to healthy women. These results highlighted the potential of VR-based body exposure as a tool for provoking fear of weight gain and other body-related disturbances in anorexia nervosa patients, suggesting its usefulness as an intervention to reduce these emotional responses and support weight recovery.

Some years later, Schroeder et al. (2023) also combined VR and ET technologies to assess the influence of body dissatisfaction on the perception of self-avatars in VR. Forty-three women with high and low levels of body dissatisfaction were immersed in a swimming pool-related virtual environment, which included locker room elements. While being exposed to the mirror of the locker room, the participants could hear the people enjoying the swimming pool. Before engaging in the mirror exposure session with their avatars, visuo-motor and visuo-tactile interactions were performed to increase embodiment. The main aim of the study was assessing whether embodying an overweight avatar intensifies body dissatisfaction and whether selective attention is drawn more towards weight-related body parts in those with high body dissatisfaction. Contrary to expectations, embodying an overweight avatar did not directly increase body dissatisfaction. However, participants with high body dissatisfaction showed a more sustained embodiment, which the authors hypothesized might relate to heightened body anxiety. On contrast, disembodiment was stronger among low body dissatisfaction participants, suggesting they might more readily detach from virtual bodies that do not align with their self-image, potentially protecting their body perception. Eye-tracking data revealed that women with high body dissatisfaction focused more on weight-related body parts when in the overweight avatar, whereas those with low body dissatisfaction did so when in the normal-weight avatar. This attentional bias highlights how individuals with high body dissatisfaction may implicitly identify with an overweight avatar, whereas those with low body dissatisfaction do not. Moreover, results indicate that selective attention, rather than embodiment, may drive body dissatisfaction.

These early studies stated the bases for using VR to simulate experiences that allow participants to view and interact with virtual representations of their bodies, helping to increase self-awareness and challenge distorted body perceptions. Eye-tracking technologies were also employed to investigate attentional biases in individuals with DEAB, revealing patterns of gaze fixation on weight-related body areas, such as the thighs and stomach. By combining VR's immersive capabilities with the precise measurements of eye tracking, researchers laid the groundwork for innovative therapeutic approaches to reduce body dissatisfaction and associated disturbances.

3.2 VR-based applications for treating body perception-related attentional bias

Addressing attentional biases is crucial in treating DEAB, as these biases contribute to the onset and persistence of these conditions (Lee and Shafran 2004). A systematic review by Matheson et al. (2019) examined the impact of cognitive bias modification on attention biases related to appearance and self-worth across different populations, including clinical, subclinical, and non-clinical groups. The review found preliminary evidence supporting the use of cognitive bias modification as a supplementary treatment for individuals at risk of or experiencing DEAB. However, it also highlighted limitations, such as the lack of real-world applicability in the studies, which were mostly conducted in controlled lab settings. The review called for more clinical trials to further explore the effectiveness of cognitive bias modification in addressing attentional biases in DEAB treatment. Similarly, attention bias modification training has been proposed as an intervention for reducing DEAB-related attentional biases. Dikstein et al. (2022) tested attention bias modification training in young women with anorexia nervosa using the dot-probe task. In this task, participants were shown pairs of words—one food or body-related (threatening) and one neutral—and had to identify the location of a probe that consistently appeared at the neutral word's location. This aimed to train participants to shift their attention away from DEAB-related cues. However, while there were some differences in attentional bias change between the treatment groups (standard treatment vs. attention bias modification training), the results did not show statistically significant reductions in DEAB-related biases. These findings point to challenges in achieving clinical improvements with attention bias modification training and suggest the need for further research to refine the procedure. Mercado et al. (2020) also explored attention bias modification training's potential in treating anorexia nervosa, using the dot-probe task to redirect attention away from food-related cues. The authors proposed that attention bias modification training could be effective by enhancing attentional control and changing how patients perceive the threat value of food, ultimately reducing food-related anxiety. Despite its promise, the authors call for further research to understand attention bias modification training's mechanisms and its clinical efficacy in treating anorexia nervosa.

VR-based interventions offer a groundbreaking approach to addressing attentional biases in DEAB by providing immersive, controlled, and interactive environments that simulate real-life scenarios, achieving ecological validity often missing in traditional therapies. Over the past decade, several studies have demonstrated the potential of VR technology for addressing critical DEAB components, such as body perception-related attentional bias and body perception disturbances (Fakrhou et al. 2024). By combining VR with ET technology, researchers have developed real-time attention bias modification training tools to guide patients in redistributing their focus from weight-related body areas to a more balanced gaze across the entire body. For instance, Meschberger-Annweiler et al. (2023) created an innovative VR-based attention bias modification training, adapted from Smeets et al. (2011), to overcome limitations of traditional Mirror Exposure Therapy, particularly its susceptibility to exacerbating body-related attentional biases in anorexia patients.

The preliminary efficacy and usability of this VR-based attention bias modification training were evaluated in a sample of 60 non-clinical female college students, using the procedure established by Porras-Garcia et al. (2019, 2020). Participants were immersed in a VR environment featuring a full-length mirror and a personalized avatar that replicated their silhouette and body mass index. Full body illusion was induced using visuo-motor and visuo-tactile stimulation before participants engaged in attention bias modification training. During the task, participants completed 300 trials in which they identified shapes or colors of geometric figures appearing on the reflection on the mirror of their avatar or the surrounding environment. As participants focused on these figures, nearby body areas gradually illuminated. If participants lost focus before maintaining their gaze for 4 seconds, the software paused the illumination until attention returned, ensuring consistent engagement. Eye-tracking data provided real-time fixation feedback, with figures appearing near weight-related body parts in 45% of trials, near non-weight-related parts in another 45%, and near neutral stimuli (i.e., cardboard boxes on the floor) in 10%. Each of the four sets of 75 trials lasted approximately 5 to 6 minutes, and attentional bias was reassessed after each set, providing five total measurements throughout the intervention. The study revealed significant reductions in attentional bias after 150 trials for both complete fixation time and number of fixations. Additionally, user experience feedback rated the intervention as moderately usable ("C" on a usability scale from "A" to "F").

Building on these findings, Miquel-Nabau et al. (2023) tested a shorter, 90-trial version of the attention bias modification training in 54 healthy women. Results confirmed the intervention's effectiveness in reducing body-related attentional biases, as participants shifted from focusing predominantly on either weight-related or non-weight-related body parts to distributing their attention more evenly across all areas. Expanding this approach to clinical populations, Ascione et al. (2023) applied a 150-trial version of the VR-based attention bias modification training to 23 female adolescents with anorexia nervosa. Personalized avatars, created using participants' photographs, were employed to ensure an individualized experience. Through visuo-motor and visuo-tactile stimulation, participants experienced an enhanced sense of body ownership, followed by attention bias modification training to reduce fixations on body areas associated with anxiety and body dissatisfaction. The intervention significantly decreased fixation time on weight-related body parts, resulting in a balanced distribution of attention across the entire body. While no significant changes were observed in the number of fixations, participants experienced a marked reduction in body dissatisfaction following the training. These results underscore the potential of VR-based attention bias modification training, integrated with eye-tracking, to modify attentional biases and improve body perceptions in individuals with anorexia nervosa, paving the way for innovative therapeutic solutions in the treatment of DEAB.

3.3 *Advantages of virtual reality in treating body perception-related attentional bias*

VR offers significant advantages in addressing body perception-related attentional biases, leveraging its immersive and adaptive capabilities. By simulating realistic environments, VR creates ecologically valid settings where individuals can engage with body perception-related stimuli in a way that feels authentic yet controlled. This is particularly beneficial for those who find traditional therapeutic approaches, such as *in vivo* exposure or guided imagery, less effective. Furthermore, VR's integration with ET technologies provides clinicians with objective measures of attentional biases, including gaze fixation and attention patterns. This allows for precise tailoring of interventions and ongoing monitoring of patient progress, enhancing treatment efficacy (Porras-Garcia et al. 2019).

The adaptability of VR extends to personalizing interventions, enabling the creation of avatars that reflect the patient's real or perceived body dimensions. Such customization supports targeted therapeutic approaches to body dissatisfaction and attentional biases (Harari et al. 2001). Moreover, VR provides a safe and controlled environment for exposure therapy, allowing patients to confront and habituate to their fears without the risks associated with real-world exposure. This reduces anxiety and avoidance behaviors, creating a supportive framework for cognitive and behavioral change (Clus et al. 2018). Furthermore, evidence supports the application of VR in addressing body perception-related issues, particularly attentional biases, in DEAB. Studies implementing attention bias modification training within VR environments report significant reductions in fixation on weight-related body parts. These changes are associated with decreased body dissatisfaction and anxiety, highlighting VR's potential as a powerful tool in cognitive-behavioral interventions (Miquel-Nabau et al. 2023). In the treatment of anorexia, VR-based therapies have shown notable success in reducing fear of gaining weight and alleviating body perception disturbances. Importantly, these interventions demonstrate promise in maintaining treatment outcomes over time, offering a durable solution for managing anorexia and related disorders (Porras-Garcia et al. 2020, 2021). These findings underscore the transformative potential of VR in enhancing therapeutic outcomes for body perception-related conditions.

3.4 Challenges and future directions

Despite its promise, the integration of VR in treating body perception-related disorders faces several challenges that must be addressed to maximize its impact. Scalability and accessibility remain key barriers, as the high cost of VR equipment and the need for specialized training limit its widespread adoption in clinical settings. Mobile VR platforms offer a potential solution, providing a more cost-effective and accessible alternative for delivering interventions (Monthuy-Blanc et al. 2022). Another pressing issue is the lack of standardized protocols across VR-based therapies, which hampers the comparability of results and the establishment of best practices. Developing universal guidelines for VR interventions in EDs is critical to advancing the field (Clus et al. 2018). Additionally, the long-term efficacy of VR therapies remains underexplored. While short-term outcomes indicate significant benefits, longitudinal studies are needed to evaluate the durability of treatment effects over time. Including follow-up assessments in future research will be essential to understanding the sustained impact of VR-based interventions on body perceptions and eating disorders (Riva et al. 2021). Addressing these challenges can pave the way for broader adoption and enhanced effectiveness of VR in clinical practice.

Conclusion

Virtual reality-based applications are transforming the treatment of body perception-related attentional biases in eating disorders. By offering immersive, personalized, and interactive environments, VR addresses the core psychological and behavioral challenges associated with DEAB. Although challenges remain in terms of accessibility and long-term validation, the integration of VR into therapeutic frameworks represents a significant advancement in the field. Future innovations in technology and research will further enhance the potential of VR to improve outcomes for individuals struggling with eating disorders.

Acknowledgements

This work was supported by the Agencia Estatal de Investigación; Ministerio de Ciencia, Inovación y Universidades. Spain (PID2019-108657RB-I00) and the Fundació la Marató de TV3 (202217-10).

References

Amir, N., C. Beard, M. Burns and J. Bomyea. 2009a. Attention modification program in individuals with generalized anxiety disorder. J. Abnorm. Psychol. 118: 28–33.

Amir, N., C. Beard, C.T. Taylor, H. Klumpp, J. Elias, M. Burns et al. 2009b. Attention training in individuals with generalized social phobia: A randomized controlled trial. J. Consult. Clin. Psychol. 77: 961–973.

Amir, N., C.T. Taylor and M.C. Donohue. 2011. Predictors of response to an attention modification program in generalized social phobia. J. Consult. Clin. Psychol. 79: 533–541.

Ascione, M., M. Carulla-Roig, H. Miquel-Nabau, B. Porras-Garcia, F. Meschberger-Annweiler, E. Serrano-Troncoso et al. 2023. Attentional bias modification training based on virtual reality and eye tracking in Anorexia Nervosa patients. J. Clin. Med. 12.

Bauer, A., S. Schneider, M. Waldorf, K. Braks, T.J. Huber, D. Adolph et al. 2017. Selective visual attention towards oneself and associated state body satisfaction: an eye-tracking study in adolescents with different types of eating disorders. J. Abnorm. Child Psychol. 45: 1647–1661.

Blechert, J., U. Ansorge and B. Tuschen-Caffier. 2010. A body-related dot-probe task reveals distinct attentional patterns for bulimia nervosa and anorexia nervosa. J. Abnorm. Psychol. 119: 575–585.

Boutelle, K.N., T. Monreal, D.R. Strong and N. Amir. 2016. An open trial evaluating an attention bias modification program for overweight adults who binge eat. J. Behav. Ther. Exp. Psychiatry 52: 138–146.

Cardi, V., M. Esposito, G. Bird, C. Rhind, J. Yiend, S. Schifano et al. 2015. A preliminary investigation of a novel training to target cognitive biases towards negative social stimuli in Anorexia Nervosa. J. Affect. Disord. 188: 188–193.

Cisler, J.M. and E.H. Koster. 2010. Mechanisms of attentional biases towards threat in anxiety disorders: An integrative review. Clin. Psychol. Rev. 30: 203–216.

Clus, D., M. Larsen, C. Lemey and S. Berrouiguet. 2018. The use of virtual reality in patients with eating disorders: Systematic review. J. Med. Internet Res. 20.

Dikstein, H., T. Gilon-Mann, R. Halevi-Yosef, A. Enoch-Levi, S. Hamdan, E. Gur et al. 2022. Attention bias modification add-on to inpatient treatment for young women with anorexia nervosa—A randomized controlled trial. Eur. Eat. Disord. Rev.

Eldar, S., A. Apter, D. Lotan, K.P. Edgar, R. Naim, N.A. Fox et al. 2012. Attention bias modification treatment for pediatric anxiety disorders: A randomized controlled trial. Am. J. Psychiatry 169: 213–220.

Fairburn, C. 1981. A cognitive behavioural approach to the treatment of bulimia. Psychol. Med. 11: 707–711.

Fairburn, C.G., R. Shafran and Z. Cooper. 1999. A cognitive behavioural theory of anorexia nervosa. Behav. Res. Ther. 37: 1–13.

Fakhrou, A., G. Avincola, G. Farruggio, I. Verduzzo and P. Caponnetto. 2024. Virtual reality as an innovative tool for eating disorders psychological treatment. Health Psychol. Res. 12.

Freeman, R., S. Touyz, G. Sara, C. Rennie, E. Gordon and P. Beumont. 1991. In the eye of the beholder: Processing body shape information in anorexic and bulimic patients. Int. J. Eat. Disord. 10: 709–714.

Gao, X., X. Deng, J. Yang, S. Liang, J. Liu and H. Chen. 2014. Eyes on the bodies: An eye tracking study on deployment of visual attention among females with body dissatisfaction. Eat. Behav. 15: 540–549.

Gao, X., Q. Wang, T. Jackson, G. Zhao, Y. Liang and H. Chen. 2011. Biases in orienting and maintenance of attention among weight dissatisfied women: An eye-movement study. Behav. Res. Ther. 49: 252–259.

Giel, K.E., H.C. Friederich, M. Teufel, M. Hautzinger, P. Enck and S. Zipfel. 2011. Attentional processing of food pictures in individuals with anorexia nervosa—An eye-tracking study. Biol. Psychiatry 69: 661–667.

Glashouwer, K.A., N.C. Jonker, K. Thomassen and P.J. de Jong. 2016. Take a look at the bright side: Effects of positive body exposure on selective visual attention in women with high body dissatisfaction. Behav. Res. Ther. 83: 19–25.

Hakamata, Y., S. Lissek, Y. Bar-Haim, J.C. Britton, N.A. Fox, E. Leibenluft et al. 2010. Attention bias modification treatment: A meta-analysis toward the establishment of novel treatment for anxiety. Biol. Psychiatry 68: 982–990.

Harari, D., M. Furst, N. Kiryati, A. Caspi and M. Davidson. 2001. A computer-based method for the assessment of body-image distortions in anorexia-nervosa patients. IEEE Trans. Inf. Technol. Biomed. 5: 311–319.

Janelle, C.M., H.A. Hausenblas, R. Ellis, S.A. Coombes and A.R. Duley. 2009. The time course of attentional allocation while women high and low in body dissatisfaction view self and model physiques. Psychol. Health 24: 351–366.

Janelle, C.M., H.A. Hausenblas, E.A. Fallon and R.E. Gardner. 2003. A visual search examination of attentional biases among individuals with high and low drive for thinness. Eat. Weight Disord. 8: 138–144.

Jansen, A., C. Nederkoorn and S. Mulkens. 2005. Selective visual attention for ugly and beautiful body parts in eating disorders. Behav. Res. Ther. 43: 183–196.

Jiang, M.Y.W. and L.R. Vartanian. 2012. Attention and memory biases toward body-related images among restrained eaters. Body Image 9: 503–509.

Jiang, M.Y. and L.R. Vartanian. 2018. A review of existing measures of attentional biases in body image and eating disorders research. Aust. J. Psychol. 70: 3–17.

Kerr-Gaffney, J., A. Harrison and K. Tchanturia. 2018. Eye-tracking research in eating disorders: A systematic review. Int. J. Eat. Disord.

Lee, M. and R. Shafran. 2004. Information processing biases in eating disorders. Clin. Psychol. Rev. 24: 215–238.

Lester, K.J. and T.C. Eley. 2013. Therapygenetics: Using genetic markers to predict response to psychological treatment for mood and anxiety disorders. Biol. Mood Anxiety Disord. 3: 4.

Lutz, H.O., C. Burmeister, L. Ferreira dos Santos, N. Morkisch, C. Dohle and J. Krüger. 2017. Application of head-mounted devices with eye-tracking in virtual reality therapy. Curr. Dir. Biomed. Eng. 3: 53–56.

Matheson, E., T. Wade and J. Yiend. 2019. Utilising cognitive bias modification to remedy appearance and self-worth biases in eating disorder psychopathology: A systematic review. J. Behav. Ther. Exp. Psychiatry 65: 101482.

Mercado, D., U. Schmidt, O. O'Daly, I. Campbell and J. Werthmann. 2020. Food related attention bias modification training for anorexia nervosa and its potential underpinning mechanisms. J. Eat. Disord. 8.

Meschberger-Annweiler, F., M. Ascione, B. Porras-Garcia, M. Ferrer-García, M. Moreno-Sánchez, H. Miquel-Nabau et al. 2023. An attentional bias modification task, through virtual reality and eye-tracking technologies, to enhance the treatment of anorexia nervosa. J. Clin. Med. 12.

Miquel-Nabau, H., N. Briseño-Oloriz, B. Porras-Garcia, M. Ascione, F. Meschberger-Annweiler, M. Ferrer-García et al. 2023. Modification of body-related attentional bias through virtual reality and eye-tracking in healthy participants: Implications for anorexia nervosa treatments. Brain Sci. 13.

Monthuy-Blanc, J., G. Corno, M. Ouellet, F. Touré, F. Bourbeau, M. Rousseau et al. 2022. eLoriCorps immersive body rating scale and eLoriCorps mobile versions: Validation to assess body image disturbances from allocentric and egocentric perspectives in a nonclinical sample of adolescents. J. Clin. Med. 11.

Mottelson, A., A. Muresan, K. Hornbæk and G. Makransky. 2023. A systematic review and meta-analysis of the effectiveness of body ownership illusions in virtual reality. ACM Trans. Comput.-Hum. Interact. 30: 1–42.

Phillipou, A., S.L. Rossell, C. Gurvich, D.J. Castle, N.F. Troje and L.A. Abel. 2016. Body image in anorexia nervosa: Body size estimation utilising a biological motion task and eyetracking. Eur. Eat. Disord. Rev. 24: 131–138.

Porras-Garcia, B., M. Ferrer-Garcia, A. Ghita, M. Moreno, L. López-Jiménez, A. Vallvé-Romeu et al. 2019. The influence of gender and body dissatisfaction on body-related attentional bias: An eye-tracking and virtual reality study. Int. J. Eat. Disord. 52: 1181–1190.

Porras-Garcia, B., M. Ferrer-García, E. Serrano-Troncoso, M. Carulla-Roig, P. Soto-Usera, H. Miquel-Nabau et al. 2021. AN-VR-BE. A randomized controlled trial for reducing fear of gaining weight and other eating disorder symptoms in anorexia nervosa through virtual reality-based body exposure. J. Clin. Med. 10.

Porras-Garcia, B., A. Ghita, M. Moreno, M. Ferrer-Garcia, P. Bertomeu-Panisello, E. Serano-Troncoso et al. 2018. Gender differences in attentional bias after owning a virtual avatar with increased weight. Annu. Rev. Cyberther. Telemed. 16: 73–79.

Reed, D.L., J.K. Thompson, M.T. Brannick and W.P. Sacco. 1991. Development and validation of the Physical Appearance State and Trait Anxiety Scale (PASTAS). J. Anxiety Disord. 5: 323–332.

Renwick, B., I.C. Campbell and U. Schmidt. 2013. Attention bias modification: A new approach to the treatment of eating disorders? Int. J. Eat. Disord. 46: 496–500.

Riva, G., C. Malighetti and S. Serino. 2021. Virtual reality in the treatment of eating disorders. Clin. Psychol. Psychother. 28: 477–488.

Rodgers, R.F. and R.H. Dubois. 2016. Cognitive biases to appearance-related stimuli in body dissatisfaction: A systematic review. Clin. Psychol. Rev. 46: 1–11.

Roefs, A., A. Jansen, S. Moresi, P. Willems, S. van Grootel and A. van der Borgh. 2008. Looking good. BMI, attractiveness bias and visual attention. Appetite 51: 552–555.

Schroeder, P.A., N.A. Gehrer, M. Reents, N. Reimer, J. Vagedes and J. Svaldi. 2023. Body dissatisfaction directs avatar perception: Embodiment and selective visual attention in body mass-modified self-avatars. Cyberpsychol. Behav. Soc. Netw. 26: 850–860.

Smeets, E., A. Jansen and A. Roefs. 2011. Bias for the (un)attractive self: On the role of attention in causing body (dis)satisfaction. Health Psychol. 30: 360–367.

Stice, E., J.M. Gau, P. Rohde and H. Shaw. 2017. Risk factors that predict future onset of each DSM-5 eating disorder: Predictive specificity in high-risk adolescent females. J. Abnorm. Psychol. 126: 38–51.

Trusheim, M.R., E.R. Berndt and F.L. Douglas. 2007. Stratified medicine: Strategic and economic implications of combining drugs and clinical biomarkers. Nat. Rev. Drug Discov. 6: 287–293.

Turton, R., V. Cardi, J. Treasure and C.R. Hirsch. 2018. Modifying a negative interpretation bias for ambiguous social scenarios that depict the risk of rejection in women with anorexia nervosa. J. Affect. Disord. 227: 705–712.

Tuschen-Caffier, B., C. Bender, D. Caffier, K. Klenner, K. Braks and J. Svaldi. 2015. Selective visual attention during mirror exposure in anorexia and bulimia nervosa. PLoS One 10: e0145886.

Vitousek, K.B. and S.D. Hollon. 1990. The investigation of schematic content and processing in eating disorders. Cogn. Ther. Res. 14: 191–214.

von Wietersheim, J., F. Kunzl, H. Hoffmann, J. Glaub, E. Rottler and H.C. Traue. 2012. Selective attention of patients with anorexia nervosa while looking at pictures of their own body and the bodies of others: An exploratory study. Psychosom. Med. 74: 107–113.

Williamson, D.A., M.A. White, E. York-Crowe and T.M. Stewart. 2004. Cognitive-behavioral theories of eating disorders. Behav. Modif. 28: 711–738.

Chapter 5

Dysfunctional Eating Attitudes and Behaviors, and Body Dysmorphia Among LGBTQ+ People

Gabriel Desjardins,[a,b,*] *Frederick Aardema*[a,c] and *Robert-Paul Juster*[a,c]

INTRODUCTION

Dysfunctional eating attitudes and behaviors (DEAB) and body perception disturbances (BPD) disproportionally affect sexually and gender diverse[1] (SGD) people (Parker and Harriger 2020). In this chapter we will use the concept of *body dysmorphia to precise the type of BPD.* However, this phenomenon is only beginning to be understood since the broader DEAB literature has historically been

[a] Montreal Mental Health University Institute Research Center, 7401, rue Hochelaga, Montréal (Québec), Canada, H1N 3MG.

[b] Department of Psychology, Université de Montréal, Pavillon Marie-Victorin 90, avenue Vincent d'Indy, Montréal (Québec), Canada, H3T 1J4.

[c] Department of Psychiatry and Addiction Medicine, Université de Montréal, Pavillon Roger-Gaudry 2900, boul. Édouard-Montpetit, bureau S-750, Montréal (Québec), Canada, H3T 1J4.

Emails: Frederick.aardema@umontreal.ca, robert-paul.juster@umontreal.ca

* Corresponding author: gabrieldesjardins.psy@gmail.com

[1] Sexually diverse people include (not exclusively) gay men, lesbian women, and bisexual people. There are other terms like pansexual and asexual. For gender diverse people, these include people with a transgender identity and nonbinary[4] people, as well as other gender identities such as agender, aromantic, etc. To sum it up, SGD people are people that are not heterosexual and/or not cisgender. Cisgender refers to people that were assigned a sex at birth (male or female) and, when they grew up, they felt comfortable with this assigned sex. Cisgender people comprise the majority of the general population.

DOI: 10.1201/9781032718125-6

female-centric,[2] contributing to the stereotype that anorexia or bulimia affect only privileged young white women (Mitchison and Mond 2015). Yet, research dating back to the 1990s has challenged this view by highlighting SGD peoples' experiences. Early studies focused primarily on gay men, who were overrepresented in eating disorder diagnoses among men. More recently, research has expanded to include lesbian women, bisexual people, and, increasingly, gender diverse people.

SGD people as a group appear particularly at risk of DEAB and BPD when compared to their cisgender heterosexual counterparts (Parker and Harriger 2020). The growing body of research on DEAB in SGD populations highlights two key issues. First, SGD people are not a homogenous group. Because DEAB research in this area remains niche and recruitment is challenging, many studies rely on broad comparisons between cisgender heterosexual and SGD groups, limiting specificity (O'Flynn et al. 2023). In fact, each SGD subgroup faces distinct but overlapping realities that are obscured when treated as a single category. Second, sexual identity is only one facet of sexuality, which also includes behaviors, attractions, attitudes, etc. (Beaulieu-Prévost and Fortin 2015). These problems have yet to be mitigated. More recently, studies show that risk levels for DEAB are not uniform but vary depending on the measurement approach and the specific identity subgroup investigated.

The first part of this chapter will discuss theories on why SGD people are at higher risk for various mental and physical health problems. The second part will provide empirical evidence supporting the overrepresentation of SGD people in DEAB and BPD. Finally, the third part will explore an integrated approach that combines theoretical and empirical foundations from research on SGD people, DEAB, BPD, and their intersections.

1. Theoretical frameworks in SGD research

1.1 Minority stress and psychological mediation

There are different conceptual frameworks that try to explain why SGD people are generally more at risk of DEAB (and other mental health problems) when compared to cisgender heterosexual people. The *minority stress model* developed by Meyer (2003) explains why sexually diverse people face health disparities. To note, this model was later enlarged to include gender diverse people by Testa et al. (2015). Here, the minority stress model will be depicted as a model explaining SGD people health disparities at large.

The minority stress model posits that SGD people encounter both distal and proximal stressors and stress processes that are based on their marginalized identity. Distal stressors refer to events of discrimination and prejudices from society at large, like knowing that there are laws being made prohibiting your freedom in your country or around the world for example. Proximal stressors refer mostly

[2] This chapter will distinguish between biological sex (or sex assigned at birth) and gender. Biological sex includes female, male, and intersex people and is based on physical characteristics. In contrast, gender refers to a social identity rather than primary and secondary sexual characteristics.

to intrapsychic stressors stemming from people in relation to their sociocultural context, like internalized homophobia or transphobia which are the interiorization of negative attitudes toward SGD people (Meyer 2003, Testa et al. 2015). Distal and proximal stress processes are intertwined. For example, a gay man with internalized homophobia can avoid holding hands with his partner in public, because of the risk of violence (distal stressor) and because of disgust at oneself (proximal stressor). These stressors add to the normal burden of life: everyone will encounter general stressors (e.g., breakups, being fired). However, in addition to these general stressors, SGD people will encounter other unique, chronic, and social stressors that are directly linked to their non-chosen identity. Indeed, being queer[3] is not a choice; only coming out of the closet is (Kornak 2015, Roselli 2018).

The minority stress model reinforces that social stigma impacts health, therefore shifting the blame on institutions rather than on marginalized people. However, social changes are protracted. When specifically addressing DEAB and BPD, we need clear clinical leverage points to help sufferers overcome their problems. *The psychological mediation framework* developed by Hatzenbuehler (2009) explains how minority stress "gets under the skin". In other words, how social stigma can negatively influence the use of psychological processes. These psychological processes are "normal" and shared by everyone, regardless of their identity. However, stigma-related stress makes them overused by SGD people as a survival response in face of hostile environments, therefore increasing the risk of psychopathological symptoms. Hatzenbuehler (2009) describes several psychological mediators that are overutilized by SGD people such as rumination, emotional (dys)regulation, social isolation, pessimism, helplessness, etc. The psychological mediation framework helps clinicians to intervene directly on these processes in psychotherapy with SGD people since they can contribute to a feedback loop reinforcing psychopathological symptoms.

1.2 Rejection sensitivity model

The literature on SGD people's mental health is currently undergoing exponential growth. As the mental health field is trying more and more to distance itself from a categorical-syndromal paradigms, we are seeing a gradual return to a more dimensional perspectives. In this spirit, a relatively new personality factor has been identified as particularly relevant for the study of SGD people: rejection sensitivity. The *rejection sensitivity model* first developed by Feldman and Downey (1994) depicts the tendency to project or introject blame in children who are victims of maltreatment from their principal attachment figures (i.e., parents or caregivers). Later, the rejection sensitivity model was extended to intimate relationships, and it is

[3] According to Kornak (2015), queer was an insult directed towards SGD people in the 70s. This term was reappropriated by SGD people to reinstate the political stance inherently tied to sexual and gender diversity in light of oppressive systems. Using the queer label can make SGD people more empowered in the face of stigma and discrimination.

now studied in various contexts, populations, and mental health conditions (Downey and Feldman 1996).

Nowadays, rejection sensitivity is conceptualized as a latent personality trait. Specifically, rejection sensitivity occurs in situations in which there is a risk of rejection from another person as well as in situations of self-vulnerability. It is crucial to understand that actual rejection does not have to occur. People sensitive to rejection may perceive subtle, irrelevant cues in interactions and interpret them as signs of potential rejection. This perception can happen even in contexts filled with acceptance and empathy, such as long-term psychotherapy with a trusted psychologist.

When the rejection sensitivity process is activated, people can: (1) be hypervigilant to possible rejection; (2) encode and perceive rejection signals easily into negative affective states, and (3) have an intense emotional and/or behavioral reaction to these perceived rejection signals. The affective reaction (3) may subsequently reinforce the cognitive components (1 and 2) because of its possible self-fulfilling prophecy. To note, rejection sensitivity exists along a continuum, with its severity and expression varying across people and contexts. In less severe forms, it may be limited to interactions with unfamiliar individuals or low-stakes social situations. In more severe cases, rejection sensitivity may extend to close relationships, including family members, romantic partners, or trusted friends. This reflects a broader and less discerning perception of social threat. Expression can also be highly context-dependent, shaped by one's developmental and attachment history—for example, manifesting predominantly in interactions with authority figures, individuals of a particular gender, or specific relational dynamics.

Case and point, imagine Jade is a rejection-sensitive person attending a party. She starts a conversation with Florence, someone she does not know well. During their exchange, Florence briefly looks away—distracted by a sudden noise Jade does not hear. Jade immediately interprets this as rejection. Her attention narrows, focused solely on being accepted, leaving little room to consider alternative explanations. Rejection sensitivity typically leads to anxious or angry reactions, depending on the individual's coping style (e.g., fight, flight, freeze, or fawn). If Jade reacts anxiously ("Why are you looking away? Do you not like me?") or angrily ("I'm talking to you—how rude!"), she risks triggering actual social rejection. This outcome reinforces her initial fear, creating a confirmation bias that strengthens the part of her that is rejection sensitive.

Rejection sensitivity is thought of as a transdiagnostic factor encompassing several mental disorders (Hsu and Jarcho 2021). Additionally, rejection sensitivity is elevated in SGD people and in people with DEAB or BPD (Gao et al. 2017, Maiolatesi et al. 2022). There are researchers specialized in SGD realities that have described rejection sensitivity as a frontrunner in clinical applications of the minority stress model (Feinstein 2020). The rejection sensitivity model is therefore a complementary paradigm through which researchers and clinicians alike can think of SGD peoples' mental health. Akin to the psychological mediation framework (Hatzenbuehler 2009), the rejection sensitivity model can help clinicians to target specific psychosocial areas to treat and help SGD people' mental health. However, the rejection sensitivity model is broader and seems to go beyond different psychological processes described in Hatzenbuehler's (2009) framework since it is grounded in personality. This aligns with the need for dimensionality as described by the DSM-5 and helps put the emphasis on the underlying pathological dynamics rather than on the discrete symptoms of a disorder (APA 2013).

More specifically, rejection sensitivity resonates across a wide range of therapeutic modalities, each offering a distinct lens to understand its origins and manifestations. In psychodynamic therapy, it may be framed through object relations, ego strength, or narcissistic vulnerability. Humanistic approaches might interpret it as a threat to self-worth or conditional regard, while cognitive-behavioral therapy may conceptualize it through maladaptive core beliefs and attentional biases toward social threat. Systemic therapies could understand rejection sensitivity within broader relational patterns—such as enmeshment, interpersonal boundaries, or intergenerational transmission of emotional invalidation or deprivation. Particularly relevant to SGD people, as well as to emerging and promising therapeutic approaches, Internal Family Systems can view rejection sensitivity as the activation of protective parts shielding exiled parts burdened with feelings of shame or fear of rejection. Crucially, rejection sensitivity is not only clinically observable but also empirically measurable—both through validated self-report instruments and experimental paradigms, such as the *Cyberball* task, which simulates social exclusion in controlled settings. This dual relevance—to both clinical insight and empirical research—makes rejection sensitivity a powerful construct for bridging theory, research, and practice.

In summary, all these conceptual frameworks help us better understand DEAB and BPD in SGD people. But why so many theories, frameworks, and models? Firstly, humans are complex, and psychopathology cannot be understood by one globalized theory. Secondly, it is important for models focused on intrapsychic realities to stay grounded in the minority stress model (Meyer 2020) when applied to DEAB and BPD. In fact, solely focusing on psychological aspects of SGD people risks reinforcing stigmatization by obscuring societies' role in mental health problems (Meyer 2020). This is partly why studying SGD people is so complex: we need leverage points for clinicians, but doing so puts the scientific field at constant risk of blaming the victims of larger and sometimes subtle oppressions.

2. Eating and body image in SGD people

Studies have compared SGD people to non-SGD people in DEAB and BPD. However, as stated earlier, doing so often lacks specificity since the SGD community is not homogenous. Early studies would show that both gay/lesbian and bisexual people were at an equivalent risk of DEAB (Matthews-Ewald et al. 2014). However, when separating gay from bisexual men, and lesbian from bisexual women, studies showed an increased risk of gay men and bisexual women when compared to their corresponding gender subgroup (Mathews-Ewald et al. 2014). Creating groups based on gender (all sexually diverse men together, and all sexually diverse women together) or worse, creating a single SGD group, are methodological practices that make us lose important information about risk and, ultimately, about possible different psychological pathways are linked to specific SGD statuses to DEAB.

2.1 Gay and bisexual cisgender men and youths

Globally, both in teenagers and young adults, sexually diverse men are significantly more at-risk of DEAB and BPD when compared to heterosexual men (Matthews-Ewald et al. 2014). However, the risk for compulsive/excessive exercise and related cognitions seems similar among men, but more studies are needed (Hallward et al. 2023). When compared to sexually diverse women, findings are mixed; however, gay teenagers appear to be at particularly elevated risk for DEAB relative to other sexually diverse subgroups (Morrison et al. 2004, Miller and Luk 2019, Cao et al. 2023).

For gay men specifically, some studies also show an increased risk of several DEAB outcomes and BPD when compared to heterosexual women, who have long-time been thought as the most at-risk subgroup. In fact, gay men are more at-risk of BPD when compared to heterosexual women (Basabas et al. 2019). However, a study showed that this was the case only at moderate and high levels of body dissatisfaction, such that gay men and heterosexual women were otherwise equivalent at low levels (Nelson et al. 2011). When looking at DEAB, however, gay men and heterosexual women are more similar than different (Meyer et al. 2001). This equivalent risk of DEAB might not be true for teenagers, since a meta-analysis showed that gay teenage boys are the most at-risk of disordered eating compared to other sexual identities (Cao et al. 2023). This is not surprising since adolescence is a critical point for identity development. Thus, gay teenage boys need not only to navigate the turbulence of puberty and individuation, but also to acknowledge their stigmatized identity. They do so while thriving for their peer acceptance and their integration in the appearance-focused gay subculture. The latter point on subculture will be explored more extensively in part 3. Relatedly, bisexual men are also more at-risk than heterosexual men to endorse DEAB or to have BPD (Morrison et al. 2004).

Some studies comparing gay to bisexual men and teenagers show that bisexual men have less BPD and DEAB (Nelson et al. 2011, Hazzard et al. 2020, Cao et al. 2023, Hallward et al. 2023). However, for BPD, a meta-analysis showed a marginally significant difference, but this could be due to equivalent levels of drive for muscularity (Ryan et al. 2010, He et al. 2020). Taken together, it seems that being gay is a specific risk factor for DEAB or BPD in men.

Nonetheless, most BP studies have grouped gay and bisexual men together, failing to recognize the dual challenge bisexual men face because of their plurisexuality (Filiault et al. 2014). A qualitative study among bisexual men showed they may have similar BP ideals than other males, while lacking the desire to engage in body modification and thinness-oriented behavior (Filiault et al. 2014). We can presume then that they share similar cognitions with gay men while being less emotionally preoccupied or behaviorally invested with appearance (Filiault et al. 2014). This may stem from the heightened pressure bisexual men face to conform to hegemonic masculinity. Internalized homophobia and the social demand to "pick a side" sexually may discourage association with traits linked to a "gay body" (e.g., thinness, visible self-modification) (Filiault et al. 2014). This reflects the double stigmatization bisexual individuals often experience: marginalization both from the heterosexual mainstream and within SGD communities. This was echoed by a quantitative study showing higher hypermasculinity in bisexual compared to gay men (Ryan et al. 2010).

2.2 Lesbian and bisexual cisgender women and youths

Studies are particularly contradictory regarding lesbian women. When compared to heterosexual women or teenage girls, some studies show lesbian women at increased risk for DEAB (Matthews-Ewald et al. 2014). Other studies show no significant differences in DEAB (Shearer et al. 2015, Luk et al. 2019, Hazzard et al. 2020), while some studies show that lesbian women are less at risk than heterosexual women on DEAB or body dissatisfaction (Meyer et al. 2001, Nelson et al. 2011). Qualitatively speaking, there might be a bias towards more recent studies pointing towards an equivalent or higher risk in lesbian women on most outcomes. In contrast, older studies seem to be putting the protective aspect of the lesbian identity front and center, stating a form of BP resilience despite sociocultural pressures for thinness targeting women. In fact, studies are generally consistent in stating that there might be some protective factors against DEAB and BPD that are related to the lesbian subculture, favoring higher body satisfaction (Meyer et al. 2001, Basabas et al. 2019). The latter point on subculture will be discussed in part 3.

For bisexual women and teenage girls, they are more similar to gay men and sexually diverse men and teenagers, being the most at-risk subgroup in most studies on DEAB and BPD. In fact, bisexual women and teenagers show increased body image distortion, and DEAB when compared to heterosexual women (Matthews-Ewald et al. 2014, Miller and Luk 2019). They seem to also be more at-risk than lesbian women and teenagers for DEAB and BPD (Nelson et al. 2011, Cao et al. 2023). As for gay and bisexual men, a meta-analysis also showed a similar pattern for BPD when comparing bisexual and lesbian women: bisexual women might have marginally higher levels of body image dissatisfaction and distortion, but this could be a trend rather than a significant difference (He et al. 2020).

2.3 Gender diverse adults and youths

Gender diverse people endorse more DEAB when compared to cisgender heterosexual people (Duffy et al. 2021). Some studies also show that gender diverse people are the most disadvantaged SGD group regarding DEAB, with higher scores than sexually diverse people (Romano et al. 2022, Hallward et al. 2023). However, one study showed no significant differences between gender diverse and sexually diverse people in DEAB, and another study showed that sexually diverse men over-exercise more in response to the COVID-19 pandemic (Krueger et al. 2021, Hart et al. 2022). What seems clearer is that gender diverse people have a higher risk of DEAB and BPD when compared to cisgender heterosexual people, despite gender diverse people receiving less eating disorder diagnoses than cisgender heterosexual women (Hallward et al. 2023). Considering minority stress, this result is unsurprising and could be explained by difficulty accessing care for gender diverse people (Hallward et al. 2023).

Few studies have disaggregated gender diverse people into different identity subgroups. In fact, there are lots of different possibilities regarding gender identity labels, but the most widespread are transgender and nonbinary. The term nonbinary is often used as an umbrella term for people whose gender identity does not align with the arbitrary binary categories of "man" or "woman".[4]

Some studies suggest a higher incidence of DEAB in transmen compared to transwomen (Romano et al. 2022). However, the literature is still scarce, and no definitive answer can be made at this time since some studies suggest no significant differences between the two (Duffy et al. 2021, Linsenmeyer et al. 2021). Relatedly, nonbinary people have not been studied much yet. We could wonder if transphobia permeates research endeavors, interpreting this underrepresentation as a reflection of the widespread difficulty to consider gender as more than binary (Maughan et al. 2022).

Compared to transmen or transwomen, nonbinary people further deconstruct the conservative view of gender as being based solely on genital parts and stereotyped performance of gender (Dembroff 2020). Nonbinary people therefore reinstate how fragile the patriarchal framework can be when it comes to institutionalized gender (Dembroff 2020). Based on this interpretation of the limited literature, nonbinary people could be even more at risk of DEAB when compared to other gender diverse people. But the few studies that have compared transgender and nonbinary people showed no differences in DEAB between the two (Duffy et al. 2021, Linsenmeyer et al. 2021). Therefore, gender diverse people are the more at-risk subgroup when compared to other SGD and cisgender people.

Few studies have taken the intersecting influence of sexual identity and gender identity in the DEAB and BPD literature. Interestingly, Hallward et al. (2022) found no significant differences in DEAB between cisgender heterosexual men and transgender heterosexual men. In contrast, two other studies suggest that heterosexual transgender individuals may be at lower risk for DEAB compared to their sexually diverse transgender counterparts—with the exception of those identifying as lesbian (Egbert et al. 2024). This result shows how intersectionality[5] can pave the way towards different types of powers, privileges, and oppressions that can co-exist inside a person, making them susceptible to different types of stressors and, consequently, different types of psychopathological profiles (Crenshaw 2013). It also reinstates the aforementioned greater BP inclusiveness of the lesbian-queer subculture.

---

[4] There are other ways to experience one's gender identity under the nonbinary umbrella term. The phenomenology of gender identities is complex and intrinsically subjective. In this chapter, nonbinary is used as an umbrella term containing all gender diverse identities but transmen or transwomen (e.g., agender, gender-neutral, genderqueer, two-spirit, gender fluid, etc.).

[5] Intersectionality theory is a framework that examines how various social identities (such as race, gender, socioeconomic class, sexual identity, bodily autonomy, etc.) intersect in a complex manner. This theory was developed by Crenshaw (2013) and highlights how individual experiences are complex and in constant interrelation with different forms of oppression not understandable in isolation from one another.

For BPD, gender diverse people can be inherently body dysphoric because of a mismatch between their biological sex and their gender identity. There are several studies on BPD in gender diverse people, but they are mostly related to gender dysphoria and not to BPD as it relates to DEAB. However, BPD and gender dysphoria can interact together and potentialize each other, culminating in DEAB as a goal or as a secondary gain to align the body to the gender identity (Campbell et al. 2024). This subject will be covered in last part.

2.4 Cisgender people unsure of their sexual identity and other sexual identities

When asked about their sexual identity, some people simply do not know, are unsure of it, or are currently questioning themselves. These people are more frequent than we think, comprising a large enough subgroup that permits analyses in many studies. Unfortunately, this heterogeneous group is often excluded from statistical analyses with only a few studies including them. Globally, this subgroup appears at an increased risk of DEAB and BPD when compared to heterosexual people, being similar in the matter to sexually diverse people (Matthews-Ewald et al. 2014, Hazzard et al. 2020, Ganson et al. 2021). We do not know much about the underlying reasons, but we can speculate that minority stressors (i.e., concealment) or identity diffusion could contribute (Parker and Harriger 2020).

Firstly, concealing one's sexual identity is a risk factor for DEAB and BPD (Parker and Harriger 2020). Secondly, navigating an identity that may be stigmatized if it reveals itself as part of sexual diversity can be stressful enough to contribute to higher DEAB or BPD risk, as in gay teenagers for example (Cao et al. 2023). Lastly, identity problems or diffusion, meaning not knowing who you really are, is a core feature of borderline personality (APA 2013). In fact, borderline personality disorder and identity diffusion itself are related to DEAB and BPD (Biberdzic et al. 2021). In a recent Canadian sample of sexually diverse teenagers, every participant that had moderate or high levels of DEAB were automatically attaining the clinical cut-off for emerging borderline personality disorder (Lee and Vaillancourt 2023).

2.5 Conclusion

In summary, it seems that being different from the sexual or gender norm confers a particular risk of DEAB and BPD. To date, what seems certain is that the magnitude of the differences in DEAB and BPD is larger between teenage boys and adult men of diverse sexual identities when compared to teenage girls and adult women of diverse sexual identities (Hazzard et al. 2020, Cao et al. 2023). Putting gender aside, it seems that heterosexual men are consistently at a lower risk of DEAB and BPD and that the long-time recognition of DEAB and body dysmorphia as a female problem is debunked by the sometimes-higher risk of gay men to the matter. Given the contradictory findings in the literature, more meta-analyses are needed to clarify differential risks across diverse identities. Our ongoing meta-analysis aims to help address this gap and provide clearer insights by 2025.

3. Integrating eating, body image, and SGD research

The current literature consistently demonstrates elevated rates of DEAB and BPD among individuals across diverse SGD identities, underscoring the heightened vulnerability of SGD populations. To contextualize these disparities, it is useful to draw from established models explaining DEAB and BPD among heterosexual women and examine how they intersect with frameworks addressing health inequities in SGD populations. Merging these theoretical perspectives—those focused on DEAB and BPD with those addressing identity-based stigma—can help clarify the unique mechanisms contributing to elevated risk of DEAB and BPD among SGD people.

In relation to the minority stress model, *the tripartite influence model* could shed light on the sociocultural climate surrounding this elevated prevalence (Tylka and Andorka 2012, Hazzard et al. 2019). This model explains how pressures stemming from family, peers, and the media can explain the incidence of DEAB and BPD. For SGD, acceptance from family and peers, and homophobic/transphobic stances sometimes propagated by the media could increase minority stress and elevated prevalences.

For sexually diverse men, the sense of belonging and connection to the gay community confers a risk for DEAB and drive for muscularity (Hunt et al. 2012). Sexually diverse men may benefit from being neutral towards their community, not too outside, and not too inside (Siconolfi et al. 2016). In fact, specific gay social media platforms (e.g., Grindr) are related to DEAB and BPD because there seems to be an emphasis placed on leanness and thinness, as well as fatphobic attitudes that are shared among users of these platforms and sexually diverse men in general (Tie et al. 2023). However, dating app usage might not be sufficient to explain the occurrences of DEAB and BPD: physical comparisons could mediate the relationship (Blassingame III 2020). This result aligns with social comparison theory (Festinger 1954), positing humans' tendency to compare themselves to others. This theory inspired researchers on DEAB and BPD to develop the *social comparison model* in which people may engage in upward appearance comparisons (e.g., comparing the bodily self to others perceived as more attractive) (O'Brien et al. 2009).

By contrast for sexually diverse women, the sense of belonging and connection to the lesbian-queer community is protective of the endorsement of DEAB (Hunt et al. 2012). This could explain why the incidence of DEAB and BPD is unclear in lesbian women specifically. There seems to be a certain acceptance of diverse bodies in the lesbian-queer community, with some aspects of this community protecting women of diverse sexual identities from damaging beauty standards (Henrichs-Beck et al. 2015). However, lesbian and bisexual women are women first and foremost, and are therefore subjugated to the same heteronormative beauty standards and pressures as are heterosexual women (Henrichs-Beck et al. 2015).

For gender diverse people, DEAB can be used to align their gender identity to their gender expression. For example, studies have shown that transwomen may restrict their caloric intake to lose body hair and muscle mass, and transmen may also restrict their caloric intake to lose their menstrual periods, their breasts, and their hips (McGuire et al. 2016). Therefore, DEAB can be a way to diminish gender dysphoria and feel more congruent with how their body looks to the outside observer and to themselves. However, studies show that DEAB and BPD are not resulting only from gender dysphoria; even after beginning hormonal treatment and seeing body changes, some transgender people still endorse BPD or DEAB (Riddle et al. 2023). In fact, hormonal treatments can cause weight gain, especially in transwomen (Riddle et al. 2023).

In the context of rejection sensitivity, SGD individuals may pursue social acceptance—and avoid rejection—by conforming to rigid societal beauty standards, as the body often feels more controllable than one's core identity. This pursuit can foster a process known as self-objectification. Body image pressures depicted in the tripartite influence models can be psychologically understood as how families, peers, and medias incite people (especially women and SGD people) to view themselves as an object whose purpose is to be appealing to people's (especially men) gazes. Combined with humans' tendency to compare themselves with one another, this can create a pervasive sociopsychological phenomena.

The objectification theory (Frederickson 1997) was initially developed for heterosexual women. This theory posits that the media portrays an overly sexualized and bodily unattainable image of women, creating a process known as self-objectification. In fact, many women see themselves as an exterior observer, evaluating their self-value solely based on their physical appearance. Self-objectification is directly linked to DEAB and BPD in heterosexual women, and more and more studies show self-objectification to be a key mediator in the endorsement of DEAB in gay and bisexual men specifically (Dakanalis et al. 2012).

This theory is also based in the evolutionary paradigm: in most cultures, men put the emphasis on physical appearance when selecting a potential sexual or romantic partner, whereas women put more emphasis on power and social status. This can explain why sexually diverse men and heterosexual women are more at risk of self-objectification when compared to heterosexual men (Dakanalis et al. 2012, Schaefer and Thompson 2018). What is interesting is that both lesbian and bisexual women also show elevated self-objectification when compared to heterosexual men (Kozee and Tylka 2006, Brewster et al. 2014). However, the association between self-objectification and DEAB is moderate in heterosexual women and gay men, low in bisexual women, and absent in lesbian women (Brewster et al. 2014, Shaefer and Thompson 2018). This is coherent with the premises of the theory: self-objectification is meant to attract the male gaze. Lesbian women could self-objectify because of their gender, but maybe they do not feel the urge to endorse DEAB and modify their appearance because of their sexual attraction, as the broader inclusivity within the lesbo-queer community may lessen this urge

In summary, SGD people are victims of broader societal systems that dehumanize them. Through the tripartite influence model, dehumanization messages are conferred to SGD people, reinforcing stigma, discrimination, and inciting them to self-objectify or compare themselves negatively. This intolerant climate pushes SGD people towards pathological psychological processes as stated by Hatzenbuehler (2009) and make them vulnerable to rejection sensitivity. In fact, human beings are inherently sociable, thriving to be accepted by peers, family, and society at large.

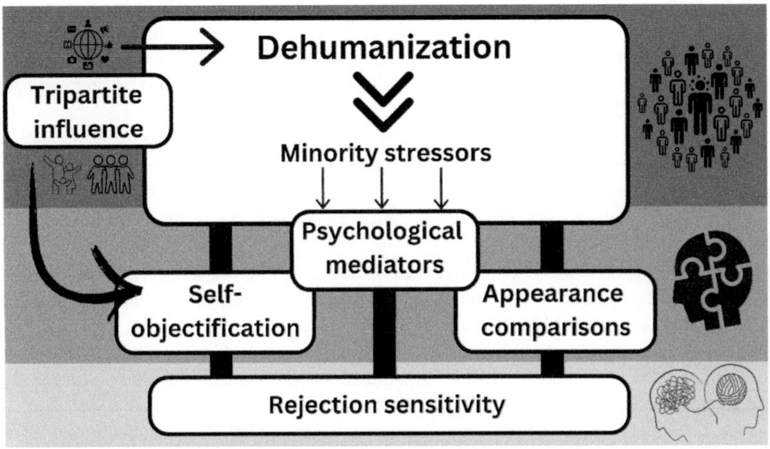

Figure 1. Integrated theoretical model of DEAB and BPD in SGD population.

Moradi (2013) has synthetized most of these theoretical models and frameworks into a larger phenomenon. *The pan-theoretical model of dehumanization* explains why SGD people are at an elevated risk of DEAB, BPD, and other mental or physical health problems (Moradi 2013). We created a figure depicting how, specifically for DEAB and BPD, the theoretical models and frameworks presented in this chapter can be understood altogether to describe SGD realities (see Figure 1).

Conclusion

In conclusion, we hope that SGD people will one day be seen as equal and deserving human beings, since sexual and gender identities are not choices, but only normal variations of human sexuality and gender. Nobody would choose to live in a world where hatred permeates against your well-being only because of who you are. SGD people are not sick because of their identities; they are sick because they are dehumanized.

References

American Psychiatric Association. 2013. Diagnostic and Statistical Manual of Mental Disorders: DSM-5. American Psychiatric Association Washington, DC.

Basabas, M.C., L. Greaves, F.K. Barlow and C.G. Sibley. 2019. Sexual orientation moderates the effect of gender on body satisfaction: Results from a national probability sample. J. Sex Res. 56: 1091–1100.

Beaulieu-Prévost, D. and M. Fortin. 2015. The measurement of sexual orientation: Historical background and current practices. Sexologies 24: e15–e19.

Biberdzic, M., J. Tang and J. Tan. 2021. Beyond difficulties in self-regulation: the role of identity integration and personality functioning in young women with disordered eating behaviours. J. Eat. Disord. 9.

Blassingame III, J.C. 2020. # Yasssforthebody: Social Media, Body Dissatisfaction, and Disordered Eating among Gay Men. Fielding Graduate University.

Brewster, M.E., B.L. Velez, J. Esposito, S. Wong, E. Geiger and B.T. Keum. 2014. Moving beyond the binary with disordered eating research: A test and extension of objectification theory with bisexual women. J. Couns. Psychol. 61: 50–62.

Campbell, L., K. Viswanadhan, B. Lois and M. Dundas. 2024. Emerging evidence: a systematic literature review of disordered eating among transgender and nonbinary youth. J. Adolesc. Health 74: 18–27.

Cao, Z., E. Cini, D. Pellegrini and K.C. Fragkos. 2023. The association between sexual orientation and eating disorders-related eating behaviours in adolescents: A systematic review and meta-analysis. Eur. Eat. Disord. Rev. 31: 46–64.

Crenshaw, K.W. 2013. Mapping the margins: Intersectionality, identity politics, and violence against women of color. pp. 93–118. In The Public Nature of Private Violence. Routledge.

Dakanalis, A., V.E. Di Mattei, E.P. Bagliacca, A. Prunas, L. Sarno, G. Riva et al. 2012. Disordered eating behaviors among italian men: objectifying media and sexual orientation differences. Eat. Disord. 20: 356–367.

Dembroff, R. 2020. Beyond binary: genderqueer as critical gender kind. Philosophers' Imprint 20.

Downey, G. and S.I. Feldman. 1996. Implications of rejection sensitivity for intimate relationships. J. Pers. Soc. Psychol. 70: 1327–1343.

Duffy, M.E., J.P. Calzo, E. Lopez, S. Silverstein, T.E. Joiner and A.R. Gordon. 2021. Measurement and construct validity of the Eating Disorder Examination Questionnaire Short Form in a transgender and gender diverse community sample. Psychol. Assess 33: 459.

Egbert, J., A. Luke and F. Qeadan. 2024. Intersectionality of demographic characteristics in self-reported anorexia nervosa, bulimia nervosa, and probable eating disorders among college students. Int. J. Eat. Disord. 57: 132–145.

Feinstein, B.A. 2020. The rejection sensitivity model as a framework for understanding sexual minority mental health. Arch. Sex. Behav. 49: 2247–2258.

Feldman, S. and G. Downey. 1994. Rejection sensitivity as a mediator of the impact of childhood exposure to family violence on adult attachment behavior. Dev. Psychopathol. 6: 231–247.

Festinger, L. 1954. A theory of social comparison processes. Hum. Relat. 7: 117–140.

Filiault, S.M., M.J.N. Drummond and E. Anderson. 2014. Bisexual men and body image. Psychol. Sex. 5: 191–200.

Frederickson, B.L. and T.-A. Roberts. 1997. Objectification Theory: Toward understanding women's lived experiences and mental health risks. Psychol. Women Q. 21: 173–206.

Ganson, K.T., R.F. Rodgers, S.B. Murray and J.M. Nagata. 2021. Prevalence and demographic, substance use, and mental health correlates of fasting among US college students. J. Eat. Disord. 9: 1–12.

Gao, S., M. Assink, A. Cipriani and K. Lin. 2017. Associations between rejection sensitivity and mental health outcomes: A meta-analytic review. Clin. Psychol. Rev. 57: 59–74.

Hallward, L., J.M. Nagata, R.F. Rodgers and K.T. Ganson. 2023. Examination of eating disorder psychopathology across sexual and gender identities among a Canadian sample. Int. J. Eat. Disord. 56: 604–615.

Hart, E.A., A. Rubin, K.M. Kline and K.R. Fox. 2022. Disordered eating across COVID-19 in LGBTQ+ young adults. Eat. Behav. 44: 101581.

Hatzenbuehler, M.L. 2009. How does sexual minority stigma "get under the skin"? A psychological mediation framework. Psychol. Bull. 135: 707–730.

Hazzard, V.M., L.M. Schaefer, K. Schaumberg, A.M. Bardone-Cone, D.A. Frederick, K.L. Klump et al. 2019. Testing the Tripartite Influence Model among heterosexual, bisexual, and lesbian women. Body Image 30: 145–149.

Hazzard, V.M., M. Simone, S.L. Borg, K.A. Borton, K.R. Sonneville, J.P. Calzo et al. 2020. Disparities in eating disorder risk and diagnosis among sexual minority college students: Findings from the national Healthy Minds Study. Int. J. Eat. Disord. 53: 1563–1568.

He, J., S. Sun, Z. Lin and X. Fan. 2020. Body dissatisfaction and sexual orientations: A quantitative synthesis of 30 years research findings. Clin. Psychol. Rev. 81: 101896.

Henrichs-Beck, C., D. Szymanski, C. Feltman and T. Batchelor. 2015. Exploring biculturality and beauty standards through breast discourse and breasted experience of sexual minority women. Psychol. Sex. Orientat. Gend. Divers. 2.

Hsu, D.T. and J.M. Jarcho. 2021. Next up for psychiatry: Rejection sensitivity and the social brain. Neuropsychopharmacology 46: 239.

Hunt, C.J., K. Gonsalkorale and B.A. Nosek. 2012. Links between psychosocial variables and body dissatisfaction in homosexual men: differential relations with the drive for muscularity and the drive for thinness. Int. J. Mens Health 11.

Kornak, J. 2015. Queer as a Political Concept. University of Helsinky.

Kozee, H.B. and T.L. Tylka. 2006. A test of objectification theory with lesbian women. Psychol. Women Q. 30: 348–357.

Krueger, E.A., J.L. Barrington-Trimis, J.B. Unger and A.M. Leventhal. 2021. Sexual and gender minority young adult coping disparities during the COVID-19 pandemic. J. Adolesc. Health 69: 746–753.

Lee, K.S. and T. Vaillancourt. 2023. Trajectories, comorbidity, and risk factors for adolescent disordered eating and borderline personality disorder features. Dev. Psychopathol.: 1–12.

Linsenmeyer, W.R., I.M. Katz, J.L. Reed, A.M. Giedinghagen, C.B. Lewis and S.K. Garwood. 2021. Disordered eating, food insecurity, and weight status among transgender and gender nonbinary youth and young adults: a cross-sectional study using a nutrition screening protocol. LGBT Health 8: 359–366.

Luk, J.W., J.M. Miller, L.M. Lipsky, S.E. Gilman, D.L. Haynie and B.G. Simons-Morton. 2019. A longitudinal investigation of perceived weight status as a mediator of sexual orientation disparities in maladaptive eating behaviors. Eat. Behav. 33: 85–90.

Maiolatesi, A.J., K.A. Clark and J.E. Pachankis. 2022. Rejection sensitivity across sex, sexual orientation, and age: Measurement invariance and latent mean differences. Psychol. Assess. 34: 431.

Matthews-Ewald, M.R., K.J. Zullig and R.M. Ward. 2014. Sexual orientation and disordered eating behaviors among self-identified male and female college students. Eat. Behav. 15: 441–444.

Maughan, L., K. Natalier and M. Mulholland. 2022. Institutional transphobia: barriers to transgender research in early years education. Gend. Educ. 34: 721–737.

McGuire, J.K., J.L. Doty, J.M. Catalpa and C. Ola. 2016. Body image in transgender young people: Findings from a qualitative, community based study. Body Image 18: 96–107.

Meyer, C., J. Blissett and C. Oldfield. 2001. Sexual orientation and eating psychopathology: The role of masculinity and femininity. Int. J. Eat. Disord. 29: 314–318.

Meyer, I.H. 2003. Prejudice, social stress, and mental health in lesbian, gay, and bisexual populations: Conceptual issues and research evidence. Psychol. Bull. 129: 674–697.

Meyer, I.H. 2020. Rejection sensitivity and minority stress: A challenge for clinicians and interventionists. Arch. Sex. Behav. 49: 2287–2289.

Miller, J.M. and J.W. Luk. 2019. A systematic review of sexual orientation disparities in disordered eating and weight-related behaviors among adolescents and young adults: Toward a developmental model. Adolesc. Res. Rev. 4: 187–208.

Moradi, B. 2013. Discrimination, Objectification, and Dehumanization: Toward a Pantheoretical Framework. In Springer New York: 153–181.

Morrison, M.A., T.G. Morrison and C.-L. Sager. 2004. Does body satisfaction differ between gay men and lesbian women and heterosexual men and women?: A meta-analytic review. Body Image 1: 127–138.

Nelson, D.L., L.G. Castonguay and B.D. Locke. 2011. Challenging stereotypes of eating and body image concerns among college students: implications for diagnosis and treatment of diverse populations. J. Coll. Couns. 14: 158–172.

O'Flynn, J.L., G.P. Nowicki, K. Laveway, A.R. Gordon and R.F. Rodgers. 2023. Toward inclusivity: A systematic review of the conceptualization of sexual minority status and associated eating disorder outcomes across two decades. Int. J. Eat. Disord. 56: 350–365.

O'Brien, K.S., P. Caputi, R. Minto, G. Peoples, C. Hooper, S. Kell et al. 2009. Upward and downward physical appearance comparisons: Development of scales and examination of predictive qualities. Body Image 6: 201–206.

Parker, L.L. and J.A. Harriger. 2020. Eating disorders and disordered eating behaviors in the LGBT population: a review of the literature. J. Eat. Disord. 8.

Riddle, M., S. Silverstein and E. Wassenaar. 2023. The care of transgender and gender diverse adolescents with eating disorders. Curr. Pediatr. Rep. 11: 148–156.

Romano, K.A., S.K. Lipson, A.L. Beccia, P.A. Quatromoni, A.R. Gordon and J. Murgueitio. 2022. Changes in the prevalence and sociodemographic correlates of eating disorder symptoms from 2013 to 2020 among a large national sample of U.S. young adults: A repeated cross-sectional study. Int. J. Eat. Disord. 55: 776–789.

Roselli, C.E. 2018. Neurobiology of gender identity and sexual orientation. J. Neuroendocrinol. 30: e12562.

Ryan, T.A., T.G. Morrison and D.T. McDermott. 2010. Body image investment among gay and bisexual men over the age of 40: A test of social comparison theory and threatened masculinity theory. Gay Lesbian Issues Psychol. 6: 4–19.

Schaefer, L.M. and J.K. Thompson. 2018. Self-objectification and disordered eating: A meta-analysis. Int. J. Eat. Disord. 51: 483–502.

Shearer, A., J. Russon, J. Herres, T. Atte, T. Kodish and G. Diamond. 2015. The relationship between disordered eating and sexuality amongst adolescents and young adults. Eat. Behav. 19: 115–119.

Siconolfi, D.E., F. Kapadia, R.W. Moeller, J.A. Eddy, S.A. Kupprat, M.J. Kingdon et al. 2016. Body dissatisfaction in a diverse sample of young men who have sex with men: The P18 Cohort Study. Arch. Sex. Behav. 45: 1227–1239.

Testa, R.J., J. Habarth, J. Peta, K. Balsam and W. Bockting. 2015. Development of the gender minority stress and resilience measure. Psychol. Sex. Orientat. Gend. Divers. 2: 65–77.

Tie, B., Y. Xu, S. Cui and J. He. 2023. Gay dating apps usage, body dissatisfaction, and disordered eating in Chinese Young Gay Men. J. Homosex.: 1–21.

Tylka, T.L. and M.J. Andorka. 2012. Support for an expanded tripartite influence model with gay men. Body Image 9: 57–67.

Chapter 6

Negative Physical Self-perception in Athletes with Dysfunctional Eating Attitudes and Behaviors

Stéphanie Mériaux-Scoffier

INTRODUCTION

Athletes' psychological well-being is of paramount importance, considering the intense pressures and demands inherent in competitive sports. The rigorous mental and physical investment required can often take a toll on athletes' mental health. The research in sport psychology has increasingly focused on the psychological well-being of athletes due to the mental and physical investment involved in a sports career and the success pressures they face. While physical activity is presented as beneficial for an individual's physical and psychological health (World Health Organization 2022), when practiced intensively, it can lead to mental health issues, especially among elite athletes (Reardon et al. 2019). A recent systematic review identified 22 studies reporting mental health symptoms among elite athletes, including 7 cross-sectional studies providing data on eating disorders (Gouttebarge et al. 2017). Eating disorders are complex issues that impact athletic performance, as well as the health and psychological well-being of athletes. However, the explanatory mechanisms are not straightforward, and the literature suggests various types of mechanisms related to the specificity of the physical, social environment, and psychological characteristics of the athlete. Understanding the variations and

University of Nice Côte d'Azur, LAMHESS, EA6312, 06205 Nice, France.
Email: stephanie.meriaux@univ-cotedazur.fr

DOI: 10.1201/9781032718125-7

psychosocial mechanisms that result from these is essential for developing effective intervention strategies aimed at promoting healthy eating behaviors among athletes, serving both their health and performance.

The etiology of dysfunctional eating attitudes and behaviors appears to be multifactorial, linked to vulnerability factors (e.g., genetic predisposition, pre-existing biological anomalies), triggering factors (e.g., strict dietary regimens, major life events, puberty), and predisposing factors (e.g., biological imbalances, relational benefits from the environment) (Jeammet 2013). Dysfunctional eating attitudes and behaviors emerge when a psychological conflict arises, combined with vulnerability factors. These behaviors appear as a solution to this impasse, an attempt to regain control, but result from a sequence of behavior due to the specific characteristics of eating disorders (Jeammet 2013). Despite the increasing research on factors influencing the emergence of dysfunctional eating attitudes and behaviors in sports, many areas remain unclear, particularly regarding the role of psychosocial factors. In this context, it is relevant to unfold the 3P model (Predisposing, Precipitating, and Perpetuating factors) adapted to the sports domain to better understand these phenomena.

Predisposing Factors: These factors increase an individual's vulnerability to developing dysfunctional eating behaviors. In sports, this may include genetic predisposition, early exposure to body image pressures, or a history of dieting and weight control behaviors. Biological imbalances, such as hormonal changes, also play a role, especially in weight-classified sports like gymnastics or wrestling. Psychological traits like perfectionism or low self-esteem can further increase susceptibility (Jeammet 2013, Vitousek et al. 2000).

Precipitating Factors: These factors trigger or provoke the onset of dysfunctional eating attitudes and behaviors. In the sports context, this could include major life events such as an injury, a change in coaching, or a decline in performance (e.g., failure in a key competition). Strict training regimens, pressure to meet specific body composition standards, or external validation through performance can act as stressors, pushing athletes toward maladaptive coping mechanisms like disordered eating. Puberty, with its associated physical changes, is also a critical period when athletes become more aware of their body image and may engage in restrictive eating practices (Smolak and Murnen 2004).

Perpetuating Factors: These are factors that maintain or exacerbate dysfunctional eating behaviors over time. In sports, these could include environmental pressures such as encouragement to maintain a certain weight class or an excessive focus on appearance in aesthetic disciplines like gymnastics or dance. The sports culture itself, often centered on performance and appearance, can reinforce dysfunctional eating behaviors (Gleaves 1996). Emotional regulation difficulties and the use of food restriction as a coping mechanism for stress or anxiety related to performance pressures can also perpetuate the behavior. Additionally, the ongoing competition or performance evaluations in sports may continually reinforce these patterns (Byrne and McLean 2001).

By integrating this adapted 3P model, we gain a more nuanced understanding of how dysfunctional eating attitudes and behaviors develop and persist in athletes. It also highlights the importance of addressing these issues through holistic interventions that consider vulnerability, triggers, and maintaining factors specific to the sports context.

Dysfunctional eating attitudes and behaviors present themselves as a solution to this impasse, as an attempt to regain control, but result from a sequence of behavior due to the specific characteristics of eating disorders (e.g., Jeammet 2013). Despite the increasing research on factors influencing the emergence of dysfunctional eating attitudes and behaviors in sports, many areas remain unclear regarding the role of psychosocial factors.

Petrie (2020) and Petrie and Greenleaf (2012, 2007) provided a conceptual model that sought to explain how eating disorders develop in male and female athletes immersed in competitive sports environments. In their model, based on non-sporting models (e.g., Stice and Bearman 2001), they conceptualized the socio-cultural multifactorial nature of eating disorder development. The six most frequently identified psychosocial factors in individuals suffering from dysfunctional eating attitudes and behaviors in sports are: (a) the pressure of the sports environment, (b) social pressure, (c) internalization of social norms, (d) body dissatisfaction, (e) negative affect, and (f) behaviors modeled by peers and family (Petrie and Greenleaf 2012, 2007). This model has not been empirically tested, and its basis is limited solely to sociocultural processes, potentially neglecting other influential factors such as personality and environmental context, as Petrie (2020) pointed out.

The various studies conducted beyond this hypothetical modeling highlight that in the sporting context, certain disciplines render athletes particularly at risk of dysfunctional eating attitudes and behaviors. These include: (a) sports in which low body weight may enhance performance (e.g., endurance), (b) weight category sports (e.g., judo, bodybuilding), and (c) aesthetic sports (e.g., figure skating, gymnastics) (Sundgot-Borgen and Torstveit 2004, Vulpinari-Grajon and Mériaux-Scoffier 2024) The dichotomy of "slimming sports" and "weight gain sports" can be problematic, as it tends to oversimplify the complex relationships athletes have with their bodies, training, and performance. Overall, while the dichotomy can be useful as a tool in specific contexts, it's important to acknowledge the underlying complexity and diversity of experiences athletes may have regarding body image and weight in relation to sport. In these disciplines, athletes face a set of norms characterized by ideals in terms of weight, body shape, and performance. Disciplines like gymnastics may convey norms related to thinness (Scoffier-Mériaux et al. 2017), while others like bodybuilding focus on muscle mass gain (Chaba et al. 2019). However, these norms are not universal and seem to fluctuate from one discipline to another. So far, the influence of body-related pressure has been demonstrated, especially in aesthetic sports (Goodwin et al. 2014), while other studies show that power and endurance sports also seem to be affected (Galli et al. 2011). Other authors highlight other risky disciplines such as technical sports or team sports (Uriegas et al. 2023). Thus, it seems challenging to generalize these conclusions as all disciplines seem to carry the risk of developing dysfunctional eating attitudes and behaviors; however, how athletes react to environmental pressures remains highly subjective and seems to involve parameters specific to everyone.

Regarding these individual factors, research from the scientific literature highlights numerous explanatory factors both included in Petrie and Greenleaf's hypothetical modeling (2007) and going beyond it. Among the most explored factors in the literature are: (a) personality, (b) anxiety, (c) social physique anxiety, (d) depression, (e) self-esteem, (f) body esteem, (g) motivation, or (h) perfectionism. This chapter delves into the specific role of athletes' self-perceptions in the emergence of dysfunctional eating attitudes and behaviors.

1. Physical self-perceptions definitions

This chapter consider physical self-perception through its perceptual, attitudinal, and behavioral components (Cash and Pruzinsky 1990, Cash 2012). In aesthetic sports, body image ideals prioritize thinness to meet performance standards (Sherman and Thompson 2009). Physical appearance plays a key role in identity and self-esteem but is only one aspect of self-concept (Fox and Corbin 1989). Cash's model (2012) highlights two attitudinal dimensions: investment (importance of appearance and internalized ideals) and evaluation (body satisfaction/dissatisfaction). In sports, self-perception includes both appearance and physical ability (Ullrich-French and Smith 2006). Body concerns involve persistent thoughts about one's image (Cash and Pruzinsky 1990, Cash 2012).

Engaging in physical activities can be effective in guarding against concerns related to body image perception and improving body satisfaction (Gualdi-Russo et al. 2022). However, within a group of aesthetic athletes, perceived physical capability was positively associated with dysfunctional eating attitudes and behaviors due to the primacy of excellence in high-level sports performance, while perceived physical appearance was not significantly related (Scoffier et al. 2010). Moreover, recent work by Carson et al. (2021) demonstrates that ideals of sports body image and power dynamics between coach and athlete can contribute to the risk of eating disorders and body image issues in female athletes. Thus, the importance placed on achieving certain body ideals in sports could contribute to disturbances in physical self-perception, particularly in terms of body dissatisfaction (e.g., Perelman et al. 2018). Specifically, several studies highlight that athletes in sports emphasizing thinness have more dissatisfaction with their body image than athletes in sports that do not emphasize it (e.g., Kong and Harris 2015, Perelman et al. 2018). Similarly to what can be observed in society at large, female athletes express more dissatisfaction with their bodies than male athletes (e.g., Milligan and Pritchard 2006, Perelman et al. 2018). Indeed, comparing one's body to those of peers or elite athletes in their specific sport can also have detrimental effects on individual body image perception (Francisco et al. 2013, Kong and Harris 2015).

The frequency of dysfunctional eating attitudes and behaviors, associated with body image issues, varies considerably among athletes, ranging from 12% to 57%. This phenomenon is more common among athletes in disciplines where implicit but rigorous norms regarding body, weight, shape, and muscle mass are particularly present, especially in aesthetic sports (e.g., Bratland-Sanda et al. 2013). Experts agree on the multidimensional aspect of inappropriate exercise, involving not only excessive duration and intensity but also qualitative characteristics such as obsessive attitudes, behavior control (i.e., loss of control, compulsive behaviors), practice conditions (e.g., even in case of fatigue or injury), its central nature (e.g., interference with personal and social activities), adverse consequences (e.g., exhaustion, discomfort, social conflicts), and withdrawal symptoms (e.g., negative mood when exercise is prevented, guilt when a session is missed) (Ouellet and Monthuy-Blanc 2020, Mountjoy et al. 2023). Thus, deepening the understanding of the concept of body image seems necessary in the sports context to better grasp its role in relation to perceived competence, sports performance, and athlete well-being.

2. Internalization of sports norms and eating attitudes

2.1 Body norms in sports

Key contributors to body satisfaction or dissatisfaction include socialization processes concerning physical appearance and the internalization of cultural standards related to the body (e.g., Swami 2015). These societal constructs are shaped by the appraisal of attributes and generate beauty ideals within a given culture (Benevides and Rodrigues 2017).

In the context of sports, body norms often revolve around ideals of athleticism, strength, and performance. Athletes are frequently expected to adhere to specific physical standards that are perceived to enhance their athletic abilities or aesthetic appeal within their respective sports. Here are some examples of body norms in various sports contexts, along with references:

- *Muscularity and leanness in bodybuilding*: Bodybuilders are typically expected to have low body fat levels and well-defined musculature to emphasize muscle size and definition (Mitchell et al. 2017).
- *Thinness and flexibility in gymnastics*: Gymnasts often strive for a lean physique and high flexibility to perform demanding routines and meet aesthetic standards associated with the sport (Sundgot-Borgen and Torstveit 2004).

These body norms can influence athletes' training methods, dietary practices, and body image perceptions, often leading to pressure to conform to specific physical ideals within their respective sports.

In sports communities where specific body standards, such as leanness or muscularity, are idealized, athletes often feel pressured to attain and maintain a certain body composition to excel in their sport (Galli and Reel 2009, Sherman and Thompson 2009). This pressure is particularly pronounced in aesthetic or weight-class sports, where body weight and shape directly influence performance outcomes (Galli and Reel 2009, Sherman and Thompson 2009). This pressure may be exerted by coaches, who may emphasize the importance of body aesthetics or performance-related physique goals, as well as teammates, who may compare their bodies to others and reinforce cultural norms of athletic appearance. Additionally, media representations of athletes, which often highlight physically fit and aesthetically pleasing bodies, can contribute to the pressure to conform to unrealistic body ideals. Furthermore, athletes may internalize these standards and impose pressure on themselves to meet or exceed expectations, driven by a desire for success and recognition within their sport (Scoffier-Meriaux et al. 2017).

2.2 Internalization of thinness norms

Internalization of thinness norms is the psychological process by which individuals adopt and integrate societal ideals of thinness into their own beliefs, attitudes, and self-perceptions, often prioritizing achieving a thin body shape or weight as a measure of attractiveness, worth, or success, regardless of its impact on their physical or mental health (Tiggemann and Slater 2014). The internalization of thinness norms, driven by societal standards of beauty, significantly influences eating attitudes in aesthetic sports (Shroff and Thompson 2006). Thinness is often portrayed as desirable in the media, leading individuals to incorporate these standards into their own self-concept and behaviors (Thompson and Stice 2001). Studies have shown a correlation between the degree of thin-ideal internalization and the severity of disordered eating pathologies (Hawkins et al. 2004). Additionally, the internalization of thinness norms mediates the relationship between sociocultural factors and eating disturbances (Keery et al. 2004, Shroff and Thompson 2006). In specific sport context such as the aesthetic sports, the internalization of thinness norms is negatively related to the self-regulation of eating attitudes in sport (Scoffier-Meriaux et al. 2015).

The influence of individual factors on the internalization of thinness norms is also notable. For instance, neuroticism has been found to mediate the relationship between self-regulation of eating attitudes and thinness norm internalization among female dancers (Scoffier-Meriaux et al. 2015). Other factors such as self-esteem, self-concept clarity, and nonconformity have also been implicated in moderating the relationship between exposure to thinness norms and disordered eating (Fingeret and Gleaves 2004, Tylka et al. 2015).

2.3 Internalization of muscular masculine norms

Participation in sports, particularly those emphasizing muscularity, can lead to the internalization of muscular masculine norms, which in turn may contribute to body dissatisfaction and eating disorders (Grieve 2007). Athletes in weight-related sports often seek to increase muscle mass, putting them at risk for body dissatisfaction and eating disorders (i.e., Cerea et al. 2018). The pursuit of muscle mass gain and the internalization of societal norms have been linked to the development of eating disorders among athletes (Doumit et al. 2018).

Media representations of muscularity and societal norms can influence body image perceptions and eating attitudes among athletes (Grossbard et al. 2013). Men may perceive a pressure to conform to a muscular ideal, driven by media portrayals and societal expectations, which can contribute to body dissatisfaction and disordered eating behaviors (Grossbard et al. 2013, Chaba et al. 2019).

By comprehensively understanding the internalization of sports norms and its implications on eating attitudes, researchers, coaches, staff, and practitioners can cultivate insights to recognize athletes at risk, acquire the skills to devise interventions, and promote healthier body image and eating behaviors among athletes.

3. Physical self-perceptions influences

3.1 Body image perceptions

Many studies investigate body image perceptions in different sport contexts. We will consider the roles of these perceptions successively in aesthetic sport context then in other specific ones. The systematic review by Berengüí et al. (2023) highlights that twenty-five studies have evaluated body image perception and the incidence of eating disorders in aesthetic sports. Studies utilizing tools to assess image perception, such as the body shape rating scale, the Figure Rating Scale (FRE), or the Stunkard Figure Rating Scale, indicate high levels of body dissatisfaction compared to other athletes in "non-aesthetic" sports (Aleksić-Veljković et al. 2020). Cheerleaders, in particular, expressed a desire to be thinner relative to their perception of body image while wearing different outfits (Torres-McGehee et al. 2012).

Based on Byrne and McLean (2001), overweight perceptions are, therefore, an additional factor to consider in the relationship between perfectionism, physique anxiety and disordered eating in female athletes. In sport contexts physical self-perceptions thus not only include perceived physical appearance but also perceived physical ability (Scoffier et al. 2010). This latter variable is recognized as being predictive of many adaptive patterns including positive affect, persistence, and performance (Duda 2001). The study of Leonkiewicz and Wawrzyniak (2022) showed a statistically significant correlation between the perception of one's own body and self and the assessment of eating behavior in female athletes. The results of González-Martí et al. (2014). showed that people suffering from Muscle Dysmorphia Symptoms, overall, have poorer physical self-concept perceptions.

3.2 Body image perception measures

Regarding the methods used to evaluate the perception of body image, the most predominant is the Body Shape Questionnaire (BSQ, Cooper et al. 2016), which is used in 39.4%. Other assessment methods have been used to evaluate other psychological aspects (self-esteem, psychological commitment to exercise, perfectionism, etc.). In each of the studies, different types of questionnaires are used to assess self-perception, which is why comparing the results obtained between the different assessment methods may lead to results of low validity and reliability. More recently, Monthuy-Blanc et al. (2020, 2022), and currently validating a second version, developed an immersive experience tested on a female athlete by Saint-Pierre et al. (2024) using the eLoriCorps IBRS 1.2 (EIE-IC; "eLoriCorps Immersive Body Rating Scale; eLoriCorps-IBRS", in revision) (cf. Figure 1), a virtual environment hosted on the In Virtuo application and created using Unity3D (Unity Technologies, San Francisco, CA). The study by Saint-Pierre et al. (2025) focusing on the evaluation of a female athlete's physical appearance through an immersive experience reveals a remarkable convergence between the evaluation performed and the importance

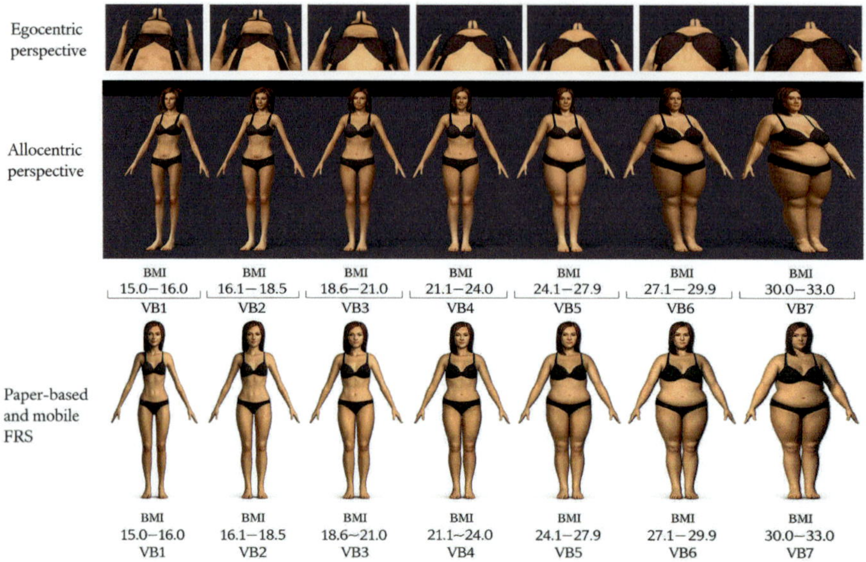

Figure 1. Egocentric and allocentric perspectives of the immersive continuum of female virtual body – eLoriCorps-IBRS 1.1 (form Monthuy-Blanc et al. 2022).

attributed to physical appearance in the athlete's discourse and immersive experience. It appears that this tool may play an important role in attenuating the social desirability bias typically associated with measures of perceived physical appearance and its sub-dimensions.

3.3 Perceived physical ability

Perceived physical ability appeared in Scoffier et al. (2010) to be positively associated with dysfunctional eating attitudes and behaviors. This relationship differed from the data of earlier studies showing that perceived physical ability was generally associated with patterns of adaptive accomplishment (Ullrich-French and Smith 2006). It differed also from the findings that positive body image and body satisfaction were protective factors regarding dysfunctional eating attitudes and behaviors, in both daily living situations and sport setting (Petrie and Greenleaf 2007). However, no significant relationship between perceived physical appearance and DEA was observed in the present study, in contrast to the findings of earlier works (Paxton et al. 1999). These discrepancies indicate the need to differentiate the variables of perceived physical appearance, body image, and body satisfaction and the concept of perceived physical ability in sport. It could be hypothesized that the primacy of excellence in performance in high-level sport and thus the purpose of demonstrating competence in such achievement contexts may account for these differences.

In basketball players, the indirect connections between physical strength/physical condition/sport competence, and bulimia/body dissatisfaction (mediated by physical self-worth) may initially seem counterintuitive, given that leanness does not directly contribute to basketball skills (Monthuy-Blanc et al. 2012). However, the observed negative indirect associations indicate that basketball players who are less content with their athletic abilities are also generally less satisfied with themselves, thus increasing the likelihood of experiencing Body dissatisfaction and resorting to bulimic strategies. This implies that when non-elite basketball players are dissatisfied with their physical prowess, they might consider extreme measures to reduce body fat levels in order to optimize their muscle-to-fat ratio.

Based on previous results, the role of the perceived physical ability seems to be ambivalent depending on the context specificities, depending on the specific body norms, and depending on other mechanisms such as the social environment influences.

3.4 *Self-perception mechanisms*

Navigating the intricate landscape of athletic performance, the influence of external factors on athletes' physical self-perception and well-being is a complex and multifaceted domain. From the feedback of coaches and parents to transitions in training or competition levels, these external forces play a pivotal role in shaping athletes' attitudes towards their bodies and their overall psychological well-being. Understanding the intricate interplay of these factors is crucial for developing targeted interventions aimed at fostering a healthier athletic community.

Influence of external factors. Negative physical self-perception in athletes with disordered eating and body image concerns can be influenced by various external factors, including coach and parental feedback, injury or illness, and transitions in training or competition levels (Abdalla et al. 2020, Ricciardelli et al. 2003, Zaccagni and Gualdi-Russo 2023). For instance, critical comments about body weight or shape from coaches or parents can exacerbate existing body image concerns and contribute to a cycle of negative self-talk and behavior (Abdalla et al. 2020). In addition to these external factors, societal pressures and cultural norms within the realm of athletics can also significantly impact an athlete's perception of their physical self. The relentless pursuit of perfection and the glorification of certain body types prevalent in sports culture can further exacerbate body image concerns and contribute to dysfunctional eating attitudes and behaviors (Abdalla et al. 2020, Ricciardelli et al. 2003, Zaccagni and Gualdi-Russo 2023). Consequently, athletes may find themselves entangled in a web of self-doubt and negative self-perception, which not only affects their performance on the field but also their overall well-being off it.

Coach-Athlete relationship and perceived physical ability. Previous research has primarily considered the coach's influence on dysfunctional eating attitudes and behaviors in terms of perceived motivational climate and coaching style (Scoffier et al. 2010). However, studies have shown that the quality of the coach-athlete relationship, including aspects such as sport friendship quality, positively influences disordered eating attitudes through perceived physical ability (Scoffier et al. 2010, Ullrich-French and Smith 2006). Perceived physical ability, in turn, is positively associated with dysfunctional eating attitudes and behaviors, although this relationship differs from earlier studies that linked perceived physical ability to patterns of adaptive accomplishment (Ullrich-French and Smith 2006). This suggests a nuanced interplay between the coach-athlete relationship, perceived physical ability, and disordered eating attitudes, highlighting the need for a more comprehensive understanding of how these factors interact to influence athletes' well-being and performance.

Body image and social environment. The surrounding social environment, including comments from coaches and family, phases of bodily changes during development, and exposure to external scrutiny in aesthetic sports, can significantly impact an athlete's body image (Ricciardelli et al. 2003). For example, negative parental perceptions of weight during adolescence are correlated with body dissatisfaction and later weight control behaviors (Abdalla et al. 2020). Additionally, constant comparisons with other athletes and pressure to conform to the thinness ideal in the sports environment contribute to body dissatisfaction and negative self-perception (Abdalla et al. 2020). These findings underscore the complex interplay between social influences, developmental factors, and sports culture in shaping athletes' body image perceptions and psychological well-being. Understanding these dynamics is crucial for developing interventions and support systems that promote positive body image and overall health among athletes.

Contextual influences. Injury or changes in body size and shape resulting from athletic events can also profoundly affect an athlete's body image and self-perception (Zaccagni and Gualdi-Russo 2023). This disruption in body image perception may lead to feelings of loss of control over one's body and impact eating behavior and psychological well-being (Zaccagni and Gualdi-Russo 2023). Moreover, the perception of body image in athletes seems to fluctuate depending on the context in which they operate, with elite athletes often experiencing more body dissatisfaction than those at lower competitive levels (Kong and Harris 2015). These fluctuations in body image perception highlight the dynamic nature of athletes' self-perception and underscore the importance of considering individual differences and contextual factors in addressing body image concerns within athletic populations. Understanding these nuances is essential for developing targeted interventions and support systems that promote positive body image and mental well-being among athletes across various competitive levels and sports disciplines.

By considering these external factors and contextual influences, researchers and practitioners can gain a deeper understanding of how self-perception mechanisms contribute to disordered eating attitudes and body image concerns among athletes.

4. Implications for prevention and intervention

Several prevention programs have been developed to address the issue of dysfunctional eating attitudes and behaviors in the sporting context. Bar et al. (2016) identified 11 such programs in their systematic review. For example, the BodySense project (Buchholz et al. 2008) aims to promote a positive body image approach. This program consists of workshops focusing on attitudes and beliefs about food, self-esteem, health, and stress management in sports practice. Conducted with 31 gymnasts, parents, and coaches, this program demonstrated a decrease in pressure regarding thinness in the group that underwent the intervention.

Although prevention programs for eating disorders and associated behaviors have shown beneficial effects among athletes, including reducing certain symptoms during and after the intervention, they also have some significant limitations. Firstly, most of these programs have not examined the long-term impact of these interventions, so it is unclear whether prevention programs can effectively address athletes' long-term issues regarding eating, weight, and body image. Secondly, current prevention programs have mainly been tested with female populations (Petrie 2020), meaning that the proposed programs may not necessarily be suitable or generalizable to men. Thirdly, these prevention programs are general and non-specific, whereas the diversity of eating disorders observed in different sports disciplines and among different athlete profiles requires more targeted and individualized approaches.

Thus, for effective and personalized management, interventions should prioritize the sporting context and consider the psychosocial and individual factors of each athlete. Consequently, a primary prevention approach should begin with a comprehensive assessment of the correlates and risk factors of eating disorders and associated behaviors in sport. This comprehensive assessment of dysfunctional eating attitudes and behaviors would then allow for better tailoring of interventions to the specific needs of athletes.

It's essential to recognize that negative physical self-perception in athletes with dysfunctional eating attitudes and behaviors is not solely a result of individual psychological factors but is often influenced by broader social and environmental contexts. Addressing these issues requires a comprehensive approach that considers both the individual athlete's experiences and the systemic factors that contribute to body dissatisfaction within the sporting community. Understanding the complex interplay between self-perceptions, societal norms, and athletic identity is crucial for designing effective prevention programs to mitigate the development of dysfunctional eating attitudes and behaviors in athletes. Targeted interventions focusing on improving athletes' body image perceptions and promoting healthier attitudes towards eating behaviors can contribute to fostering a positive sport environment conducive to athletes' well-being.

Conclusion

In conclusion, negative physical self-perception among athletes with dysfunctional eating attitudes and behaviors stands as a significant issue, profoundly impacting their mental health, performance, and overall well-being. By delving into the underlying factors fueling these negative self-perceptions, coaches, healthcare professionals, and sports organizations can collaborate to cultivate supportive environments fostering positive body image and psychological resilience among athletes.

Throughout this chapter, we've highlighted the intricate relationship between athletes' self-perceptions and dysfunctional eating attitudes and behaviors. By dissecting the multifaceted nature of body image perceptions and their influence on eating behaviors, researchers and practitioners can craft comprehensive strategies aimed at cultivating healthier attitudes and behaviors in sports.

It's evident that athletes face pressures to conform to specific body ideals within their respective sports, often leading to adverse effects on their psychological well-being. The pervasive internalization of thinness norms, particularly prominent in aesthetic sports, underscores the urgency for targeted interventions addressing body image concerns among athletes.

Looking ahead, further research is imperative to explore the nuanced interactions between sports norms, self-perceptions, and eating behaviors. Moreover, the development of effective intervention strategies is paramount to promoting positive body image and psychological well-being among athletes. By tackling these issues holistically, we can establish a nurturing and empowering environment conducive to the holistic health of athletes across all levels of competition.

References

Abdalla, D.R., H.P. Gomide, R.N. Chaves, E.F. Pereira and R.R. Luiz. 2020. Associations between body image dissatisfaction and depressive symptoms in early adolescence. J. Pediatr. Psychol. 45: 804–813.

Aleksić-Veljković, A., D. Đurović, M. Biro, M. Stojanović and D. Ilić. 2020. Comparison of body dissatisfaction among female athletes and non-athletes from Serbia. Facta Univ. Ser. Phys. Educ. Sport 18: 427–440.

Arcelus, J., G.L. Witcomb, A. Mitchell and H. Turner. 2015. Prevalence of eating disorders amongst dancers: a systematic review and meta-analysis. Eur. Eat. Disord. Rev. 23: 92–101.

Bar, R., S.E. Cassin, M.M. Dionne and M. Israel. 2016. Prevention programs for body image and eating disorders on university campuses: a review of large, controlled interventions. Eat. Disord. 24: 369–382.

Benevides, R.T.F. and D.L. Rodrigues. 2017. Body image and self-esteem in adolescents. Rev. Psicol. Criança Adolesc. 8: 51–60.

Berengüí, R., S. Angosto, A. Hernández-Ruiz, M. Rueda-Flores and M.A. Castejón. 2023. Body image perception and eating disorders incidence in aesthetic sports: a systematic review. J. Sports Sci. 41: 250–267.

Bratland-Sanda, S. and J. Sundgot-Borgen. 2013. Eating disorders in athletes: overview of prevalence, risk factors, and recommendations for prevention and treatment. Eur. J. Sport Sci. 13: 499–508.

Bravata, D.M., C. Smith-Spangler, V. Sundaram, A.L. Gienger, N. Lin, R. Lewis et al. 2003. Using pedometers to increase physical activity and improve health: a systematic review. J. Am. Med. Assoc. 289: 2296–2304.

Buchholz, A., H. Mack, G.L. McVey, S. Feder and N. Barrowman. 2008. An evaluation of the prevention project BODYSENSE: a positive body image initiative for female athletes. Eat. Disord. J. Treat. Prev. 16: 308–321.

Byrne, S. and N. McLean. 2001. Eating disorders in athletes: a review of the literature. Journal of Science and Medicine in Sport 4(2): 145–159. https://doi.org/10.1016/s1440-2440(01)80025-6.

Carson, F., D.L. Paulhus and Z. Huang. 2021. Interpersonal manipulation in eating disorder pathology. Eat. Behav. 41: 101498.

Cash, T.F. 2012. Cognitive-behavioral perspectives on body image. Encycl. Body Image Hum. Appear. 1: 334–342.

Cash, T.F. and T. Pruzinsky. 1990. Body Images: Development, Deviance, and Change. Guilford Press, New York.

Cerea, S., A.I. Sanz-Vergel, F.J. Gracia and D. Sánchez-Oliva. 2018. Psychosocial factors related to eating disorders among bodybuilders. J. Health Psychol. 25: 1535–1545.

Chaba, L., C. Soares and P. Santos. 2019. Eating disorders in male bodybuilders: a review. Sport Sci. Health 15: 265–273.

Cooper, P.J., M.J. Taylor, Z. Cooper and C.G. Fairburn. 2016. The development and validation of the Body Shape Questionnaire. Int. J. Eat. Disord. 6: 485–494.

Doumit, R., G. Halawi and E. Hassan. 2018. Eating disorders among the Lebanese athletic population. J. Eat. Disord. 6: 1–6.

Duda, J.L. 2001. Achievement goal research in sport: pushing the boundaries and clarifying some misunderstandings. Adv. Motiv. Sport Exerc. 13: 129–182.

Fingeret, M.C. and D.H. Gleaves. 2004. Sociocultural influences on body image concerns of young African American and European American women. Sex Roles 53: 701–715.

Fox, K.R. and C.B. Corbin. 1989. The physical self-perception profile: development and preliminary validation. J. Sport Exerc. Psychol. 11: 408–430.

Francisco, R., M. Alarcão and I. Narciso. 2013. Self-esteem and body image in adolescents. Int. J. Dev. Educ. Psychol. 1: 463–470.

Galli, N. and J.J. Reel. 2009. A comparison of body dissatisfaction among female college athletes and non-athletes. Meas. Phys. Educ. Exerc. Sci. 13: 186–202.

Galli, N., T.A. Petrie, C.A. Greenleaf and J.J. Reel. 2011. Mediators of weight-based stigmatization in physical activity settings. J. Health Psychol. 16: 812–821.

Gleaves, D.H. 1996. The role of sports culture in eating disorders: a review of the literature. J. Appl. Sport Psychol. 8: 204–221.

Goodwin, H., E. Haycraft, L. Taranis and C. Meyer. 2014. Psychosocial factors associated with disordered eating in men and women. Int. J. Eat. Disord. 47: 611–618.

Gouttebarge, V., G. Kerkhoffs and M. Lambert. 2017. Prevalence and determinants of symptoms of common mental disorders in retired professional Rugby Union players. Eur. J. Sport Sci. 17: 992–1001.

Grieve, F.G. 2007. A conceptual model of factors contributing to the development of muscle dysmorphia. Eat. Disord. 15: 63–80.

Grossbard, J.R., C.M. Lee, C. Neighbors, C.S. Hendershot and M.E. Larimer. 2013. Body image concerns and contingent self-esteem in male and female college students. Sex Roles 69: 235–249.

Homan, K.J., S.L. Crowley and L.A. Sim. 2019. Motivation for sport participation and eating disorder risk among female collegiate athletes. Eat. Disord. 27: 369–383.

Jeammet, J.-L. 2013. L'adolescence et ses enjeux. Presses Universitaires de France (PUF), Paris.

Kong, P. and L.M. Harris. 2015. The sporting body: body image and eating disorder symptomatology among female athletes from leanness focused and nonleanness focused sports. J. Psychol. 149: 141–160.

Leonkiewicz, M. and A. Wawrzyniak. 2022. The relationship between rigorous perception of one's own body and self, unhealthy eating behavior and a high risk of anorexic readiness. J. Eat. Disord. 10: 48.

Milligan, B. and M. Pritchard. 2006. The relationship between gender, type of sport, body dissatisfaction, self-esteem and disordered eating behaviors in division I athletes. Athl. Insight 8: 32–46.

Mitchell, L., S.B. Murray, S. Cobley, D. Hackett, J. Gifford, L. Capling et al. 2017. Muscle dysmorphia symptomatology and associated psychological features in bodybuilders and non-bodybuilder resistance trainers: a systematic review and meta-analysis. Sports Med. 47: 233–259.

Monthuy-Blanc, J., S. Bouchard, M. Ouellet, G. Corno, S. Iceta and M. Rousseau. 2020. Eloricorps immersive body rating scale: exploring the assessment of body image disturbances from allocentric and egocentric perspectives. J. Clin. Med. 9: 2926.

Monthuy-Blanc, J., G. Corno, M. Ouellet, F. Touré, F. Bourbeau, M. Rousseau et al. 2022. Eloricorps immersive body rating scale and mobile versions: validation to assess body image disturbances in adolescents. J. Clin. Med. 11: 1156.

Monthuy-Blanc, J., C. Maïano, A.J. Morin and Y. Stephan. 2012. Physical self-concept and disturbed eating attitudes and behaviors in French adolescent girls. Body Image 9: 373–380.

Morrison, T.G., R. Kalin and M.A. Morrison. 2004. Body-image evaluation and investment among adolescents: a test of sociocultural and social comparison theories. Adolescence 39: 571–592.

Mountjoy, M., K.E. Ackerman, D.M. Bailey, L.M. Burke, N. Constantini, A.C. Hackney et al. 2023. 2023 International Olympic Committee's (IOC) consensus statement on relative energy deficiency in sport (REDs). Br. J. Sports Med. 57: 1073–1097.

Ouellet, M. and J. Monthuy-Blanc. 2022. Quand bouger n'est plus synonyme de santé: une recension des traitements de l'exercice physique pathologique en troubles des conduites alimentaires. Ann. Médico-Psychol. 180: 862–874.

Paxton, S.J., H.K. Schutz, E.H. Wertheim and S.L. Muir. 1999. Friendship clique and peer influences on body image concerns, dietary restraint, extreme weight-loss behaviors, and binge eating in adolescent girls. J. Abnorm. Psychol. 108: 255.

Perelman, H., J. Buscemi, E. Dougherty and A. Haedt-Matt. 2018. Body dissatisfaction in collegiate athletes: differences between sex, sport type, and division level. J. Clin. Sport Psychol. 12: 718–731.
Petrie, T.A. 2020. Eating disorders in sport. pp. 694–710. *In*: Tenenbaum, G., R.C. Eklund and N. Boiangin (eds.). Handbook of Sport Psychology. John Wiley & Sons.
Petrie, T.A. and C. Greenleaf. 2012. Eating disorders in sport. pp. 635–659. *In*: Murphy, S. (ed.). Oxford Handbook of Sport and Performance Psychology. Oxford University Press.
Petrie, T.A. and C.A. Greenleaf. 2007. Eating disorders in sport: from theory to research to intervention. pp. 352–378. *In*: Tenenbaum, G., R.C. Eklund and N. Boiangin (eds.). Handbook of Sport Psychology. John Wiley & Sons.
Reardon, C.L., B. Hainline, C.M. Aron, D. Baron, A.L. Baum, A. Bindra et al. 2019. Mental health in elite athletes: International Olympic Committee consensus statement. Br. J. Sports Med. 53: 667–699.
Ricciardelli, L.A., M.P. McCabe, K.E. Holt and J. Finemore. 2003. A biopsychosocial model for understanding body image and body change strategies among children. J. Appl. Dev. Psychol. 24: 475–495.
Scoffier, S., C. Maïano and F. d'Arripe-Longueville. 2010. Social relationships and acceptance in disturbed eating attitudes in elite adolescent female athletes: mediating role of physical self-perceptions. Int. J. Eat. Disord. 43: 65–71.
Scoffier-Mériaux, S., C. Falzon, P. Lewton-Brain, E. Filaire and F. d'Arripe-Longueville. 2015. Big five personality traits and eating attitudes in intensively training dancers. J. Sports Sci. Med. 14: 627.
Scoffier-Mériaux, S., C. Ferrand and F. d'Arripe-Longueville. 2017. The internalisation of sociocultural and thin-ideal standards in sports scale: development and validation. Int. J. Sport Exerc. Psychol. 15: 370–378.
Smolak, L. and S.K. Murnen. 2004. Body image and disordered eating in childhood and adolescence. J. Early Adolesc. 24: 197–218.
St-Pierre, M.J., G. Corno, S. Meriaux and J. Monthuy-Blanc. 2025. Dysfunctional eating attitudes and behaviors among athletes: the role and potential of virtual reality. L'Encéphale.
St-Pierre, M.J., J. Monthuy-Blanc, F. Bourbeau, G. Corno and S. Mériaux-Scoffier. 2024. Percevoir l'image de son corps sportif autrement: apport innovant de la réalité virtuelle chez une sportive en natation artistique. Cah. Nutr. Diét. 59: 247–258.
Stice, E. and S.K. Bearman. 2001. Body-image and eating disturbances predict depressive symptoms in adolescent girls: a growth curve analysis. Dev. Psychol. 37: 597.
Stice, E. and H.E. Shaw. 2002. Role of body dissatisfaction in the onset and maintenance of eating pathology: a synthesis of research findings. J. Psychosom. Res. 53: 985–993.
Swami, V. 2015. Cultural influences on body size ideals. Eur. Psychol. 20: 44–51.
Thompson, J.K. and E. Stice. 2001. Thin-ideal internalization: evidence for a new risk factor for body-image disturbance. Curr. Dir. Psychol. Sci. 10: 181–183.
Torres-McGehee, T.M., E.V. Monsma, T.P. Dompier and S.A. Washburn. 2012. Eating disorder risk and the role of clothing in collegiate cheerleaders' body images. J. Athl. Train. 47: 541–548.
Tylka, T.L. and N.L. Wood-Barcalow. 2015. The Body Appreciation Scale-2: item refinement and psychometric evaluation. Body Image 12: 53–67.
Vitousek, K., M. Manke and K. Wilkins. 2000. Perfectionism and eating disorders: implications for treatment. J. Clin. Psychol. 56: 981–994.
Vulpinari-Grajon, B. and S. Mériaux-Scoffier. 2024. Enhanced risk of disordered eating in female athletes: contribution of sport types and competitive levels. Perform. Enhanc. Health 12: 100277.
Zaccagni, L. and E. Gualdi-Russo. 2023. The impact of sports involvement on body image perception and ideals: a systematic review and meta-analysis. Int. J. Environ. Res. Public Health 20: 5228.

Chapter 7

Beyond the Mirror

Exploring Body Image in Individuals with Obesity

Giuseppe Riva,[1,2,3,*] *Fabio Frisone*[1,2,3] and *Giulia Brizzi*[2,3]

INTRODUCTION

Obesity is abnormal or excessive fat accumulation that presents a health risk. Globally, obesity has reached epidemic proportions, with rates continuing to rise across all age groups and socioeconomic status (Schwartz and Brownell 2004). Defined by a body mass index (BMI) of 30 or higher, obesity is not merely an aesthetic concern (World Health Organization 2020). Still, it is associated with numerous chronic diseases, including type 2 diabetes, cardiovascular diseases, and certain types of cancer (Safaei et al. 2021). The condition results from an intricate interplay of different factors, such as genetic, behavioral, psychological, and socio-cultural (Safaei et al. 2021). This multifaceted nature makes obesity a public health challenge to prevent and treat (Safaei et al. 2021). The role of the body in obesity extends far beyond its physical and metabolic dimensions; it is central to the condition due to its profound impact on body image. Indeed, body image plays a critical role in shaping the psychological and emotional experience of individuals with obesity, influencing self-perception, mental health, and the ability to engage in effective long-term weight management. We know that individuals affected by obesity suffer from heightened body dissatisfaction, exacerbated by societal stigma and weight bias (Sarwer et al. 2005), but the story might be more complex.

[1] Applied Technology for Neuro-Psychology Lab, IRCSS Istituto Auxologico Italiano, Via Pelizza da Volpedo 41, 20149, Milano, Italy.
[2] Humane Technology Lab., Università Cattolica del Sacro Cuore, Largo Gemelli 1, 2013, Milano, Italy.
[3] Department of Psychology, Università Cattolica del Sacro Cuore, Largo Gemelli 1, 2013, Milano, Italy.
Emails: fabio.frisone@unicatt.it, giulia.brizzi@unicatt.it
* Corresponding author: giuseppe.riva@unicatt.it

DOI: 10.1201/9781032718125-8

1. The role of the body in obesity

In modern societies, the body plays a central role as both a personal identity marker and a social symbol, often reflecting cultural ideals of beauty, health, and status, while also shaping individual self-esteem and social interactions. Especially in Western cultures, most women tend to be dissatisfied with their bodies: data revealed that one adolescent girl out of two reports body dissatisfaction (Makinen et al. 2012). Recent studies highlighted that sociocultural pressure to be thin is central to the development of negative feelings about the body, which are recognized as a critical risk factor for the emergence of overweight and obesity (Puhl and Heuer 2009).

1.1 The self-objectification theory

Objectification Theory (Calogero et al. 2010), offers a psycho-social framework for understanding the development of eating and weight disorders. According to this theory, societal and cultural norms impose a self-evaluation model that shapes individuals' emotional and behavioral responses to their bodies. The theory emphasizes the existence of an objectified societal ideal of beauty, mainly focused on physical appearance and aesthetics (Brizzi et al. 2024). Such an ideal is transmitted through various socio-cultural channels (e.g., advertising, media) and is then internalized by individuals by continuous implicit and explicit exposure (Calogero et al. 2010). It follows that satisfaction (or dissatisfaction) with their own body relates to the extent to which individuals meet (or fail to meet) this ideal. This leads people to a self-objectification process. Individuals who engage in self-objectification tend to evaluate themselves primarily based on their physical appearance and conformity to cultural standards of attractiveness (Dakanalis et al. 2015). This leads them to adopt an observer's perspective of their own body, viewing it as an object with the primary purpose of being "beautiful (Brizzi et al. 2024, Calogero et al. 2010). As a result, they often experience increased body surveillance, body shame, and appearance-related anxiety, which contributes to the onset of disordered eating and body dissatisfaction (Dakanalis et al. 2015). Even if self-objectification can be a critical risk factor for the development of obesity and overweight through its link with teasing, body image dissatisfaction, and unhealthy weight control behaviors, the Objectification Theory is still not able to answer two critical questions (Riva and Dakanalis 2018): Why do not all the individuals experiencing self-objectification develop EDs? What is the role of body experience in the etiology of obesity?

1.2 The contribution of neuroscience

Here we will embrace an emerging field of neuroscience—the multisensory integration of bodily representations and signals (Tsakiris 2017)—to answer the above questions. Multisensory body integration is a critical cognitive and perceptual process that allows individuals to protect and extend their boundaries at both the homeostatic and psychological levels (Riva 2018). To achieve this goal, the brain integrates sensory data arriving from real-time multiple sensory modalities and internal bodily information with predictions made using the stored information about the body from conceptual, perceptual, and episodic memory (Shriver et al. 2019). In this view, the emotional (Shriver et al. 2019), motor (Fink et al. 2019), proprioceptive (Garner et al. 1983), and interoceptive (Simmons and DeVille 2017) deficits reported by many authors in individuals with obesity may reflect a broader impairment in multisensory integration processing (Brizzi et al. 2023). Specifically, it can affect the individual's abilities (Tsakiris 2017): (a) to identify the relevant interoceptive signals that predict potential pleasant (or aversive) consequences; (b) to modify/correct the autobiographical allocentric (observer view) memories of body-related events (self-objectified memories).

The first effect of impaired multisensory body integration is a prospective aversive body state (Brizzi et al. 2023). This situation makes it difficult for obese individuals to obtain and regulate a sense of self and could contribute to problems with body image and self-disturbance. The second effect of impaired multisensory body integration is that obese patients may be locked to an allocentric disembodied negative memory of the body that is not updated even after a demanding diet and significant weight loss (Scarpina et al. 2016). Therefore, successful dieting attempts cannot improve body dissatisfaction, and subjects may either start more radical dieting attempts or, at the opposite end, engage in "disinhibited" eating behaviors (Riva 2012).

Confirming this idea, a first longitudinal study (Quick et al. 2013) used data from a prospective study of 496 adolescent girls who completed a baseline assessment at age 11–15 years and 4 annual follow-ups to test whether behavioral and psychological risk factors predict the onset of obesity during adolescence and to compare the predictive power of these factors with that of parental obesity. Contrary to original hypotheses, elevated intake of high-fat foods, binge eating, and exercise did not predict obesity onset: the most important predictor was elevated dietary restraint scores associated with maladaptive compensatory behaviors for weight control, such as vomiting or laxative abuse. Moreover, a second study (Puhl et al. 2017) tried identifying 10-year longitudinal predictors of overweight incidence during the transition from adolescence to young adulthood using a population-based cohort (N = 2,134). At a 10-year follow-up, 51% of young adults were overweight (26% increase from baseline). Among females and males, higher levels of body dissatisfaction, weight concerns, unhealthy weight control behaviors (e.g., fasting, purging), dieting, binge eating, weight-related teasing, and parental weight-related concerns and behaviors during adolescence and/or increases in these factors over the study period predicted the incidence of overweight at 10-year follow-up. Finally, a third longitudinal study (Stice et al. 2005) explored whether weight-based teasing in adolescence predicts adverse eating and weight-related outcomes 15 years later. The results are quite clear: weight-based teasing in adolescence predicted higher BMI and obesity 15 years later. For women, these longitudinal associations occurred across peer and family-based teasing sources, but for men, only peer-based teasing predicted higher BMI.

While body image dissatisfaction plays a significant role in the development of obesity, it is important to acknowledge that obesity is also closely tied to how individuals feed their bodies. Beyond self-perception issues, eating behaviors are shaped by a complex interplay of psychological, emotional, and environmental factors. Stress and negative emotions have been shown to significantly influence eating habits, often leading to overeating as a maladaptive coping strategy (Macht 2008). According to the theory of emotional eating (Macht 2008), some people use eating to regulate or escape negative emotions, a behavior associated with both obesity and binge eating disorders. Macht identified five classes of emotion-induced changes in eating, which include: (i) emotional control of food choice, (ii) emotional suppression of food intake, (iii) impairment of cognitive eating controls, (iv) eating to regulate emotions, and (v) emotion-congruent modulation of eating (Macht 2008). This emotion-driven overeating is not merely about hunger but is instead a response to emotional distress, where food serves as a temporary escape or source of comfort. As a result, stress and emotional turmoil can create a harmful cycle in which negative feelings perpetuate unhealthy eating patterns, further contributing to weight gain and obesity (Macht 2008).

In addition to its impact on eating behavior, emotional distress can also reduce motivation to engage in physical exercise, a critical component in obesity prevention and treatment. When individuals experience high-stress levels, body dissatisfaction, or other emotional challenges, their willingness to participate in physical activity may decrease, as exercise is often perceived yet another overwhelming task. Moreover, negative body image can make individuals feel self-conscious about exercising in public or participating in physical activities, reinforcing sedentary behaviors. This emotional barrier to exercise, combined with maladaptive eating habits, perpetuates the cycle of weight gain, making it harder for individuals to adopt healthier lifestyles.

These preliminary observations indicate that obesity is a complex phenomenon centered on the relationship between the individual and their body. Experiencing one's body not as an ally but as an adversary in achieving personal goals can lead to psychological and physical discomfort that is challenging to address. Considering this data, obesity needs holistic prevention and treatment approaches that can consider the role of the body in the onset and maintenance of the condition. Then, a critical question becomes: how can we reshape the body experience?

2. Virtual reality to reshape body image in obesity

Technology is offering new tools and methods for addressing obesity-related issues (Riva et al. 2004). Between them, an emerging trend is the use of Virtual Reality (VR; Brizzi and Riva 2024, Di Natale et al. 2024) (see also Chapter 3). Psychology and neuroscience define VR as (Schultheis and Rizzo 2001) "an advanced form of human-computer interface that allows the user to interact with and become immersed in a computer-generated environment in a naturalistic fashion" (p. 82). This is because, as recently suggested (Brizzi and Riva 2024), VR shares the same basic mechanisms of our brain: embodied simulations. According to neuroscience, our brain creates an embodied simulation of the body in the world used to represent and predict actions, concepts, and emotions. Similarly, the VR experience attempts to predict the sensory consequences of the individual's movements, providing them with the same scene they will see in the real world (Brizzi and Riva 2024). This transforms VR into an experiential technology that can target both the body and the mind at the same time (Brizzi and Riva 2024). Because of this unique property, several meta-reviews found VR as a powerful clinical tool for behavioral health, providing assessment and treatment options for different mental health problems (Eijler et al. 2019, Riva et al. 2016).

Starting from all these premises, the chapter will present how we can use VR to achieve successful obesity treatment, targeting the body at different levels: namely, cognitive, emotional, and perceptual levels. In particular, we will discuss how we can use VT to reshape body image by working on multisensory integration, emotion regulation, and physical activity.

2.1 Reshape the body by working on multisensory integration

As a multisensory technology, VR allows targeting an impaired multisensory body integration through two different strategies—"reference frameshifting" (Akhtar et al. 2017, Riva 2011) and "body swapping" (Brizzi and Riva 2024, Brizzi et al. 2023, Di Natale et al. 2024)—that can be integrated within a classical Cognitive-Behavioral Training (CBT) for obesity.

Reference frameshifting method. The first method, "reference frameshifting" (Akhtar et al. 2017, Riva 2011), structures the individual's bodily self-consciousness (see Table 1) through the focus and reorganization of its contents.

To achieve it, the subject re-experiences in VR a negative situation related to the body (e.g., teasing) both in first-person and in third person (e.g., seeing and supporting their avatar in the VR world) integrating the therapeutic methods used by Butter and Cash (1987) and Wooley and Wooley (1985). Specifically, VR situations are used in the same way as guided imagery (Leuner 2985) is used in the cognitive and visual/motorial approach. In general, the therapist asks the patient to give detailed descriptions of the virtual experience, and the feelings associated with it. Furthermore, the patient is taught how to cope with them using different techniques (see Table 1). This approach has been successfully used in different randomized trials with obese patients (Cesa et al. 2013, Manzoni et al. 2016), allowing both to update the contents of their body memory and to improve the clinical outcomes over traditional CBT.

Body swapping method. In the second strategy—"body swapping" (Brizzi and Riva 2024, Brizzi et al. 2023, Di Natale et al. 2024)—VR is used to induce the illusion of ownership of a virtual body with a different shape and/or size. Since the publication by Botvinick and Cohen (1998) revealing that it is simple to generate in people the illusion that a rubber hand is part of their body (Rubber Hand Illusion), there has been increasing interest in the study of bodily illusions. Specifically, this term refers to the controlled illusory generation of unusual bodily feelings, such as the feeling of ownership over a rubber hand that affects the experience of a body part or the entire body (i.e., a body-swap illusion).

More recently, an increasing body of pioneered research conducted by Riva and colleagues (Serino et al. 2019, Serino et al. 2016a) revealed that the embodiment in a virtual body that substitutes the own body in virtual reality with visuo-tactile stimulation (body-swap illusion) alters body percept (i.e., participants

Table 1. The adapted VR body image rescripting protocol.

Phase 1 - Interview	
 **Figure 1**	During a clinical interview, the patient is asked to relive the contents of the allocentric negative body image and the situation/s in which it was created and/or reinforced (e.g., being teased by my boyfriend at home) in as much detail as possible. The meaning of the experience for the patient is also elicited (Figure 1).
Phase 2- VR scene development	
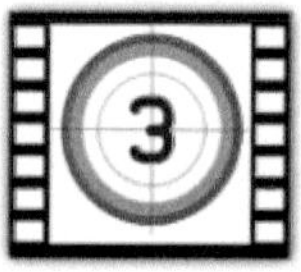 **Figure 2**	The clinician reproduces the setting of the identified situation (e.g., the corridor of the classroom where my boyfriend teased me) using the VR development toolkit (Figure 2).
Phase 3 - Egocentric VR experience	
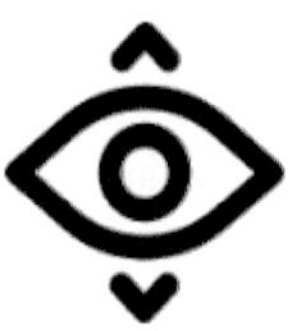 **Figure 3**	The patient is asked to re-experience the event in VR from a first-person perspective (the patients do not see their body in the scene) expressing and discussing their feelings. They are then asked what needs to happen to change the feelings in a positive direction (Figure 3). The main cognitive techniques used in this phase, if needed, are: • Countering: Once a list of distorted perceptions and cognitions is developed, the process of countering these thoughts and beliefs begins. • Label Shifting: The patients first try to identify the kinds of negative words they use to interpret situations in their life, such as bad, terrible, obese, inferior, and hateful. The situations in which these labels are used are then listed. The patient and therapist replace each emotional label with two or more descriptive words.
Phase 4 - Allocentric VR experience	
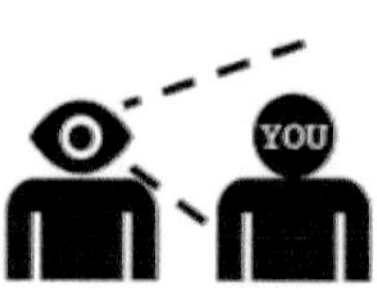 **Figure 4**	The patient is asked to re-experience the event in VR from a third-person perspective (the patients see their body in the scene) intervening to calm and reassure their virtual avatar and counter any negative evaluation (Figure 4). The therapist follows the Socratic approach, for example "What would need to happen for you to feel better? How does it look through the eyes of a third person? Is there anything you as a third person like to do? How do the other people respond?" The main cognitive techniques used in this phase, if needed, are: • Alternative Interpretation: The patient learns to stop and consider other interpretations of a situation before proceeding to the decision-making stage. • Deactivating the Illness Belief: The therapist first helps the patient list her beliefs concerning weight and eating.

are significantly fatter or thinner than they are) suggesting, among others, that virtual reality is more than a way of placing people in a simulated world (i.e., manipulating their sense of place). A first study (Serino et al. 2016b) showed that the body-swap illusion can induce an update of the negative stored representation of the body. In particular, it has been found that after embodying a virtual body with a skinny belly there was an update of the "remembered body", with women reporting a significant (post-illusion) decrease in their body-size distortion. Consistent with this perspective, Brizzi et al. (2024) and Preston et al. (2014) induced illusory ownership over a slimmer mannequin by synchronously stroking the mannequin body and the corresponding part of the participant's body. It has been found that illusory ownership over a slimmer body decreases significantly participants' perceived body size but also significantly increases participants' body satisfaction.

Support for the use of bodily illusions to alter the dysfunctional experience of the body in obesity comes for instance from the study by Serino et al. (2016b). The study observed that swapping in a slimmer body as compared to the real one was able to increase body satisfaction and reduce body-size distortion in a non-operable super-super obese patient (i.e., with BMI > 60 kg/m^2). In addition, the illusion was able to increase the patient's motivation to maintain healthy eating behaviors. While no studies to date have directly exploited the capability of the bodily illusions in obese treatment in proper randomized controlled trials, the evidence deriving from the extant experimental studies suggests (a) a direct link between perceptual (described as an inability to accurately estimate body size) and affective (described as subjective body-dissatisfaction) body components, and (b) a positive perceptual and affective response after body illusion in terms of body perception and motivation to change eating behaviors (Serino et al. 2016b).

2.2 *Reshape the body working on emotion regulation*

Different studies suggest the use of VR to address emotion regulation in obesity. Indeed, through VR it is possible to modulate food craving, i.e., the intense desire to consume a specific food. According to Jansen (1998), once eating behavior has been established, exposure to specific food cues—i.e., cues systematically associated with food intake such as the presence of high-calorie food—induces a conditioned response (hyperinsulinemia), which thus activates a hypoglycemic compensatory response. This biochemical response is experienced as a food craving and may lead to an eating episode.

By exposing participants to these cues, Cue Exposure Therapy is designed to break the mental links that typically precede using progressively. For example, in Cue Exposure Therapy (CET) (Figure 5), an obese individual may be exposed to a chocolate cake or any other high-calorie food. Initially, the exposure to the cue prompts the brain to "expect" consumption. However, frequent exposure to different cues—without eating—reduces the likelihood of cue-induced eating in the future by desensitizing the brain's reaction. VR is perfect for CET. On one side, as demonstrated by Gorini et al. (2010), real food and virtual food induced a comparable emotional reaction in patients, that is higher than the one elicited by photos of the same food. Moreover, unlike exposure to photographs, *in vivo* exposure, and guided

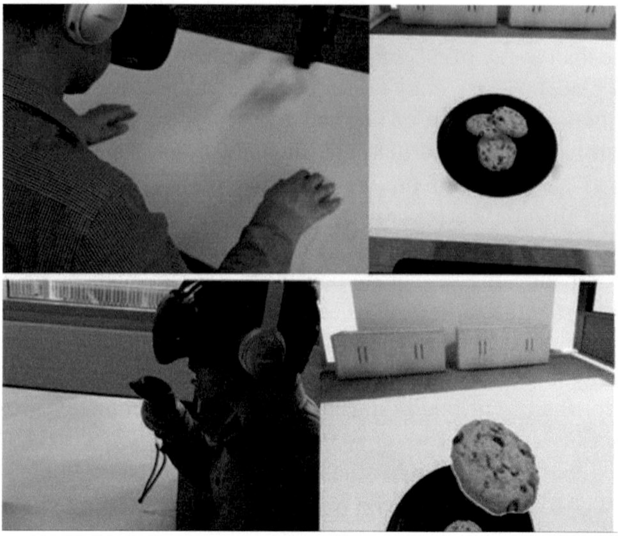

Figure 5. Example of VR-CET paradigm (image from Harris et al. 2023).

imagination, VR offers good ecological validity, and also fair internal validity, while allowing strict control over the variables. On the other side, several studies support the ability of food-related VR environments to induce food craving (Ferrer-Garcia et al. 2013, Gorini et al. 2010, Gutierrez-Maldonado et al. 2017, Pla-Sanjuanelo et al. 2015, Pla-Sanjuanelo et al. 2017). Their results suggest that craving experienced in VR environments incorporating cues and contexts related to binging behavior was consistent with trait and state craving assessed outside the VR environments. In addition, participants with the highest scores on trait and state craving also experienced cravings when exposed to food in VR. Finally, scores on questionnaires assessing trait and state craving were able to predict the average craving experienced in VR.

These results provide a clear rationale for VR-CET use to manage obesity, and different studies are providing experimental support to this claim. Specifically, VR CET can potentially lead to improved body image as obese individuals gain confidence in their ability to navigate challenging food situations without excessive emotional eating or negative self-perception.

A first study assessed the efficacy of CET based on VR (VR-CET) as a second-level treatment in patients with Bulimia Nervosa and Binge Eating Disorders (Gutierrez-Maldonado et al. 2017). 64 patients diagnosed with Bulimia Nervosa or Binge Eating resistant to treatment (i.e., binge episodes persisted after CBT) were randomly assigned to one of two conditions: VR-CET (experimental) and CBT (control) booster sessions.

Both groups were proposed with CBT booster sessions consisting of six 60-minute sessions held twice weekly over 3 weeks. Over the six sessions, participants in the experimental group were exposed to different VR environments related to binge behaviors in which patients faced high-risk situations and handled the virtual foods using a computer mouse. Exposure ended after a significant reduction in the level of anxiety, or after 60 minutes. Data showed a significant interaction between groups and time (before and after sessions), revealing a significantly higher reduction in binges, purges, bulimia symptoms, craving for food, and anxiety in the experimental group as compared to the control one. Moreover, a follow-up study showed that the VR-CET group maintained the results also after six months (Ferrer-Garcia et al. 2017).

In sum, these results support the use of VR-CET as an effective way to reduce food cravings and related behaviors in eating and weight-disordered individuals (Figure 2).

In addition, Manzoni et al. (2009) evaluated the efficacy of a 3-week relaxation protocol enhanced by VR in reducing emotional eating in a sample of 60 female inpatients with obesity who reported emotional eating. To reach this goal they used a three-arm exploration randomized controlled trial with 3 months of follow-up. The intervention included 12 individual relaxation training sessions provided traditionally (imagination condition) or supported by VR (VR condition). Control participants received only standard hospital-based care. Their data showed that VR-enhanced relaxation training was effective in reducing eating emotional episodes, and depressive and anxiety symptoms, and in improving perceived self-efficacy for eating control at a 3-month follow-up after discharge. The virtual reality condition proved better than the imagination condition in emotional eating reduction. Weight decreased in subjects in all three conditions without significant differences between them, probably due to the common treatment all inpatients received. Considering this, VR-enhanced relaxation training is a useful tool for reducing emotional eating episodes and thereby reducing weight and obesity.

2.3 Reshape the body working on physical activity

The term "exergames", originated from the fusion of the words "exercise" and "gaming", and indicates video games that provide a form of exercise. As explained by Rizzo et al. (2011), "the core concept of exergaming rests on the idea of using vigorous body activity as the input for interacting with engaging digital game content with the hope of supplanting the sedentary activity that typifies traditional game interaction that relies on keyboards, gamepads, and joysticks" (p. 259).

Exergames encourage regular physical activity, which can lead to improvements in fitness and body composition. As individuals become more physically active and see positive changes in their bodies, their body image improves. This is supported by research such as the study by Staiano et al. (2017) which found that exergaming interventions led to improvements in body composition and self-esteem in overweight and obese adolescents.

By creating engaging digital gaming interactions via body movements, the motivation to participate in calorie-burning cardiovascular exercise activities is increased. In particular, the three factors influencing motivation and compliance (Staiano et al. 2017)—feedback, challenge, and rewards – are all supported by virtual reality experiences, enabling effective intervention in obesity management.

Feedback is a critical part of physical exercise because it offers informative and evaluative suggestions on skill development and progress, allowing the perceptions of competence and the identification of possible errors or shortcomings. Typically, feedback can be visual, auditory, or sensory, but in VR their integration and multiple uses are possible. For example, we can use a progress bar with the remaining time and tasks, physical indications in the player avatar (stumbling, showing a slower pace, etc.), a sound to indicate the amount of exercise left, other avatars (e.g., the virtual coach) commenting on the performance, etc.

According to the theory of "Flow" introduced by Csikszentmihalyi (1990), an optimal match between skill and challenge is critical to achieving an intrinsically motivating experience. In this view, the ability of the exergame to assess the skill of the user and to provide a level of challenge matched to it is required to guarantee compliance and motivation.

Using VR, it is possible to develop exergames in which subjects experience themselves as competent and efficacious. Specifically, the VR experience can offer different difficulty levels—from easy tasks to very difficult ones—offering a controlled setting in which the individual can develop new skills through trial and error. Using this approach, the level of challenge can be balanced with the skill of the user so that failures can support perceived relatedness and competence without reducing perceived competence (Staiano et al. 2017).

The final component for the success of exergames is the reward. It is well known that external rewards support behavior as long as the rewards are present, but intrinsically motivated activity is more likely to produce long-term change (Ryan et al. 1983). Again, VR supports the provision of effective reward, by allowing two different types of reward (Staiano et al. 2017): controlling rewards that are task- and performance-contingent, and autonomy-supportive rewards that are verbal and task-noncontingent. In particular, VR allows the use of embodiment as a form of autonomy-supportive reward through specific poses and ballets that can be replicated and shared by users. Differently from non-VR videogames, the use of embodied avatars with normal body size has the potential to increase the effectiveness of exergames among overweight children as demonstrated by a recent study (Lwin and Jung 2014).

These principles have been used in different successful exergames (Farič et al. 2019, Farrow et al. 2019, Finkelstein et al. 2011). For example, Astrojumper is an immersive virtual reality exergame used to engage children and adults in rigorous, full-body exercise (Finkelstein et al. 2011). The overall goal of these exergames is relatively easy: users fly through an immersive, stereoscopic outer space environment in first-person perspective, and they have to avoid or grab the different virtual planets that are speeding toward them. A critical feature of Astrojumper is that feedback, challenges, and rewards are calibrated to optimize motivation. As the authors explain (Finkelstein et al. 2011): "To make sure that Astrojumper would be playable for users at all levels of physical fitness, Astrojumper begins very slowly, providing all users with a warm-up phase. After this phase is complete, planets will begin to gradually come out at a slightly faster rate. If the player is successfully able to avoid these planets, the speed will continue to increase. If the player starts to collide with the planets, their speed will be reduced. This back-and-forth adjustment finds a speed where the player can avoid almost all of the planets and will continuously update throughout the game" (p.87).

The results achieved support this approach. A study involving 30 subjects (10 participants were children and 20 were adults) demonstrated that Astrojumper is an effective way to provide a workout, motivating both children and adults to exercise through immersive VR (Finkelstein et al. 2011).

Up to now the most significant barrier to the wide use of VR exergames is the cost (Farič et al. 2019). However, the appearance of cheaper standalone VR devices associated with successful commercial VR exergames like Beat Saber or Dance Central may improve the use of this approach in the prevention and treatment of obesity.

Conclusions

Most clinicians and patients consider obesity a problem of energy input and expenditure: more energy input than expenditure. However, clinical practice and epidemiological data clearly show that obesity is more complex than this simple equation would suggest and highlight how socio-cultural pressures to conform to a certain body shape play a key role in the development of negative feelings about the body, which is a critical risk factor for the development of overweight and obesity (Weinberger et al. 2019).

In this chapter, we underlined the potential of VR in the management of body image in obesity by discussing different applications: body swapping and reference frameshifting, emotion regulation, and exergames. These aspects can play a fundamental role in the autobiographical reconstruction of patients with eating disorders (Frisone et al. 2023), allowing them to manage their condition from different parameters.

The available clinical results suggest the added value of VR as part of an integrated obesity treatment targeting both the physical and the psychological side of the problem. However, longer follow-up data and multi-centric trials are required to investigate the possible effects of behavioral, emotional, and body image changes on the long-term maintenance of weight loss.

Acknowledgments

The work in this paper was supported by the project Arcadia VR - Assistenza e Riabilitazione del Comportamento Alimentare tramite Dispositivi basati sull'Intelligenza Artificiale e sulla Realtà Virtuale (Assistance and Rehabilitation of Eating Behavior through Devices Based on Artificial Intelligence and Virtual Reality) - MINISTERIAL DECREE DECEMBER 31, 2021 - INNOVATION AGREEMENTS and by the Italian Ministry of Health.

References

Akhtar, S., L.V. Justice, C. Loveday and M.A. Conway. 2017. Switching memory perspective. Conscious Cogn. 56(Supplement C): 50–57.

Botvinick, M. and J. Cohen. 1998. Rubber hands 'feel' touch that eyes see. Nature 391: 756.

Brizzi, G. and G. Riva. 2024. Playing with spatial frames: altering the body matrix through multisensory egocentric and allocentric body illusions. Hum. Behav. Emerg. Technol. 2024: 7316063.

Brizzi, G., F. Frisone, C. Rossi and G. Riva. 2024. Gender differences in bodily experience: Insights from virtual reality body illusion. Acta Psychol. 249: 104386.

Brizzi, G., M. Sansoni, D. Di Lernia, F. Frisone, C. Tuena and G. Riva. 2023. The multisensory mind: a systematic review of multisensory integration processing in Anorexia and Bulimia Nervosa. J. Eat. Disord. 11: 204.

Butters, J.W. and T.F. Cash. 1987. Cognitive-behavioral treatment of women's body image satisfaction: A controlled outcome-study. J. Consult. Clin. Psychol. 55: 889–897.

Calogero, R.M., S. Tantleff-Dunn and J.K. Thompson. 2010. Self-Objectification in Women: Causes, Consequences, and Counteractions. American Psychological Association, Washington, DC.

Cesa, G.L., G.M. Manzoni, M. Bacchetta, G. Castelnuovo, S. Conti, A. Gaggioli et al. 2013. Virtual reality for enhancing the cognitive behavioral treatment of obesity with binge eating disorder: randomized controlled study with one-year follow-up. J. Med. Internet Res. 15: e113.

Csikszentmihalyi, M. 1990. Flow: The Psychology of Optimal Experience. HarperCollins, New York.

Dakanalis, A., G. Carrà, R. Calogero, R. Fida, M. Clerici, M.A. Zanetti et al. 2015. The developmental effects of media-ideal internalization and self-objectification processes on adolescents' negative body-feelings, dietary restraint, and binge eating. Eur. Child Adolesc. Psychiatry. 24: 997–1010.

Di Natale, A.F., S.F.M. Pizzoli, G. Brizzi, D. Di Lernia, F. Frisone, A. Gaggioli et al. 2024. Harnessing immersive virtual reality: a comprehensive scoping review of its applications in assessing, understanding, and treating eating disorders. Curr. Psychiatry Rep. 1–17.

Eijlers, R., E.M. Utens, L.M. Staals, P.F. de Nijs, J.M. Berghmans, R.M. Wijnen et al. 2019. Systematic review and meta-analysis of virtual reality in pediatrics: effects on pain and anxiety. Anesth. Analg. 129: 1344–1353.

Farič, N., E. Yorke, L. Varnes, K. Newby, H.W.W. Potts, L. Smith et al. 2019. Younger adolescents' perceptions of physical activity, exergaming, and virtual reality: qualitative intervention study. JMIR Serious Games 7: e11960.

Farrow, M., C. Lutteroth, P.C. Rouse and J.L.J. Bilzon. 2019. Virtual-reality exergaming improves performance during high-intensity interval training. Eur. J. Sport Sci. 19: 719–727.

Ferrer-Garcia, M., J. Gutierrez-Maldonado and J. Pla. 2013. Cue-elicited anxiety and craving for food using virtual reality scenarios. Stud. Health Technol. Inform. 191: 105–109.

Fink, P.W., S.P. Shultz, E. D'Hondt, M. Lenoir and A.P. Hills. 2019. Multifractal analysis differentiates postural sway in obese and nonobese children. Mot. Control. 23: 262–271.

Finkelstein, S., A. Nickel, Z. Lipps, T. Barnes, Z. Wartell and E.A. Suma. 2011. Astrojumper: Motivating exercise with an immersive virtual reality exergame. presence: teleoperators. Virtual Environ. 20: 78–92.

Frisone, F., G. Brizzi, M. Sansoni, A.F. Di Natale, S.F.M. Pizzoli, G. Stanghellini et al. 2023. Autobiographical memory in feeding and eating disorders: a systematic review. Psychopathology 1–25.

Gardner, R.M., V. Salaz, B. Reyes and S.J. Brake. 1983. Sensitivity to proprioceptive feedback in obese subjects. Percept. Mot. Skills 57: 1111–1118.

Gorini, A., E. Griez, A. Petrova and G. Riva. 2010. Assessment of the emotional responses produced by exposure to real food, virtual food and photographs of food in patients affected by eating disorders. Ann. Gen. Psychiatry 9: 30.

Gutiérrez-Maldonado, J., M. Ferrer-García, A. Dakanalis and G. Riva. 2017. Virtual reality: Applications to eating disorders. pp. 146–161. *In*: Agras, S.W. and A. Robinson (eds.). The Oxford Handbook of Eating Disorders, Second Edition. Oxford University Press, Oxford, UK.

Harris, N.M., R.W. Lindeman, C.S.F. Bah, D. Gerhard and S. Hoermann. 2023. Eliciting real cravings with virtual food: Using immersive technologies to explore the effects of food stimuli in virtual reality. Front. Psychol. 14: 956585.

Jansen, A. 1998. A learning model of binge eating: cue reactivity and cue exposure. Behav. Res. Ther. 36: 257–272.
Leuner, H. 1969. Guided affective imagery: a method of intensive psychotherapy. Am. J. Psychother. 23: 4–21.
Makinen, M., L.R. Puukko-Viertomies, N. Lindberg, M.A. Siimes and V. Aalberg. 2012. Body dissatisfaction and body mass in girls and boys transitioning from early to mid-adolescence: additional role of self-esteem and eating habits. BMC Psychiatry 12: 35.
Manzoni, G.M., G.L. Cesa, M. Bacchetta, G. Castelnuovo, S. Conti, A. Gaggioli et al. 2016. Virtual reality-enhanced cognitive-behavioral therapy for morbid obesity: a randomized controlled study with 1 year follow-up. Cyberpsychol. Behav. Soc. Netw. 19: 134–140.
Manzoni, G.M., F. Pagnini, A. Gorini, A. Preziosa, G. Castelnuovo, E. Molinari et al. 2009. Can relaxation training reduce emotional eating in women with obesity? An exploratory study with 3 months of follow-up. J. Am. Diet. Assoc. 109: 1427–1432.
Macht, M. 2008. How emotions affect eating: A five-way model. Appetite. 50: 1–11.
Makinen, M., L.R. Puukko-Viertomies, N. Lindberg, M.A. Siimes and V. Aalberg. 2012. Body dissatisfaction and body mass in girls and boys transitioning from early to mid-adolescence: additional role of self-esteem and eating habits. BMC Psychiatry 12: 35.
Pla-Sanjuanelo, J., M. Ferrer-García, F. Vilalta-Abella, G. Riva, A. Dakanalis, J. Ribas-Sabaté et al. 2019. Testing virtual reality-based cue-exposure software: Which cue-elicited responses best discriminate between patients with eating disorders and healthy controls?. Eating and Weight Disorders-Studies on Anorexia, Bulimia and Obesity 24: 757–765.
Pla-Sanjuanelo, J., M. Ferrer-García, J. Gutierrez-Maldonado, G. Riva, A. Andreu-Gracia, A. Dakanalis et al. 2015. Identifying specific cues and contexts related to bingeing behavior for the development of effective virtual environments. Appetite 87: 81–89.
Preston, C. and H.H. Ehrsson. 2014. Illusory changes in body size modulate body satisfaction in a way that is related to non-clinical eating disorder psychopathology. PLoS ONE 9.
Puhl, R.M., M.M. Wall, C. Chen, S. Bryn Austin, M.E. Eisenberg and D. Neumark-Sztainer. 2017. Experiences of weight teasing in adolescence and weight-related outcomes in adulthood: A 15-year longitudinal study. Prev. Med. 100: 173–179.
Puhl, R.M. and C.A. Heuer. 2009. The stigma of obesity: A review and update. Obesity 17: 941–964.
Quick, V., M. Wall, N. Larson, J. Haines and D. Neumark-Sztainer. 2013. Personal, behavioral and socio-environmental predictors of overweight incidence in young adults: 10-yr longitudinal findings. Int. J. Behav. Nutr. Phys. Act. 10: 37.
Riva, G. 2011. The key to unlocking the virtual body: virtual reality in the treatment of obesity and eating disorders. J. Diabetes Sci. Technol. 5: 283–292.
Riva, G. 2012. Neuroscience and eating disorders: The allocentric lock hypothesis. Med. Hypotheses 78: 254–257.
Riva, G. 2018. The neuroscience of body memory: from the self through the space to the others. Cortex. 104: 241–260.
Riva, G. and A. Dakanalis. 2018. Altered processing and integration of multisensory bodily representations and signals in eating disorders: a possible path toward the understanding of their underlying causes. Front. Hum. Neurosci. 12: 49.
Riva, G., R.M. Baños, C. Botella, F. Mantovani and A. Gaggioli. 2016. Transforming experience: the potential of augmented reality and virtual reality for enhancing personal and clinical change. Front. Psychiatry 7: 164.
Riva, G., F. Vatalaro, F. Davide and M. Alcañiz. 2004. Ambient Intelligence: The Evolution of Technology, Communication and Cognition Towards The Future of Human-Computer Interaction. IOS Press, Amsterdam. Online: http://www.emergingcommunication.com/volume6.html.
Rizzo, A.S., B. Lange, E.A. Suma and M. Bolas. 2011. Virtual reality and interactive digital game technology: new tools to address obesity and diabetes. J. Diabetes Sci. Technol. 5: 256–264.
Ryan, R.M., V. Mims and R. Koestner. 1983. Relation of reward contingency and interpersonal context to intrinsic motivation: A review and test using cognitive evaluation theory. J. Pers. Soc. Psychol. 45: 736.

Safaei, M., E.A. Sundararajan, M. Driss, W. Boulila and A. Shapi'i. 2021. A systematic literature review on obesity: Understanding the causes & consequences of obesity and reviewing various machine learning approaches used to predict obesity. Comput. Biol. Med. 136: 104754.

Sarwer, D.B., J.K. Thompson and T.F. Cash. 2005. Body image and obesity in adulthood. Psychiatr. Clin. North Am. 28: 69–87.

Scarpina, F., D. Migliorati, P. Marzullo, A. Mauro, M. Scacchi and M. Costantini. 2016. Altered multisensory temporal integration in obesity. Sci. Rep. 6: 28382.

Schultheis, M.T. and A.A. Rizzo. 2001. The application of virtual reality technology in rehabilitation. Rehabil. Psychol. 46: 296–311.

Schwartz, M.B. and K.D. Brownell. 2004. Obesity and body image. Body Image 1: 43–56.

Serino, S., E. Pedroli, A. Keizer, S. Triberti, A. Dakanalis, F. Pallavicini et al. 2016a. Virtual reality body swapping: a tool for modifying the allocentric memory of the body. Cyberpsychol. Behav. Soc. Netw. 19: 127–133.

Serino, S., F. Scarpina, A. Keizer, E. Pedroli, A. Dakanalis, G. Castelnuovo et al. 2016b. A novel technique for improving bodily experience in a non-operable super-super obesity case. Front. Psychol. 7: 837.

Shriver, L.H., J.M. Dollar, M. Lawless, S.D. Calkins, S.P. Keane, L. Shanahan et al. 2019. Longitudinal associations between emotion regulation and adiposity in late adolescence: indirect effects through eating behaviors. Nutrients 11: 517.

Simmons, W.K. and D.C. DeVille. 2017. Interoceptive contributions to healthy eating and obesity. Curr. Opin. Psychol. 17: 106–112.

Staiano, A.E., R.A. Beyl, D.S. Hsia, P.T. Katzmarzyk and R.L. Newton Jr. 2017. Twelve weeks of dance exergaming in overweight and obese adolescent girls: Transfer effects on physical activity, screen time, and self-efficacy. J. Sport Health Sci. 6: 4–10.

Stice, E., K. Presnell, H. Shaw and P. Rohde. 2005. Psychological and behavioral risk factors for obesity onset in adolescent girls: a prospective study. J. Consult. Clin. Psychol. 73: 195–202.

Tsakiris, M. 2017. The multisensory basis of the self: From body to identity to others. Q. J. Exp. Psychol. 70: 597–609.

Weinberger, N.A., A. Kersting, S.G. Riedel-Heller and C. Luck-Sikorski. 2016. Body dissatisfaction in individuals with obesity compared to normal-weight individuals: A systematic review and meta-analysis. Obes. Facts 9: 424–441.

WHO. 2020. World Health Organization. Air Quality Guidelines for Europe. World Health Org., Eur. Ser. 91.

Wooley, S.C. and O.W. Wooley. 1985. Intensive out-patient and residential treatment for bulimia. pp. 120–132. *In*: Garner, D.M. and P.E. Garfinkel (eds.). Handbook of Psychotherapy for Anorexia and Bulimia. Guilford Press, New York, USA.

Younbo, J., J.L.B. and L.M. O. 2014. Wii, Myself, and Size: The influence of proteus effect and stereotype threat on overweight children's exercise motivation and behavior in exergames. Games Health J. 3: 40–48.

Part II

… To Practical Applications in Sociocultural Contexts

Chapter 8

Prevention of Dysfunctional Eating Attitudes and Behaviors Focusing on Body Image

*Isabelle Carrard** and *Sophie Bucher Della Torre*

INTRODUCTION

According to Monthuy-Blanc et al. (2023), described in the Preface, every eater falls on a continuum of profiles ranging from functional to completely dysfunctional. Dysfunctional eating attitudes and behaviors (DEAB) include eating disorders and disordered eating, now recognized by researchers as serious but still socially normalized (Neumark-Sztainer 2005). Body perception disturbances (BPD), including body dissatisfaction, represent a breaking point on the continuum and indicate the need for intervention. Addressing body image, a risk factor for unhealthy eating and physical activity behaviors, and depression enables integrated prevention efforts for DEAB, obesity, and poor mental health while avoiding potentially conflicting or iatrogenic messages (Irving and Neumark-Sztainer 2002, Mond et al. 2013). In this chapter, we highlight how focusing on body image can help prevent DEAB and promote healthy behaviors. We also describe the major existing prevention interventions, discuss our specific context, and explore future prospects for other studies in this area.

Department of Nutrition and Dietetics, Geneva School of Health Sciences (HEdS-GE), HES-SO University of Applied Sciences and Arts, Western Switzerland, Rue des Caroubiers 25, 1227 Carouge-Geneva, Switzerland.

Email: sophie.bucher@hesge.ch

* Corresponding author: isabelle.carrard@hesge.ch

DOI: 10.1201/9781032718125-10

1. Conceptual framework

1.1 Body image

The conceptualization of body image used in most current research is based on the cognitive and behavioral model designed by Cash (2011). This integrated model combines the multiple influences that shape body image attitudes, including evaluation and investment schemas. Evaluation refers to body satisfaction or dissatisfaction with how one looks and results from a comparison between how individuals perceive their own body and the beauty ideals they value (Cash 2011). Investment refers to the importance of appearance to self-worth and of having an attractive appearance.

1.2 Sociocultural models

Because BPD play a major role in DEAB, understanding the factors that contribute to their development provides valuable guidance for intervention. Sociocultural models, such as the tripartite influence model (Thompson et al. 1999) or the dual pathway model (Stice 2001), highlight the added effects of cultural pressures and personal factors on the development of BPD. The tripartite influence model postulates that external pressures from the media, family, and peers influence body satisfaction through the mediation of beauty ideal internalization and social comparison. Beauty ideal internalization is defined as the endorsement of societal ideals of attractiveness and engaging in behaviors designed to achieve them. Social comparison is the unfavorable comparison of one's appearance with that of others. The resulting BPD then influence DEAB and global psychological functioning. Originally developed to explain DEAB in young women, the tripartite influence model has been refined to integrate the internalization of the mesomorphic ideal and concerns about muscularity and body fat that characterize men's body image and DEAB (Tylka 2011).

In addition to the influence of mass media on body dissatisfaction, which has been experimentally linked to body dissatisfaction in girls and women by conveying Western cultural ideals of beauty through photoshopped images, movies, and television shows (Groesz et al. 2002), sociocultural models also emphasize the role of family and peers. This influence often manifests in behaviors such as fat talk and teasing. Fat talk among peers, a self-deprecating type of weight and shape talk often considered normative for women, is associated with increased BPD (Sharpe et al. 2013). Similarly, hearing family members participate in fat talk is negatively associated with mindful eating and body appreciation (Webb et al. 2018). Direct criticism and teasing about appearance and weight from family and peers have also been strongly associated with BPD and DEAB (Menzel et al. 2010).

1.3 Socio-ecological model

Given the pervasive societal messages linking thinness to beauty, health, and self-control, effectively addressing BPD requires targeting not only individuals but also the various contexts that transmit and perpetuate the factors leading to BPD and DEAB. To this end, several authors have used a socio-ecological framework that features the various levels that influence individual development, from the more proximal to the more distal. This model accounts for personal characteristics, family and peer influences, school and other institutional factors, community factors, as well as societal factors (Neumark-Sztainer 2005). Accordingly, prevention interventions should target not only individuals, but also their inter-individual contexts (e.g., parents, siblings, peers, coaches), their immediate environment (e.g., policies in schools, sports facilities, living spaces), and the larger environment or societal context (e.g., legislation).

1.4 Objectification theory

In parallel, one research trend has focused on the asymmetrical prevalence of DEAB between men and women, underscoring that societal pressures linking appearance to social worth differ by gender. Women face not only unattainable beauty ideals but also sexual objectification, as present in regular social interactions and the media (Fredrickson and Roberts 1997). Objectification theory posits that women are socialized to internalize an external view of their bodies, leading to possible body surveillance, decreased interoceptive awareness, anxiety, difficulty experiencing flow, body shame, and ultimately DEAB, sexual dysfunction, and depression. A meta-analysis by Schaefer and Thompson (2018) found a positive relationship between self-objectification and DEAB, with a stronger relationship in women compared to men. Following this societal vision, DEAB prevention interventions should aim to transform the social environment that shapes gendered experiences of the body rather than focus solely on individuals to mitigate risk factors.

1.5 Protective factor models

Historically, body image has been studied empirically in relation to psychopathology and poor mental health, with an emphasis on disorders and how to reduce distress. Recently, however, interest has shifted to protective factors. Two partially overlapping lines of research have given new impetus to body image research: the developmental theory of embodiment and positive body image.

The developmental theory of embodiment. The developmental theory of embodiment describes the loss of body connection that occurs in girls during adolescence, which can lead to DEAB or self-harm, linking these issues to social structures rather than individual psychology. The concept of embodiment itself, as advocated by Piran (2016), includes (a) an attunement to inner states, (b) an experiential breadth, and (c) a relationship with social structures. Piran (2016) also explored the experience of embodiment in a large-scale qualitative program involving women of all ages and identified five dimensions: (1) body connection and comfort; (2) agency and functionality; (3) experience and expression of desire; (4) attuned self-care; and (5) inhabiting the body as a subjective site and resisting objectification. These dimensions range on a continuum from embodiment (body connection and comfort, embodied agency and passion, and attuned self-care) to disembodiment (disrupted body connection and discomfort, restricted agency and passion, and self-neglect or harm; Piran 2018).

Positive body image. Positive body image research has evolved with the rise of positive psychology (Tylka and Wood-Barcalow 2015b). Positive body image is not seen as the opposite of negative body image on the same continuum, but as a distinct and inversely correlated dimension. Menzel and Levine (2011) proposed three essential components of positive body image: (a) appreciation of body appearance and function, (b) awareness of and attention to body experiences, and (c) positive cognitions for coping with interpersonal challenges to a healthy body image. The Body Appreciation Scale (BAS; Avalos et al. 2005) and its revised version (BAS-2; Tylka and Wood-Barcalow 2015a) are the main instruments used to assess positive body image. A systematic review of 240 articles found that body appreciation was consistently associated with lower DEAB and higher well-being (Linardon et al. 2022). Importantly, these associations were maintained after controlling for the influence of negative body image, reinforcing that positive body image is distinct from negative body image and requires its own measurement tools and interventions.

In sum, the concept of positive body image offers a new framework for developing DEAB prevention interventions by focusing on protective as well as risk factors. As the next section demonstrates, interventions that target risk factors have had the benefit of time to prove their effectiveness, but those that focus on protective factors offer promising new avenues.

2. Empirical and clinical support

In their reviews of the effectiveness of eating disorder prevention interventions, Watson et al. (2016) and Le et al. (2017) identified media literacy as the most effective approach for universal prevention, that is, interventions aimed at the general population, regardless of individual risk levels. For selective prevention, which targets individuals with at least one specific risk factor but no symptoms, the systematic reviews revealed cognitive dissonance, healthy lifestyle interventions, and cognitive behavioral therapy to be effective. For indicated prevention, consisting of interventions that include participants with multiple signs or symptoms of eating disorders, only cognitive behavioral therapy was evaluated. However, in their meta-analysis, Le et al. (2017) determined that the evidence was too insufficient to conclude on its effectiveness.

In the last ten years, interventions developed to improve body image have shifted from a focus on DEAB prevention toward protective factors and promoting positive body image (Halliwell 2015). This section first focuses on the main universal and selective prevention interventions developed for DEAB, then presents examples of emerging interventions targeting dimensions of positive body image.

2.1 Universal prevention

Media literacy is effective for universal audiences, particularly in school settings, and is one of the few approaches suitable for young children. It targets media-driven pressure by promoting analytical and critical thinking about media messages, educating individuals about media manipulation, and encouraging the rejection of unrealistic body standards. Media Smart is the media literacy intervention program with the longest follow-up assessment, with findings supporting the program's effectiveness in helping young people critically evaluate the media's promotion of a single beauty ideal and the gender stereotypes it perpetuates (Wilksch and Wade 2009). However, media literacy faces the new challenge of addressing social media. Social media have been identified as key contributors to BPD and DEAB, both through passive exposure to idealized body images and active engagement with appearance-related content, such as liking or posting pictures (Revranche et al. 2022, Rousefell et al. 2020). Scholars have recommended integrating social media into theoretical DEAB models to better inform targeted interventions, as current media literacy interventions show limited effectiveness (Tylka et al. 2023, Yager 2024).

Classroom-based body image interventions are the easiest way to disseminate universal prevention to children and adolescents. Yager et al. (2013) reviewed such interventions and found seven that showed significant pre-post improvements in body image. All used a combination of approaches, but the main constant was media literacy, used in six effective interventions. These successful approaches also included self-esteem activities and discussions about peer influence. In contrast, psychoeducation, that is, informing about body image and BPD, did not stand out as an effective method. More recently, Yager et al. (2024) listed some "well-intended" approaches that can be iatrogenic, arguing that practices such as weighing students, recording food intake and calculating calories, teaching directly about eating disorders, using popular media and magazines, or showing images of thin people should be avoided in curriculum-based activities in schools. Experts have noted that some interventions still lack theoretical underpinnings and that it would be preferable to replicate and disseminate interventions that have already been shown to be effective rather than develop new ones (Yager 2024).

In line with the socio-ecological model, "whole school" approaches have been developed. In addition to formal curriculum activities, these interventions include greater teacher, student, and other key stakeholder participation to change the school culture, improve the physical environment, and adapt school policies. Despite some positive outcomes, overall evaluations of these interventions have been disappointing, especially considering the important resources required (Yager 2024). One promising example is Piran's (2018) intervention in a residential dance school, a high-risk setting for the development of DEAB. Through a participatory process, the school environment was reshaped to promote greater equity. Girls had the opportunity to engage with their bodies in a safe, respectful space where open expression, freedom from appearance pressures, and honoring personal needs supported healthy embodiment.

2.2 Selective prevention

Cognitive dissonance is likely the most evaluated approach to DEAB selective prevention for individuals with BPD. The principles of cognitive dissonance, as coined by Festinger (1957), suggest that when individuals act in ways that contradict their beliefs, they experience discomfort (dissonance) that they then attempt to reduce by changing their beliefs or acts. In this line of thinking, the Body Project, originally developed by Stice and colleagues (2000), consists of three interactive group sessions with activities in which participants publicly speak against the thin ideal or practice responding to fat talk. The Body Project primarily aims to reduce thin-ideal internalization, a risk factor upstream of BPD (Stice 2001, Thompson et al. 1999) and its effectiveness has been successfully evaluated with young women who reported BPD (Stice et al. 2019).

Initially developed as an inactive control for the Body Project, the Healthy Weight Program unexpectedly also proved effective in reducing BPD (Stice et al. 2001). In this group intervention, participants are encouraged to implement healthy lifestyle changes to promote good health and well-being rather than for appearance reasons using behavior change techniques, principles of social psychology, and interactive psychoeducation. Since its development, the Healthy Weight Program has evolved to shift from an emphasis on weight maintenance to one on health and well-being promotion (Becker et al. 2010). In the Healthy Weight Program, participants receive an alternative to dieting and dietary restriction by implementing small, manageable, and concrete lifestyle changes. In addition, group support and learned problem-solving techniques increase participants' self-efficacy and promotes empowerment. A recent meta-analytic review confirmed that the Body Project and the Healthy Weight Program, alongside an intervention aimed at increasing self-esteem and self-efficacy, were among the few that significantly reduced the risk of future eating disorder onset (Stice et al. 2021a).

In Switzerland, our own research team aimed to assess the Body Project and the Healthy Weight Program in the French-speaking part of the country (Carrard and Bucher Della Torre 2021). Both interventions were of interest: While the Body Project had the largest effect sizes and was the most widely evaluated, the Healthy Weight Program offered integrated DEAB prevention, promoted healthy behaviors, and seemed to be better accepted by certain subgroups, such as athletes (Becker et al. 2012). For this project called HEIDI, which targeted young women with BPD aged 18–25, we used the validated French version of the Body Project. We translated the Healthy Weight Program and adapted it to align with Swiss health recommendations. Forty participants were randomized into three groups (Body Project, Healthy Weight, and a control group). The results showed high acceptability and significant decreases in BPD, dietary restraint, and improvements of mental health, with effects maintained after one month (Carrard et al. 2023). Despite these encouraging results, participant recruitment was challenging, in part due to the COVID-19 pandemic. Feedback from the recruitment process also revealed that many young women struggled to recognize that it was not their bodies that needed to change, but rather their BPD, reflecting the strong internalization of societal pressures around appearance. Building on this initial experience, our team will continue the HEIDI project to explore complementary new intervention approaches that enhance protective factors.

2.3 Interventions to promote a positive body image

As prevention strategies have shifted to promoting positive body image rather than decreasing BPD, new targets have emerged, such as body functionality, body appreciation, body esteem or body image flexibility. These protective factors have expanded prevention options to include self-compassion, yoga, exercise, gratitude, intuitive eating, or a combination of these (Guest et al. 2019, Rupani et al. 2024). In this section, we describe interventions based on three especially active ingredients: body functionality, yoga and exercise, and self-compassion. These have shown promising effects and can be theoretically related to the three dimensions of positive body image defined by Menzel and Levine (2011): (a) appreciation of body appearance and function, (b) awareness of and attention to body experiences, and (c) positive cognitions for coping with interpersonal challenges to a healthy body image.

Body functionality is an aspect of positive body image that refers to everything that the body can do. This includes body functions related to physical capacities, but also internal processes, senses, creativity, self-care, and communication with others (Alleva et al. 2015). Focusing on body functionality rather than body appearance has been associated with greater body satisfaction and appreciation. In addition, focusing on body functionality is also a way to decrease self-objectification and self-surveillance, by encouraging women to think of their bodies as active, dynamic, and instrumental, as opposed to passive, static, and aesthetic (Alleva et al. 2015). An online, writing-based functionality intervention called Expand Your Horizon was found to have a positive impact on body appreciation, body esteem, and satisfaction with functionality and had the best evidence of effectiveness in a review of interventions aimed at promoting positive body image in adults (Alleva et al. 2018, Guest et al. 2019).

Yoga has the potential to enhance the overall experience of embodiment by positively impacting dimensions such as body connection, agency and functionality, attuned self-care, and resistance to objectification (Piran and Neumark-Sztainer 2020). When yoga instruction emphasizes mindfulness rather than appearance, it fosters more positive affect and better embodiment experiences (Cox et al. 2020). Therefore, yoga could improve body image through interoceptive changes, increased gratitude for one's body, perceived accomplishment, self-confidence, and seeing diverse body types in practice. However, it could also negatively impact body image if participants engage in social comparison or self-criticism (Neumark-Sztainer et al. 2018). In a systematic review of 17 yoga intervention studies focused on adults in universal or indicated prevention, at least half found significant improvements after the intervention compared to the baseline (Rupani et al. 2024). More generally, in cross-sectional studies among children and adolescents, more physical activity is generally associated with less BPD (Gualdi-Russo et al. 2022). However, some appearance- or leanness-oriented sports are associated with a higher risk of DEAB among participants (Chapa et al. 2022), and body image issues remain one of the reasons for girls' early disengagement from sports (Matheson et al. 2023).

Lastly, self-compassion is a promising approach to promoting positive body image. In addition to being an effective strategy against BPD (Braun et al. 2016), self-compassion supports body appreciation and body image flexibility by encouraging individuals to interpret social comparisons and self-criticism with more balance and empathy. It also offers alternative ways for people to value themselves, shifting the focus away from societal body ideals. Several studies, mostly on adult women, have tested self-compassion. For example, Albertson et al. (2015) found that a three-week intervention consisting of listening to a self-compassion podcast improved self-compassion and body appreciation and reduced BPD compared to waitlist participants. In adolescents, some programs such as Be Real's BodyKind (Mahon et al. 2023) or Digital SMART (Mahon and Hevey 2023) have shown promising results.

Considering well-established interventions, such as those targeting risk factors and BPD, and more recent developments, there is now a wide range of interventions available to promote improved body image. However, further evaluation of these programs can enhance their effectiveness by, for example, assessing protective factors in the delivery of well-established interventions or longer follow-up for the more recent developments.

3. Applications to the sociocultural context

3.1 The place of body image in DEAB prevention in Switzerland

Health promotion in Switzerland reflects the decentralized organization of the country. The federal government decides on national strategies and coordinates health promotion campaigns, while the twenty-six cantons are responsible for developing and implementing these efforts in their regional context. A key organization in the country is the foundation Swiss Health Promotion. This foundation coordinates programs with the cantons to promote healthy eating, physical activity, and mental health among children, adolescents, and seniors. Since 2017, Swiss Health Promotion and the cantons have funded action plans to promote a healthy body image, complementing existing measures that support healthy eating and physical activity among children and adolescents.

Switzerland's French-speaking cantons have collaborated to develop body positive actions for three settings: schools, out-of-school settings, and media. Inspired by socio-ecological interventions, we intervened in out-of-school settings in particular to educate adults in contact with young people, especially social workers and sports instructors, about the importance of a healthy body image. More precisely, we targeted the representations and attitudes of the adults with whom young people were in contact in their out-of-school environment. We give here a brief description of the developments of these actions and their evolution.

3.2 How to train adult actors in out-of-school settings

First, we conducted qualitative interviews with sports instructors to better understand their perceived needs and potential misconceptions and unhelpful attitudes. Based on this first step and a literature review (Carrard et al. 2019), we concluded that the positive body image framework (Tylka and Wood-Barcalow 2015b) provided an appropriate perspective for addressing body image in a health promotion context.

We next designed a training course for social workers and sports instructors that focused on how to develop a positive body image for themselves and as role models for the young people they work with. Our aim was to help these adults change their attitudes about body weight and shape that could be harmful to young people and to debunk misconceptions about what constitutes a healthy body image, healthy eating, and adaptive movement. The participants were also encouraged to analyze their personal and professional environment and elaborate on concrete strategies to foster a positive body image. The three components of a positive body image were presented and then practiced in everyday life situations.

After disseminating the training to the target population in our canton, the demand for training in other cantons quickly exceeded our resources. For this reason, we decided to formalize the training into a Massive Open Online Course (MOOC) that was first launched in fall 2022. The MOOC, entitled "A Positive Body Image for Everyone: Understanding and Taking Action," is divided into four weeks of content. The MOOC is in French and represents about 15 hours of work. Each week includes theory capsules, educational exercises, videos, a cartoon summary, an audio file, and an evaluation quiz. In addition, the MOOC's design was based on cognitive behavioral principles, such as exposure, and addressed DEAB risk factors identified in sociocultural models, such as the internalization of beauty ideals, social comparison, fat talk, and criticism from caregivers or friends. New developments in positive body image research, such as self-compassion (Neff 2023), were also incorporated in the MOOC to address self-criticism.

As with any health promotion initiative, the challenge is to evaluate the impact of such a program. While the benefits to young people cannot be directly measured, we collected pre-post data from the MOOC participants to assess whether the MOOC achieved its goal of changing youths' environment. Data on knowledge, beliefs, practices, and body appreciation, as assessed by the BAS-2, will be analyzed and published. To date, we have achieved approximately 350 subscriptions per opening, with an average completion rate of 34%. This is a respectable completion rate since a major drawback of MOOCs is their high participant dropout rate, which usually reaches 90% (Bezerra and Silva 2017). This MOOC, which has the strength to be based on theoretical frameworks, appears as a promising strategy to create numerous ambassadors of positive body image and improve youths' environment.

Conclusion

This chapter reviewed the evolution of research on the concept of body image as a valuable target for the integrated prevention of DEAB, obesity and poor mental health.

Effective prevention for the whole population requires a combination of universal and selective interventions. In addition to universal prevention interventions, equity requires that subgroups in need of prevention interventions receive interventions specifically designed for them. This has contributed to our reflection on the HEIDI project's development to cover the specific needs of population subgroups in effective, culturally adapted interventions, in addition to the universal dimension ensured by the MOOC on positive body image.

An important challenge remains the dissemination of effective interventions. However, some inspiring examples have been reported, for example, a successful collaboration with sororities was able to disseminate the Body Project (Becker et al. 2017b). Widespread dissemination requires that the intervention be delivered without the need for a researcher or caregiver. To this end, the Body Project and a modified version of the Healthy Weight Program delivered by peers were found to be valuable options (Becker et al. 2008, Becker et al. 2010). The dissemination of effective interventions to more diverse populations also merits further investigation. In particular, most preventive interventions have shown reduced efficacy in boys, who experience different sociocultural pressures on appearance and new forms of DEAB (Nagata et al. 2020). Finally, since various racial/ethnic groups and gender and sexual minorities also show increased prevalence of DEAB (Cheng et al. 2019, Nagata et al. 2024), further prevention efforts are needed to assess whether effective interventions are reaching them (Stice et al. 2021b). These populations may also need tailored interventions that promote greater embodiment, as they often experience stigma, trauma, lack of agency, and lack of safety (Meyer 2003). Other issues may also come into play, such as food insecurity, which is highly associated with DEAB (Becker et al. 2017a).

The landscape of interventions reported in this chapter highlights how the individual is currently the primary target of prevention efforts, while the socio-ecological model proposes acting at the levels of the individual's environment, such as family and schools, and of society to protect the individual from culturally prevalent pressures, beliefs, and attitudes. No single intervention will solve this problem, which is rooted in deep societal influences. Multiple initiatives are necessary to transform the social environment that shapes gendered experiences of the body (Yager 2024), thereby empowering individuals who experience pressure and objectification to protect themselves from the cultural conditions that create BPD rather than internalizing these pressures, which can lead to the development of DEAB or other mental health problems.

Acknowledgments

We thank the Health Promotion Switzerland and the Geneva Department of Health and Mobility for supporting our MOOC's development and implementation.

References

Albertson, E.R., K.D. Neff and K.E. Dill-Shackleford. 2015. Self-compassion and body dissatisfaction in women: A randomized controlled trial of a brief meditation intervention. Mindfulness 6: 444–454.

Alleva, J.M., P.C. Diedrichs, E. Halliwell, C. Martijn, B.G. Stuijfzand, G. Treneman-Evans et al. 2018. A randomised-controlled trial investigating potential underlying mechanisms of a functionality-based approach to improving women's body image. Body Image. 25: 85–96.

Alleva, J.M., C. Martijn, G.J. Van Breukelen, A. Jansen and K. Karos. 2015. Expand your horizon: A programme that improves body image and reduces self-objectification by training women to focus on body functionality. Body Image 15: 81–89.

Avalos, L., T.L. Tylka and N. Wood-Barcalow. 2005. The body appreciation scale: Development and psychometric evaluation. Body Image 2: 285–297.

Becker, C., S. Bull, K. Schaumberg, A. Cauble and A. Franco. 2008. Effectiveness of peer-led eating disorders prevention: A replication trial. J. Consult. Clin. Psychol. 76: 347–354.

Becker, C., K. Middlemass, B. Taylor, C. Johnson and F. Gomez. 2017a. Food insecurity and eating disorder pathology. Int. J. Eat. Disord. 50: 1031–1040.

Becker, C., M. Perez, L.S. Kilpela, P.C. Diedrichs, E. Trujillo and E. Stice. 2017b. Engaging stakeholder communities as body image intervention partners: The body project as a case example. Eat. Behav. 25: 62–67.

Becker, C., C. Wilson, A. Williams, M. Kelly, L. McDaniel and J. Elmquist. 2010. Peer-facilitated cognitive dissonance versus healthy weight eating disorders prevention: A randomized comparison. Body Image 7: 280–288.

Becker, C.B., L. McDaniel, S. Bull, M. Powell and K. McIntyre. 2012. Can we reduce eating disorder risk factors in female college athletes? A randomized exploratory investigation of two peer-led interventions. Body Image 9: 31–42.

Bezerra, L.N. and M.T. Silva. 2017. A review of literature on the reasons that cause the high dropout rates in the moocs. Rev. Espacios 38: 11.

Braun, T.D., C.L. Park and A. Gorin. 2016. Self-compassion, body image, and disordered eating: A review of the literature. Body Image 17: 117–131.

Carrard, I. and S. Bucher Della Torre. 2021. A study protocol for a preliminary randomised controlled trial assessing the acceptability and effectiveness of two eating disorders prevention interventions in switzerland: The HEIDI BP-HW project. PLoS One 16: e0259796.

Carrard, I., S. Bucher Della Torre and M. Levine. 2019. [Promoting a positive body image in young people.]. Santé Publique. 31: 507–515. (La promotion d'une image corporelle positive chez les jeunes.)

Carrard, I., S. Cekic and S. Bucher Della Torre. 2023. A randomized controlled trial to evaluate the acceptability and effectiveness of two eating disorders prevention interventions: The HEIDI BP-HW project. BMC Womens Health 23: 446.

Cash, T.F. 2011. Cognitive-behavioral perspectives on body image. pp. 39–47. *In*: Cash, T.F. and L. Smolak (eds.). Body Image. A Handbook of Science, Practice, and Prevention 2nd ed. The Guilford Press.

Chapa, D.A.N., S.N. Johnson, B.N. Richson, K. Bjorlie, Y.Q. Won, S.V. Nelson et al. 2022. Eating-disorder psychopathology in female athletes and non-athletes: A meta-analysis. Int. J. Eat. Disord. 55: 861–885.

Cheng, Z.H., V.L. Perko, L. Fuller-Marashi, J.M. Gau and E. Stice. 2019. Ethnic differences in eating disorder prevalence, risk factors, and predictive effects of risk factors among young women. Eat. Behav. 32: 23–30.

Cox, A.E., S. Ullrich-French, C. Cook-Cottone, T.L. Tylka and D. Neumark-Sztainer. 2020. Examining the effects of mindfulness-based yoga instruction on positive embodiment and affective responses. Eat. Disord. 28: 458–475.

Festinger, L. 1957. A Theory of Cognitive Dissonance. Stanford University Press.

Fredrickson, B.L. and T.-A. Roberts. 1997. Objectification theory: Toward understanding women's lived experiences and mental health risks. Psychol. Women Quart. 21: 173–206.

Groesz, L.M., M.P. Levine and S.K. Murnen. 2002. The effect of experimental presentation of thin media images on body satisfaction: A meta-analytic review. Int. J. Eat. Disord. 31: 1–16.

Gualdi-Russo, E., N. Rinaldo and L. Zaccagni. 2022. Physical activity and body image perception in adolescents: A systematic review. Int. J. Environ. Res. Public Health. 19.

Guest, E., B. Costa, H. Williamson, J. Meyrick, E. Halliwell and D. Harcourt. 2019. The effectiveness of interventions aiming to promote positive body image in adults: A systematic review. Body Image 30: 10–25.

Halliwell, E. 2015. Future directions for positive body image research. Body Image 14: 177–189.

Irving, L.M. and D. Neumark-Sztainer. 2002. Integrating the prevention of eating disorders and obesity: Feasible or futile? Prev. Med. 34: 299–309.

Le, L.K., J.J. Barendregt, P. Hay and C. Mihalopoulos. 2017. Prevention of eating disorders: A systematic review and meta-analysis. Clin. Psychol. Rev. 53: 46–58.

Linardon, J., Z. McClure, T.L. Tylka and M. Fuller-Tyszkiewicz. 2022. Body appreciation and its psychological correlates: A systematic review and meta-analysis. Body Image 42: 287–296.

Mahon, C., D. Hamburger, Z. Yager, M. Almaraz, J. Mooney, T. Tran et al. 2023. Pilot feasibility and acceptability trial of be real's bodykind: A universal school-based body image intervention for adolescents. Body Image 47: 101636.

Mahon, C. and D. Hevey. 2023. Pilot trial of a self-compassion intervention to address adolescents' social media-related body image concerns. Clin. Child Psychol. Psychiatry 28: 307–322.

Matheson, E.L., J. Schneider, A. Tinoco, H. Silva-Breen, N.M. LaVoi and P.C. Diedrichs. 2023. How can we help you? A global investigation into girls' body image experiences in sport and intervention preferences. Body Image 46: 265–279.

Menzel, J.E. and M.P. Levine. 2011. Embodying experiences and the promotion of positive body image: The example of competitive athletics. pp. 163–186. *In*: Calogero, R.M., S. Tantleff-Dunn and J.K. Thompson (eds.). Self-objectification in Women: Causes, Consequences, and Counteractions. American Psychological Association.

Menzel, J.E., L.M. Schaefer, N.L. Burke, L.L. Mayhew, M.T. Brannick and J.K. Thompson. 2010. Appearance-related teasing, body dissatisfaction, and disordered eating: A meta-analysis. Body Image 7: 261–270.

Meyer, I.H. 2003. Prejudice, social stress, and mental health in lesbian, gay, and bisexual populations: Conceptual issues and research evidence. Psychol. Bull. 129: 674–697.

Mond, J., D. Mitchison, J. Latner, P. Hay, C. Owen and B. Rodgers. 2013. Quality of life impairment associated with body dissatisfaction in a general population sample of women. BMC Public Health. 13: 920.

Monthuy-Blanc, J., U. Faghihi, M.N.G. Fardshad, G. Corno, S. Iceta, M.-J. St-Pierre et al. 2023. When eating intuitively is not always a positive response: Using machine learning to better unravel eaters profiles. J. Clin. Med. 12: 5172.

Nagata, J.M., K.T. Ganson and S.B. Murray. 2020. Eating disorders in adolescent boys and young men: An update. Curr. Opin. Pediatr. 32: 476–481.

Nagata, J.M., E. Stuart, J.O. Hur, S. Panchal, P. Low, A.V. Chaphekar et al. 2024. Eating disorders in sexual and gender minority adolescents. Curr. Psychiatry Rep. 26: 340–350.

Neff, K.D. 2023. Self-compassion: Theory, method, research, and intervention. Annu. Rev. Psychol. 74: 193–218.

Neumark-Sztainer, D. 2005. Preventing the broad spectrum of weight-related problems: Working with parents to help teens achieve a healthy weight and a positive body image. J. Nutr. Educ. Behav. 37: S133–S139.

Neumark-Sztainer, D., A.W. Watts and S. Rydell. 2018. Yoga and body image: How do young adults practicing yoga describe its impact on their body image? Body Image 27: 156–168.

Piran, N. 2016. Embodied possibilities and disruptions: The emergence of the experience of embodiment construct from qualitative studies with girls and women. Body Image 18: 43–60.

Piran, N. 2018. Journeys of Embodiment at the Intersection of Body and Culture: The Developmental Theory of Embodiment. Academic Press, Elsevier.

Piran, N. and D. Neumark-Sztainer. 2020. Yoga and the experience of embodiment: A discussion of possible links. Eat. Disord. 28: 330–348.

Rupani, N., J. Miller, J.A. Renteria and K.E. Kaliebe. 2024. The impact of yoga on body image in adults: A systematic review of quantitative studies. Body Image 51: 101772.

Schaefer, L.M. and J.K. Thompson. 2018. Self-objectification and disordered eating: A meta-analysis. Int. J. Eat. Disord. 51: 483–502.

Sharpe, H., U. Naumann, J. Treasure and U. Schmidt. 2013. Is fat talking a causal risk factor for body dissatisfaction? A systematic review and meta-analysis. Int. J. Eat. Disord. 46: 643–652.

Stice, E. 2001. A prospective test of the dual-pathway model of bulimic pathology: Mediating effects of dieting and negative affect. J. Abnorm. Psychol. 110: 124–135.

Stice, E., A. Chase, S. Stormer and A. Appel. 2001. A randomized trial of a dissonance-based eating disorder prevention program. Int. J. Eat. Disord. 29: 247–262.

Stice, E., C.N. Marti, H. Shaw and P. Rohde. 2019. Meta-analytic review of dissonance-based eating disorder prevention programs: Intervention, participant, and facilitator features that predict larger effects. Clin. Psychol. Rev. 70: 91–107.

Stice, E., L. Mazotti, D. Weibel and W.S. Agras. 2000. Dissonance prevention program decreases thin-ideal internalization, body dissatisfaction, dieting, negative affect, and bulimic symptoms: A preliminary experiment. Int. J. Eat. Disord. 27: 206–217.

Stice, E., Z.A. Onipede and C.N. Marti. 2021a. A meta-analytic review of trials that tested whether eating disorder prevention programs prevent eating disorder onset. Clin. Psychol. Rev. 87: 102046.

Stice, E., Z.A. Onipede, H. Shaw, P. Rohde and J.M. Gau. 2021b. Effectiveness of the body project eating disorder prevention program for different racial and ethnic groups and an evaluation of the potential benefits of ethnic matching. J. Consult. Clin. Psychol. 89: 1007–1019.

Thompson, J.K., L.J. Heinberg, M.N. Altabe and S. Tantleff-Dunn. 1999. Exacting Beauty: Theory, Assessment and Treatment of Body Image Disturbance. American Psychological Association.

Tylka, T.L. 2011. Refinement of the tripartite influence model for men: Dual body image pathways to body change behaviors. Body Image 8: 199–207.

Tylka, T.L., R.F. Rodgers, R.M. Calogero, J.K. Thompson and J.A. Harriger. 2023. Integrating social media variables as predictors, mediators, and moderators within body image frameworks: Potential mechanisms of action to consider in future research. Body Image 44: 197–221.

Tylka, T.L. and N.L. Wood-Barcalow. 2015a. The body appreciation scale-2: Item refinement and psychometric evaluation. Body Image 12: 53–67.

Tylka, T.L. and N.L. Wood-Barcalow. 2015b. What is and what is not positive body image? Conceptual foundations and construct definition. Body Image 14: 118–129.

Watson, H.J., T. Joyce, E. French, V. Willan, R.T. Kane, E.E. Tanner-Smith et al. 2016. Prevention of eating disorders: A systematic review of randomized, controlled trials. Int. J. Eat. Disord. 49: 833–862.

Webb, J.B., C.B. Rogers, L. Etzel and M.P. Padro. 2018. "Mom, quit fat talking—i'm trying to eat (mindfully) here!": Evaluating a sociocultural model of family fat talk, positive body image, and mindful eating in college women. Appetite 126: 169–175.

Wilksch, S.M. and T.D. Wade. 2009. Reduction of shape and weight concern in young adolescents: A 30-month controlled evaluation of a media literacy program. J. Am. Acad. Child Adolesc. Psychiatry 48: 652–661.

Yager, Z., P.C. Diedrichs, L.A. Ricciardelli and E. Halliwell. 2013. What works in secondary schools? A systematic review of classroom-based body image programs. Body Image 10: 271–281.

Yager, Z. 2024. Something, everything, and anything more than nothing: Stories of school-based prevention of body image concerns and eating disorders in young people. Eat. Disord. 32: 727–745.

Chapter 9

Body Experience in Eating Disorders

Clinical Guidelines

Michel Probst

INTRODUCTION

In severe dysfunctional eating attitudes and behaviours (DEAB) as eating disorders, body perception disturbances (BPD) are an important aspect highlighted in diagnostic criteria. Bruch (1962) was the pioneer in describing "the perceptual and conceptual" disturbances present in anorexia nervosa, delineating (1) BP disturbances reaching delusional proportions, (2) difficulties in perceiving internal sensations like hunger, satiety, or affective states accurately, and (3) a pervasive sense of personal ineffectiveness. Subsequently, she underscored the significance of addressing dysfunctional body perception a key-component in treating DEAB effectively (Bruch 1973). Since Bruch's seminal work, a body of literature examining BPD in DEAB has emerged over the past 60 years. The prognostic significance of BP was later corroborated (Danielsen and Ro 2012, Exterkate et al. 2009, McLean and Paxton 2019). Given its prognostic importance, addressing negative body attitudes should be prioritized in treating this disorder. The question then becomes: how? This chapter provides practical clinical guidelines for addressing BPD in DEAB based on clinical and research findings. The content draws from 35 years of clinical and research experience as a physiotherapist/body-oriented therapist in an eating disorder unit in Belgium.

Treuveld 8, B-3080 Tervuren, Belgium.
Email: Michel.probst@kuleuven.be

DOI: 10.1201/9781032718125-11

1. Conceptual framework

The notion of body image is a widely employed concept across various disciplines such as psychiatry, psychology, and the social sciences. The interpretation varies depending on the specific field of study. The origins of the concept of body image, in this chapter called more broadly body perception (BP), can be traced back to neurology, as discussed by Head and Gerstman, has been a subject of psychoanalytic thought (e.g., by Reich and Schilder), phenomenological inquiry (e.g., Merleau Ponty), and other philosophical reflections (e.g., Sartre, Spinoza, Kant), and has undergone extensive psychological research (e.g., Kolb, Cash). Initially, BP was conceived as a singular construct. Schilder (1950) introduced BP as the mental representation of one's body. Research data unequivocally suggests that the concept of BP has evolved into a more multidimensional construct, incorporating at least three aspects: neurophysiological, psychological, and behavioural dimensions (Cash 2004). The neurophysiological aspect involves various perceptual experiences including visual spatial perceptions, sensory judgments, physical sensations, body awareness, body recognition, physical appearance, and body size and shape. The psychological aspect encompasses cognitive processes such as thought patterns and styles, as well as subjective experiences like feelings, emotions, affect, and mood. The behavioural component, for instance avoidance and checking behaviour, may be a consequence of both neurophysiological and psychological aspects (Cash and Smolak 2011, Probst et al. 2013, Probst and Diedens 2018). Body perception is subjective, varies from person to person, and can be influenced by various factors, including societal standards of beauty, cultural norms, media representation, personal experiences, and interactions with others. Positive BP involves feeling comfortable and confident in one's own body, accepting its natural shape, size, and imperfections, having positive self-esteem and having good mental health. On the other hand, negative BP can lead to dissatisfaction, low self-esteem, and even mental health issues such as DEAB or depression (see Table 1).

In summary, BP image embodies a person's "inner view" of their body: their emotions, perceptions, thoughts, and beliefs about their body that influence their behaviours toward it (Cash 2004). This term encompasses different aspects, including physical appearance, embodiment (how a person uses their body to engage with the world), and also emphasizes (and appreciates) body functionality. To illustrate the complexity of the concept of BP, an interesting task is offered (Table 2).

Table 1. A more concrete example of positive versus negative vicious circle of body perception.

	Positive vicious circle	**Negative vicious circle**
Body perception	"I am comfortable with my appearance and understand that one's looks do not determine their worth or abilities"	"I am dissatisfied with my appearance"
Self-esteem	"I respect myself"	"I doubt my adequacy"
Mental health	"It's okay if things aren't always perfect"	"If things aren't perfect, it's a complete disaster"

Table 2. *"People don't believe what they see, they see what they believe"*

The "waist circumference estimation with a rope" exercise explores how individuals perceive their own bodies through a series of estimation tasks. Using a 120 cm rope, they estimate:

- A neutral object
- Their own waist
- Another person's waist
- Their ideal waist size
- They then measure in standing position their actual waist using the rope.

Estimates are compared with actual measurements to explore perception rather than accuracy.

Key clinical findings include:

- Neutral objects are estimated accurately
- The own waist is overestimated
- The estimation of other persons are perceived accurately
- Ideal waist is often larger than actual
- Actual measurements often surprise participants

Conclusion: Self-perception is frequently distorted by unconscious assumptions and based on flawed assumptions (Probst and Diedens 2018).

2. Empirical and clinical support

2.1 Clinical manifestations of body perception in DEAB

Patients with DEAB often exhibit unrealistic perceptions of their body size, commonly viewing themselves as overweight. Research indicates a notable contrast between how they perceive their own bodies and how they perceive others'. Despite accurately estimating the body size of fellow patients, they fail to recognize similar characteristics in themselves, sometimes even perceiving themselves as larger or less attractive. This overestimation may be localized to specific body parts, such as the stomach or thighs. The cognitive and affective components of BP disturbance involve extreme forms of self-criticism or occasionally exaggerated admiration for certain body parts. Patients express dissatisfaction with body areas such as hips, thighs, abdomen, and legs, often perceiving them as ugly or fat. Individuals with DEAB commonly harbor a fear of unattractiveness and are preoccupied with perceived defects in particular body parts. Patients with anorexia nervosa simultaneously deny the abnormalities of their emaciated bodies. This disconnection between perception and reality often leads to a BPD, with some individuals experiencing a sense of detachment or depersonalization from their bodies. Paradoxically, some may even take pride in their emaciated appearance. The pursuit of an unrealistic ideal, characterized by extreme thinness, is prevalent among individuals with DEAB. Behavioural manifestations of BPD include avoidance behaviours such as avoiding mirrors, social activities, triggering situations, and physical intimacy, as well as engaging in excessive and compulsive physical activities. Patients may establish rigid rules or standards regarding their bodies, such as insisting on visible ribs or thighs not touching when standing. Poor BP is associated with overall low self-esteem in early adolescence, encompassing physical, social, and academic domains. Individuals with DEAB often lack confidence in their bodies, feel physically insecure, and experience negative self-worth. They frequently have conflicting perspectives regarding their appearance, internalizing societal beauty standards, and projecting inaccurate perceptions onto others. Additionally, they may hold unrealistic beliefs regarding the effects of food intake, dieting, or exercise on their body structure. Abnormal eating behaviors lead to disturbances in gastric motility. These physiological reactions to eating may be misinterpreted by patients with DEAB as discomfort, fat, or swelling, which exacerbate psychological distress surrounding food, weight, and appearance.

2.2 Assessment of body perception

BP assessment involves evaluating an individual's perception and feelings about their own body. The literature offers various methods and tools. The most commonly used are self-report questionnaires and interviews. Because patients have to repeat their story over and over again to the point of annoyance, two alternative options are offered, which are presented in Tables 3 and 4.

Table 3. *"My Hand, My Life Guide" and "Discover Yourself".*

During an initial consultation, patients are asked to express their viewpoints based on their hand: • The thumb represents the talents, competences, skills, and positive characteristics. • The index finger indicates the direction in which the subject aspires to go with their life and what they want to achieve. • The middle finger symbolizes irritations or frustrations. • The ring finger signifies principles, dedication, and what is important in their lives. • The little finger reflects insecurities. • The high five corresponds to what they realize or achieve in their lives.

Table 4. Discover Yourself - "Crossing the Threshold".

"Crossing the Threshold" In this exercise, the patient stands on one side of the room, which is divided into five areas representing different percentages (0% –25% –50% –75% –100%). A series of general, non-binding statements, followed by more personal ones, are provided. The patient responds by standing on the appropriate line corresponding to their answer, crossing the line if necessary. Statements may include: • Sometimes singing in the shower. • Enjoying challenges. • Feeling dissatisfied with their body or a part of their body. • Hiding their body.

Many questionnaires are available to assess the different components of BP, which might be included in a BP assessment: assessing the level of dissatisfaction with one's body, such as overall appearance, weight, shape, and specific body parts, determining how accurately individuals perceive their own body size, and shape, compared to their actual physical characteristics. Other important topics are evaluating emotional responses (feelings of happiness, sadness, anxiety shame), examining thoughts and beliefs about one's body, observing checking and avoidance behaviours as well as the physical activity levels. Assessing the impact of social interactions, peer comparisons, media exposure, and cultural influences and identifying signs of other mental health conditions are also relevant (Sanchez et al. 2023).

2.3 Therapeutic approaches

Currently, literature predominantly reveals three therapeutic approaches—verbal, non-verbal, or mixed therapies—largely based on cognitive behavioural therapy that focus on BP and more precisely the bodily experience within therapeutic contexts: (1) cognitive-behavioural therapy; (2) body-oriented therapy (Probst and Maïano 2020a, b, Probst and Maïano 2022). Body-oriented therapy is extensively discussed in the third part of this chapter.

Cognitive-behavioural therapy (CBT). It has become integral in treating DEAB and BP issues. It aims to alter dysfunctional cognitions. Disturbed BP stem from irrational thoughts, unrealistic expectations, and misinterpretations.

The objective of this therapy is to challenge these interpretations through cognitive restructuring. This involves, for instance, diminishing the overemphasis on weight and physical appearance while highlighting alternative lifestyles. In this therapy, professionals assist individuals with DEAB in identifying dysfunctional cognitions, breaking them down, and seeking counterarguments and alternative perspectives (examples are provided in Tables 5 and 6). Virtual reality exposure therapy is a CBT-based approach which could be also useful (see Chapter 3).

Table 5. Examples of Negative Thinking and Alternative Perspectives.

Negative Thought Example: "My stomach is fat." Alternative Thinking Examples: "My stomach isn't bloated; perhaps I'm mistaken." "My weight is low, so my stomach can't be fat." "My dress size is small, so I can't have a bloated stomach." "Others have never commented on my belly." "Maybe I'm overly critical about my appearance."

Table 6. Overview of the distorted strategies, cognitive errors related to BP (adapted form Cash and Pruzinky 1995).

Concept	Explanation
Beauty or beast	Dichotomous thinking: Seeing things as either black or white, attractive or ugly.
Unreal ideal	Comparing ourselves against unrealistic standards leading to feelings of despair and self-devaluation.
Unfair to compare	Comparing ourselves to others, which is unfair and can lead to negative self-perception.
Magnifying glass	Selective attention, focusing disproportionately on flaws or imperfections.
Blind mind	Minimizing positive characteristics and focusing solely on perceived shortcomings.
Ugly by association	Overgeneralizing discontent, engaging in biased fault-finding with various aspects of one's appearance.
Blame game	Arbitrarily inferring that one's appearance caused an unwanted event or outcome.
Mind misreading	Projecting negative BP thoughts onto others, assuming what they must think.
Misfortune telling	Believing that one's looks will lead to specific negative consequences in the future.
Beauty bound	Concluding that one's appearance limits or prevents participation in certain activities.
Feeling ugly	Emotional reasoning that feeling ugly confirms one's actual appearance.
Moody mirror	Generalizing negative thoughts and moods from non-appearance events to body experience.

3. Applications to the social cultural context

Body-oriented therapy represents a unique, holistic mixed therapy approach, incorporating both verbal and non-verbal experiences to connect individuals with DEAB to their bodies and inner selves. It acknowledges that emotional distress often manifests physically. Its primary goal is to enhance well-being, autonomy, and empowerment by fostering sensory, bodily, and movement awareness, as well as physical activity and exercise in all their dimensions, bridging physical and mental aspects. This approach is heavily influenced by CBT and acknowledges that emotional distress often manifests physically. Body-oriented therapy aims to understand one's own patterns of functioning, identify and address needs, become aware of and develop potential and resources, learn to experience emotions, build or rebuild self-confidence, and explore new possibilities in life and relationships. It utilizes three types of techniques: (1) psychosensory techniques, involving introspective exploration of one's senses (e.g., relaxation, massage, breathing exercises, mirror exercises, etc.); (2) expressive techniques, emphasizing gestures and movements to express internal content externally (e.g., dance, theatrical techniques like mime and role play, spontaneous play, etc.); and (3) perceptual-motor techniques, focusing on dynamics and movement production (e.g., yoga, tai chi Chuan, physical and sporting activities). The verbal aspect of body-oriented therapy entails expressing thoughts and emotions related to the exercises offered, in a respectful manner, in the here and now. Body-oriented therapy emerges as a potent clinical complement to standard treatments, aimed at restoring a realistic self-concept.

3.1 Body-oriented treatment in DEAB

Body-oriented therapy for patients with DEAB focuses on the body and movement, aiming to transform distorted BP into a more positive and realistic attitude through confrontation and understanding of the body. This therapy involves interventions centred around the body, movement, and senses, with the goal of fostering a meaningful and positive personal identity. The diversity of exercises, encompassing various aspects including physical, cognitive, affective, and social elements, serves as a natural and powerful strategy for improving BP. The approach comprises three levels:

- The physical health-related approach aims to enhance the overall physical health and functioning of individuals with DEAB.
- The psycho-social related approach emphasizes the obtaining of mental and physical skills related to bodily movement. Fostering personal growth aids in improving individuals' capacity to operate autonomously within society.
- The psychotherapeutic related approach utilizes the motor domain to improve the social and affective functioning of individuals. Therapists create an environment conducive to initiating and facilitating a process in the patient, employing specific methods to help patients access their inner world, step out of their comfort zones, and explore new experiences, thoughts (obsession, perfectionism, worrying) and many emotions (depressive feelings, fear, guilt,

anger, stress, feelings of unease, estrangement, and dissatisfaction) (Probst and Diedens 2018).

The foundation of this approach lies in the non-academic self-concept of the transtheoretical theory, which includes the "Physical self-concept," "Psychological self-concept," and "Social self-concept" (Marsh and Shavelson 1985). Concrete goals of body-oriented therapy include rediscovering the body, reducing psychological and physical tension through relaxation techniques, enhancing biopsychosocial well-being, increasing awareness of bodily sensations, improving psychological flexibility, understanding bodily communication, modifying distorted BP, and cultivating self-acceptance and recognition of uniqueness.

To achieve these goals, various interventions are employed, including posture and postural awareness, relaxation techniques, breathing exercises, touch based activities, interventions focused on self-perception, sensory awareness, and physical activities such as exercise and sports, and guided imagery exercise. These interventions are designed to be concrete and simple, integrating seamlessly into daily life. The proposed bodily activities aim to encourage patients with severe DEAB to engage in new experiences, develop a gentle and respectful attitude toward their bodies, and find enjoyment in being in their bodies.

Posture interventions. Proper posture and postural awareness have been shown to alleviate physical symptoms and enhance self-esteem. Postural abnormalities resulting from weakened muscles can lead to musculoskeletal compensations such as scoliosis and low back pain.

Relaxation techniques. Relaxation techniques have demonstrated effectiveness in reducing perceived stress and anxiety levels, as well as salivary cortisol levels. Achieving a harmonious balance between sympathetic and parasympathetic nervous system activities is crucial. Techniques such as progressive relaxation, autogenic training, yoga, and biofeedback exercises can stimulate the parasympathetic nervous system, thereby mitigating stress responses (Mayer et al. 2017). Breathing exercises, focusing on reducing breathing frequency, emphasizing abdominal breathing, and prolonging exhalation, aim to enhance diaphragmatic breathing and body awareness. Although pulmonary complications related to breathlessness or rapid breathing have not been extensively studied (Nitsch et al. 2023).

Touch-based exercises. Touch-based exercises, such as massage (including both relaxing and active techniques applied to the back and legs with or without instruments, along with passive limb mobilization) or somatic experiencing, can help individuals reconnect with their bodies in a safe and nurturing environment. By fostering a sense of safety and embodiment, touch-based therapies can support individuals in raising their well-being, alleviating pain, reducing anxiety, releasing tension, improving body awareness, and enhancing self-esteem. Therapists have to take into account that many patients with DEAB have a fear of touch, proximity, and closeness. The therapist is responsible for maintaining the delicate balance between positive and negative reactions.

Interventions targeting self-perceptions. Interventions targeting self-perception aim to enhance awareness of one's bodily appearance through mirror exercises and body estimation techniques (Griffen et al. 2018, Ormondi and Freysteinson 2021, Probst et al. 2008). Mirrors play a significant role in the lives of individuals with DEAB, akin to the importance of scales in measuring weight. Scientific and clinical evidence supports the use of mirror exercises as an effective treatment for negative BP. Mirror exercises aim to address BP concerns, change the way individuals use mirrors, and manage associated emotions constructively. Regular mirror exposure promotes habituation, reducing body dissatisfaction and anxiety. With mirror exercises, the avoidance is broken, and the disgust will disappear through habituation. This habituation process encourages more appropriate behaviour and, in some cases, feelings of success. During the exercise, the subject is instructed to observe and describe their body in a neutral, objective, respectful, mild, and curious manner, from head to toe, while a therapist is present. Various styles of mirror exercises are described in the literature. Mirrors can be used effectively when combined with visualization, CBT, and mindfulness-based approaches. Research suggests that mirror exposure increases BP satisfaction, reduces BP avoidance and checking behaviours, and improves awareness of body-related cognitive errors. Patients in inpatient treatment programs often value mirror exercises highly, with some considering them essential components of the treatment program.

Interventions targeting body awareness. Fogel (2009) cited body awareness as "the ability to pay attention to ourselves to feel our sensations and movements online, along with the motivational and emotional feelings that accompany them in the present moment, without the mediating influence of judgmental thoughts". Sensory, body, and movement awareness interventions aim to explore the body through sensory experiences, tactile awareness, movement exploration, and internal sensory experiences (e.g., body journey). Numerous exercises inspired by practices such as Qi Gong, Tai Chi, Pilates, mindfulness (the body scanning), and Feldenkrais are available. The competition between different methods often aims to demonstrate the superiority of a particular approach; however, studies have shown minimal differences in treatment outcomes. It is crucial for therapists to exercise caution in adopting techniques, as the positive effects of awareness may be exaggerated, and not all studies are equally reliable (Vancampfort et al. 2023a, b, Olsen et al. 2023). Similarly, the hype surrounding mindfulness should be critically evaluated (Kral et al. 2022, Van Dam et al. 2018). Despite academic discussions, clinical practice indicates that enhancing bodily awareness enables patients to challenge negative assumptions about their bodies and promotes increased bodily acceptance. Given the absence of a superior treatment approach, considering the patient's preferences is crucial for treatment success.

Physical activities. In terms of physical activities, providing supervised sessions including fitness, resistance and strength exercises, aerobic exercises, calisthenics, Pilates, sports, and gymnastics is essential. However, the role of physical activity in the treatment of DEAB remains controversial, as it may potentially interfere with treatment goals. Current clinical experience and research suggest that restricting physical activity may not be advisable unless there are medical or therapeutic reasons. Guided, supervised, and adapted physical activity is considered an important therapeutic intervention without significant side effects. In some cases, addressing the absence of physical activity itself can be a therapeutic intervention (Probst 2018, Probst et al. 2020, Mathisen et al. 2023). The practice of adapted and controlled physical activities reduces the risk of a hidden practice and makes it possible to prevent excessive physical activity and to canalize the urge to be physically active. It offers the patient the feeling that the goal of the treatment is not only to gain weight. Adapted physical activities positively influence the physical and psychological well-being of the person suffering from DEAB and allow people with DEAB to learn how to exercise responsibly and safely for their health.

Guided imagery. Guided imagery is a widely employed and potent therapeutic intervention, backed by research, particularly beneficial for individuals facing challenges in articulating their inner experiences solely through verbal communication (Krau 2020). By harnessing the power of mental imagery, guided imagery activates the mind-body connection, thereby augmenting an individual's overall sense of well-being while simultaneously mitigating stress and anxiety levels. One example presented in Table 7 illustrates the role of guided imagery.

In the "Utopia" guided imagery exercise, the concept of "dream body" can be addressed. The concept of a "dream body" may reflect societal standards of beauty and perfection, which can be unrealistic and harmful. Exploring the motivations behind desiring a different body can uncover deeper insecurities and psychological issues. Discussing alternative ways to achieve desired benefits without changing the body can promote self-acceptance and holistic well-being. Recognizing and challenging societal norms and pressures related to BP can foster a healthier relationship with one's own body. Open communication and support from partners or trusted individuals can facilitate constructive dialogue and reflection on BP issues.

Expressive writing. Expressive writing, defined as writing about thoughts and feelings related to personally stressful or traumatic experiences, is applicable to individuals with DEAB. Writing a letter enables reflection without the need for verbal communication, providing a safe and private setting for expressing emotions. It helps individuals who struggle with verbal expression confront their distressing emotions and personal experiences. Expressive writing can facilitate cognitive change and flexibility, potentially impacting rigid thinking styles. A systematic review (Ramsey-Wade et al. 2020) suggests that expressive writing improves quantitative outcomes such as self-esteem, BP, mood, and disordered eating. Qualitative analysis of 428 letters from females with DEAB (between 16 and 35 years old) reveals various attitudes towards their bodies, ranging from negative to positive actions, beliefs, feelings, and thoughts. Many letters initially express negative emotions but transition to a more positive perspective, focusing on topics such as self-care, hope, self-respect, acceptance, gratitude, and intrinsic motivation for recovery (VDT unpublished data). An example of expressive writing is provided in Table 8.

Table 7. Utopia: going to buy a new body!

The goal of this guided imagery exercise "Utopia" is to help patients gain insight into their own thoughts and to open the way for more introspection.
The exercise consists of five steps. The subject is invited to write their thoughts and feelings step by step.
Step 1: Identifying the ideal body: Imagine that you could go to a store to buy a "dream body". What would this dream body look like?
Step 2: Comparing the ideal body and the actual body: To what extent does this dream body differ from the actual body?
Step 3: Reflecting on the ideal body: To what extent are those differences important for you? How does this body look different than yours?
Step 4: Discussing the advantages of the dream body: What would be the benefits of this new body? How important are these benefits?
Step 5: Searching for alternatives: Instead of thinking about what must or should change, think of other ways to get these same benefits without changing your body.

Table 8. Expressive Writing – An old school Letter to Your Body.

The idea of writing a letter to one's own body originates in narrative therapy. It is a guided imagery exercise where the subject writes a letter to their body or a specific body part, as they would to a family member. This task allows individuals to express feelings and thoughts in a non-verbal manner. In a later phase, they may be asked to respond to the letter from the body or body part.

Psychoeducation. Psychoeducation points out the process of providing education and information to patients (and their family members) on topics related to the body, serving as vital aspect of the therapy program. This approach assists individuals in taking ownership of their health and body. Incorporating a psychoeducation component on bodily functions becomes crucial. For example, explaining the functioning of the respiratory system during breathing exercises, clarifying the function of body fat highlighting that weight gain is not synonymous with feeling "fat" or "bloated", but rather relates to health, attractiveness, expressiveness, and new life experience they may not have encountered before. Other pertinent topics encompass basic anatomy and physiology, osteoporosis, body and sensory awareness, discerning bodily sensation and states, managing stress, anxiety, developing coping strategies, distinguishing healthy and maladaptive or dysfunctional physical activity, and comprehending the impact of media on socio-cultural ideals.

Further considerations. In addition, the therapist must help strengthen internal and avoid external control. Listen to the patient's story, explore the BP and self-esteem, and guide the subject in discovering positive qualities and becoming aware of the body. Recognize and correct cognitive errors or irrational thoughts and encourage a dialogue with their body. This approach is inspired by CBT and also includes elements of therapeutic support and education on the themes of maladaptive ideas concerning the functioning of the body and physical activity, essential physiological needs, the process of empowerment to act (or empowerment) and the development of action strategies focused on relapse prevention. It goes without saying that during these activities, the person with DEAB will encounter inadequate cognitive and psychological processes (for example, attention, interpretation and selective remembering; overestimation of threats and consequences; comparison, etc.) and its main cognitive distortions related to a negative BP (e.g., social comparison, emotional or sensory reasoning, all-or-nothing thinking, etc.).

Individual versus group approach. Both individual and group approaches have advantages and disadvantages. On one hand, individual therapy is characterized by personalized attention, greater confidentiality, flexibility, a higher focus on individual goals, and likely a deeper exploration. On the other hand, a group approach offers social support, a diversity of perspectives, skill-building opportunities, normalization, cost-effectiveness. Patients can learn from each other in a group setting. To illustrate two group exercises related to BP are presented in Tables 9 and 10.

Table 9. "*I Don't need Attention*".

The focus lies in exploring self-awareness in relation to others. Body awareness, self-esteem, coping with stress, being seen, and non-verbal communication are important aspects. Participants sit close to each other in a circle. They are invited one by one to enter the middle of the group without speaking for sixty seconds. It is up to the participant to decide what to do during their turn. The therapist observes and allows both the participant and group members to express their experiences and feelings.

Table 10. The labyrinth; "Life's Risks".

This exercise focuses on coping with pressure, fear of failure, anxiety, and stress, by employing problem-solving strategies, cognition, and memory. Participants must navigate an unknown route marked out in advance by the therapist on a board divided into 100 equal squares. The route starts on one side and ends on the other. Only one person can be in the labyrinth at a time. After each step, the player receives either a message to continue or that they've made a wrong move. After two wrong steps, the player must backtrack. The game ends when all group members reach the other side. Various adaptations are possible. This exercise not only addresses cognitive and emotional aspects but also has a symbolic dimension open for discussion during evaluation. Life can be likened to a labyrinth; sometimes, risks must be taken. Making decisions is often easier when viewed from the outside of a problem. Accepting help and facing problems together can make problem-solving easier. Listening to others and believing in oneself are essential. Trying to solve problems alone often leads to repeated mistakes.

Some therapeutic guidelines. Patients are empowered to take responsibility, becoming the architects of their therapeutic journey. Therefore, it's crucial to consider the individual preferences of individuals with DEAB. By acknowledging and respecting their uniqueness unconditionally, feelings of self-worth can be elevated. Body oriented therapy exercises aren't inherently therapeutic in themselves. It is not one specific exercise that causes a positive effect, but the combination of exercise and the patient's experience and perception play a central role. Therapy unfolds gradually, step by step, with small increments. Through repeated exposure to body-oriented situations enable patients to explore changing attitudes during exercises and become accustomed to these changes (Probst et al. 1995). The core message underlying all exercises and discussions is self-respect, fostering a sense of love and appreciation for one's body. During sessions, patients should recognize that outward appearance isn't the sole determinant of value; other personal aspects hold equal importance in life. The experiences and ideas elaborated during body-oriented therapy are a valuable clinical addition to available treatments. Patients are continuously confronted with their bodies, often after years of struggle and self-loathing. It is essential to provide a secure and well-structured therapeutic framework, respecting privacy and maintaining transparent communication about the content in which the therapist constantly provides information about who, what, why, and how are explained. Clear explanations of objectives, procedures, and expectations, ensuring everyone understands their roles, are imperative. During body-oriented interventions, patients gain access to alternative experiences, fostering a safe environment for emotional exploration and behavioural development. Exercises should ideally be designed for application outside therapy sessions, either individually or with a partner, facilitating continuity and integration of learning.

Throughout body-oriented interventions, an alternative frame of experience becomes available. The possibility experiencing feelings in a safe environment allows patients to connect with their inner world and develop behaviours they might not have otherwise. Whenever possible, exercises should be designed for application outside therapy session, either individually or with a partner. This can be successfully achieved through breathing exercises, relaxation training, mirror exercises, and coping strategies. The therapist opts for encouraging rather than interfering, offering support rather than advice, maintaining clear boundaries rather than none, scheduling clear appointments rather than vague ones, and maintaining a proper distance rather than excessive proximity.

3.2 Body-oriented therapy: does it help?

Research on the effectiveness of body-oriented therapy for DEAB is still ongoing. Today, both quantitative and qualitative research are limited. Body-oriented therapy tends to improve physical and mental capacity and therefore increase quality of life (Vancampfort et al. 2014a, b, c, d). Follow-up data shows that patients with DEAB still tend to have a negative BP compared to non-clinical subjects. However, long-term follow-ups indicate improvement in BP after six months, with consistency thereafter (Probst et al. 1999). More specific, objective data are required. Is it reasonable to suppose "normalization"? Altering body attitudes is a gradual process that requires time. Numerous individuals with DEAB will preserve a special affinity with their bodies throughout their lives (Probst et al. 1999, Geerdens et al. 2012).

Based on qualitative studies assessing patients' opinions and experiences regarding the recovery process and clinical experience, there is evidence to suggest that body-oriented therapy provides valuable insights.

Some patient statements include:

- "Body-oriented therapy has helped me tremendously."
- "I want to thank the body-oriented therapist for his guidance. He taught me a lot and encouraged me to see myself differently."
- "Although body-oriented therapy wasn't always easy, I learned a lot from it."
- "I feel more confident and willing to take risks thanks to body-oriented therapy. I appreciate the therapist's patience and interest in me."
- "Therapy was challenging at times, but it helped me reach a point of self-acceptance."
- "The therapy sessions were confronting, but they helped me accept myself more fully."
- "I struggled with self-reflection, but therapy helped me overcome it."
- "The therapy wasn't always easy, but the therapist's support made it worthwhile. I now view my body differently."

These statements align with previous research (Probst 2007) but should be interpreted carefully. They were collected during discharge interviews, in the therapist's presence, which might influence responses due to the "hello-goodbye effect." Supplementing qualitative remarks with objective evaluations and observations from other team members provides a clearer picture of the value of body-oriented therapy for certain patients. However, the effectiveness of therapy can vary depending on individual factors (type and severity, the therapist's expertise, and the patient's willingness to engage in the therapeutic process). Body-oriented therapy is perceived as effective in improving self-awareness, both physically and mentally. It fosters a closer connection with one's body, enhances BP and self-esteem, and helps in recognizing distorted thinking patterns. The role of the therapist, peer support, individual motivation, openness, and time are considered essential elements of body-oriented therapy. These results should be further investigated with larger sample sizes.

Conclusion

Overall, body-oriented therapy offers a holistic approach to treating DEAB, recognizing the interconnectedness of the mind, body, and emotions. Body-oriented therapy for weight, eating, and trauma-related disorders focuses on facilitating dialogue between patients and their bodies rather than providing a solution. Body-oriented therapy is often used as a complementary or adjunctive approach rather than a standalone treatment. By incorporating bodily techniques into treatment, the subjects become aware of different physical sensations (increasing body awareness), interpret these signals without negative thoughts and concomitant feelings (decreasing catastrophizing) and use this information from the body to act accordingly (increasing self-efficacy). The subjects are empowered to cultivate a deeper sense of self-awareness, self-compassion, and acceptance, laying the foundation for lasting recovery and a more harmonious relationship with food and their bodies. Through a combination of bodily oriented techniques and traditional psychotherapy modalities, individuals are supported in processing past experiences, challenging negative beliefs, and developing healthier coping mechanisms. While body-oriented therapy may be helpful for some individuals, it may not be as effective for others, depending on their unique needs and circumstances. Therefore, a qualified therapist, a broad assessment, and a tailored approach to meet the specific preferences of the individual are necessary conditions for an optimal outcome.

References

Bruch, H. 1962. Perceptual and conceptual disturbances in anorexia nervosa. Psychol. Med. 24: 187–194.

Cash, T. and T. Pruzinksy. 1990. Body Images. Development, Deviance and Change. Guilford, New York.

Cash, T. 1995. What Do You See When You Look in the Mirror? Helping Yourself to a Positive BP. Bantam Books, New York.

Cash, T. 2004. Editorial Body Image: past, present, and future. Body Image 1–5.

Cash, T. and L. Smolak. 2011. Body Image. A Handbook of Science, Practice and Prevention. Guilford, New York.

Danielsen, M. and Ø Rø. 2012. Changes in body image during inpatient treatment for eating disorders predict outcome. Eat. Disord. 20: 261–275.

Exterkate, C.C., P. Vriesendorp and C. De Jong. 2009. Body attitudes in patients with eating disorders at presentation and completion of intensive outpatient day treatment. Eat. Behav. 10: 16–21.

Fogel, A. 2013. Body Sense: The Science and Practice of Embodied Self-Awareness. W. W. Norto, New York.

Geerdens, C., J. Vanderlinden, G. Pieters, A. De Herdt and M. Probst. 2012. Missing data in long-term follow-up of patients with eating disorders using the Body Attitude Test. European Eat. Disord. Rev. 21: 224–229.

Griffen, T.C., E. Naumann and T. Hildebrandt. 2018. Mirror exposure therapy for Body image disturbances and eating disorders: A review. Clin. Psychol. Rev. 65: 163–174.

Keel, P., D. Dorer, D. Franko, S. Jackson and D. Herzog. 2005. Postremission predictors of relapse in women with eating disorders. Am. J. Psychiat. 162: 2263–2268.

Kral, T., K. Davis, C. Korponay, M. Hirshberg, R. Hoel, L. Tello et al. 2022. Absence of structural brain changes from mindfulness-based stress reduction: two combined randomize controlled trials. Sci. Adv. 20: 8.

Krau, S. 2020. The multiple uses of guided imagery. Nurs. Clin. North. Am. 55: 467–474.

Marsh, H.W. and R. Shavelson. 1985. Self-concept: its multifaceted hierarchical structure. Educ. Psychol. 20: 107–123.

Mathisen, T., P. Hay and S. Bratland-Sanda. 2023. How to address physical activity and exercise during treatment from eating disorders: a scoping review. Curr. Opin. Psychiatr. 36: 427–437.

Mayer, G., M. Arzt, B. Braumann, J. Ficker, I. Fietze, H. Frohnhofen et al. 2017. Sleep-related breathing disorders in adults. Somnologie 21: 290–301.

McLean, S. and S. Paxton. 2019. Body image in the context of eating disorders. Psychiat. clin. 42: 145–156.

Nitsch, A., M. Kearns and P. Mehler. 2023. Pulmonary complications of eating disorders: a literature review. J. Eat. Disord. 11: 12.

O'Dea, J.A. 2012. Body image and self-esteem. pp. 141–147. *In*: Cash, T.F. (ed.). Encyclopedia of Body Image and Human Appearance. Elsevier Academic Press, New York.

Olsen, A., D. Catalan-Matamoros, L. Danielsson, L. Hedlund and A. Gyllensten. 2023. Comment to efficacy of basic body awareness therapy on functional outcomes: A systematic review and meta-analysis of randomized controlled trials. Physiother. Res. Int. 28: e1994.

Ormondi, H. and W. Freysteinson. 2022. The mirror and obesity: a systematic review on the effects of mirror exposure on behaviour and obese individuals. J. Clin. Nurs. 31: 2367–2376.

Probst, M., W. Vandereycken, H. Van Coppenolle and G. Pieters. 1999. Body experience in eating disorders before and after treatment: a follow-up study. Eur. Psychiat. 14: 333–340.

Probst, M. 2007. Onderzoek in de psychomotorische therapie: de perceptie van de psychomotorische therapie door patiënten met eetstoornissen [Perception of psychomotor therapy in patients with eating disorders]. pp. 133–151. *In*: Simons, J. (ed.). Actuele themata uit de psychomotorische therapie. Acco, Leuven.

Probst, M., G. Pieters, D. Vancampfort and J. Vanderlinden. 2008. Body experience and mirror behaviour in female eating disorders patients and non-clinical subjects. Psihologijske Teme [Psychological Topics]. 17: 335–348.

Probst, M., M. Majeweski, M. Albertsen, D. Catalan-Matamoros, M. Danielsen, A. De Herdt et al. 2013. Physiotherapy for patients with anorexia nervosa. Adv. Eat. Disord. 1: 224–238.

Probst, M. and J. Diedens. 2018. The body in movement, a clinical approach. pp. 215–236. *In*: Jáuregui Lobera, I. (ed.). Eating Disorders - A Paradigm of the Biopsychosocial Model of Illness. Intech, Zagreb.

Probst, M. 2018. Eating disorders and exercise, a challenge. pp. 170–188. *In*: Stubbs, B. and S. Rosenbaum (eds.). Exercise-Based Interventions for People with Mental Illness. Elsevier: London.

Probst, M. and Maïano, C. 2020a. La thérapie à médiation corporelle dans le traitement des troubles de santé mentale: « Du corps perdu au corps retrouvé ». Rev Francophone de Cliniques Comportementales et Cognitives. 25: 37–46.

Probst, M. and C. Maïano. 2020b. Les thérapies corporelles. pp. 409–423. *In*: Aimé, A., C. Maïano and M.-M. Ricard (eds.). Les troubles des conduites alimentaires : Du diagnostic aux traitements. Presses de l'Université de Montréal, Montréal.

Probst, M., A. Aimé and C. Maiano. 2020. Troubles des conduites alimentaires et activités physiques adaptées. pp. 339–356. *In*: Maïano, C., O. Hue, G. Moullec and V. Pepin (eds.). Guide d'intervention en activités physiques adaptées à l'intention des kinésiologues. Presses de l'université du Quebec, Quebec.

Probst, M. and C. Maiano. 2022. Les pratiques psychocorporelles. pp. 225–234. *In*: Aimé, A., J. Dion and C. Maiano (eds.). L'image corporelle sous toutes ses formes. Presses de l'université du Québec, Québec.

Schilder, P. 1950. Image and Appearance of the Human Body. International Universities Press, New York.

Smith, L., L. Sanchez, E. Fernandze-Egea, T. Ford, C. Parris and B. Underwood. 2023. Eating disorders and physical multimorbidity in the English general population. Eat. Weight Disord. 28: 72.

Ramsey-Wade, C., H. Williamson and J. Meyrick. 2021. Therapeutic writing for disordered eating: A systematic review. J. Creativity in Mental Health. 16: 59–76.

Utay, J. and M. Miller. 2006. Guided imagery as an effective therapeutic technique: A brief review of its history and efficacy research. J. Instructional Psychol. 33: 40–43.

Vancampfort, D., J. Vanderlinden, M. De Hert, A. Soundy, M. Adámkova, L. Skjaervenv et al. 2014a. A systematic review of physical therapy interventions for patients with anorexia and bulimia nervosa. Disabil. Rehabil. 36: 628–634.

Vancampfort, D., A. De Herdt, J. Vanderlinden, M. Lannoo, A. Soundy, G. Pieters et al. 2014b. Health related quality of life, physical fitness and physical activity participation in treatment-seeking obese persons with and without binge eating disorder. Psychiat. Res. 216: 97–102.

Vancampfort, D., M. Probst, A. Adriaens, G. Pieters, M. De Hert, B. Stubbs et al. 2014c. Changes in physical activity, physical fitness, self-perception and quality of life following a 6-month physical activity counseling and cognitive behavioral therapy program in outpatients with binge eating disorder. Psychiat. Res. 219: 361–366.

Vancampfort, D., M. Probst, A. Adriaens, G. Pieters, M. De Hert, A. Soundy et al. 2014d. Clinical correlates of global functioning in obese treatment seeking persons with binge eating disorder. Psychiatr. Danubina. 26: 256–260.

Vancampfort, D., E. Brunner, T. Van Damme and B. Stubbs. 2023a. Efficacy of basic body awareness therapy on functional outcomes: A systematic review and meta-analysis of randomized controlled trials. Physiother. Res. Int. 28: e1975.

Vancampfort, D., E. Brunner, T. Van Damme and B. Stubbs. 2023b. Basic body awareness therapy within physiotherapy: more clarity abouts its core concepts and more scientific evidence is needed. Physiother. Res. Int. 28: e1995.

Van Dam, N., K. van Vugt, D. Vago, L. Schmalzl, C. Saron and A. Olendzki. 2018. Mind the hype: a critical evaluation and prescriptive agenda for research on mindfulness and meditation. Perspect. Psychol. Sci. 13: 36–61.

Chapter 10

Dysfunctional Eating Attitudes and Behaviours, Meaningful Occupations and Perceptual Disturbances

A Multidimensional Perspective

Marie-Josée St-Pierre,[1,2,3,*] *Anick Sauvageau*[2] and *Émie Therrien*[3]

INTRODUCTION

Eating, an act as natural as it is essential, goes far beyond the simple need to nourish the body (Pollan 2009, Monthuy-Blanc et al. 2025). Eating is an occupation, just like all other occupations surrounding food and drink intake (St-Pierre et al. 2022, Sorlie et al. 2020). This chapter examines the conceptualization of eating from an occupational perspective, encompassing all eating-related occupations. From preparing to sharing a meal, every aspect of these occupations carries symbolic value and personal meaning (Lock and Pépin 2019). Eating-related occupations are multifaceted experiences that intertwine physical, cognitive, emotional, social, cultural, and even spiritual dimensions. These deeply meaningful occupations contribute to individual

[1] Montreal Mental Health University Institute Research Center, 7401, rue Hochelaga, H1N 3MG, Montréal, QC, Canada.
[2] Department of Occupational Therapy, Université du Québec à Trois-Rivières, Trois-Rivières, QC, Canada.
[3] Research Unity Loricorps, Montreal Mental Health University Institute Research Center, 7401, rue Hochelaga, H1N 3MG, Montréal, QC, Canada.
Emails: Anick.Sauvageau@uqtr.ca, Emie.Therrien@uqtr.ca
* Corresponding author: Marie-Josee.St-Pierre@uqtr.ca

DOI: 10.1201/9781032718125-12

and collective health, identity, and social cohesion, profoundly shaping our daily lives. They also reflect personal choices, cultural norms, and social interactions. All of which can vary depending on individual circumstances, societal values, and available resources (Hasselkus and Dickie 2024).

This chapter presents an occupational analysis of eating-related occupations. It provides a conceptual framework for exploring how these occupations can either promote well-being or present challenges, depending on the context. The first section establishes the foundational concepts for the framework. To understand how eating-related occupations may shift from a source of meaningful engagement to one of distress, the initial part focuses on the mobilization and meaning in the context of perceptual disturbances. Dysfunctional eating attitudes and behaviours (DEAB) are regarded as the "dark side of occupations" within a continuum of commitment to eating-related occupations, emphasizing their dysfunctional influence on other daily occupations (St-Pierre et al. 2022, 2023). The second section lays out the essential theoretical underpinnings necessary for a systematic and in-depth occupational analysis.

The third and final section explores eating-related occupations through the lens of occupational analysis, with a particular focus on their cultural and contextual dimensions. The section begins by outlining the key theoretical foundations that support a structured and comprehensive analysis of these occupations. It then examines the multidimensional and complex nature of eating-related occupations, illustrating the embedded demands across tasks structured within an occupational sequence.

Finally, the chapter concludes with a clinical case study that demonstrates how practitioners can use occupational analysis in real-life situations. This practical example underscores the significance of this method in promoting well-being and deepening our understanding of eating-related occupations as a universal yet deeply personal human experience.

1. Conceptual framework

1.1 Perceptual disturbances and the context of eating-related occupations

Body perceptual disturbances are central to dysfunctional eating attitudes and behaviours (DEAB) and arise from a complex interplay between internal perceptions and external influences. According to Lock and Pépin (2019), family functioning is a key predisposing factor, while cognitive biases influence how individuals with DEAB perceive social interactions and self-image. Cultural and societal ideals, especially the valorization of thinness, are further reinforced by family pressure and media exposure (Farooq and Zareef 2025, Jiotsa et al. 2021). Social media and communication technologies exacerbate these disturbances by promoting body dissatisfaction and unrealistic beauty standards (Aparicio-Martinez et al. 2019, Alleva and Tylka 2021). These influences often disrupt family dynamics, causing caregivers to experience distress that limits their ability to fulfil their social and occupational roles (Clark and Nayar 2012). At the individual level, DEAB has a profound impact on one's relationship with their body and occupations involving eating, physical presence, or appearance (Quiles-Cestari and Ribeiro 2012, St-Pierre et al. 2022). This gap between perceived and ideal body image often leads to avoiding occupations that involve physical engagement or bodily exposure (St-Pierre et al. 2022, 2023). Emotional and cognitive challenges such as low self-esteem, poor social skills, memory issues, and anxiety further impair occupational participation, often reinforcing cycles of body perceptual disturbances and eating preoccupation (Mack et al. 2023, Clark and Nayar 2012). The need for control usually manifests through ritualistic behaviours or perfectionism. Some individuals may adopt excessive exercise routines as a means of asserting control, while perfectionism can present as either heightened engagement in certain occupations or complete avoidance (Vansteelandt et al. 2007). Physical symptoms, such as fatigue and pain, also limit daily functioning (Pawaskar et al. 2017, Striegel et al. 2012). These disturbances are dynamic and influenced by context and emotional states (Espeset et al. 2012, Glashouwer et al. 2019). Emotional factors, such as anxiety about social interactions or a lack of motivation, exacerbate the difficulties faced by individuals with DEAB (Crouch and Alers 2014, Pettersen et al. 2013). Inadequate coping strategies also contribute to challenges in balancing symptom-related occupations with those that promote overall well-being (Singlehurst et al. 2007, Taylor 2017). Time use often becomes rigid and centred on eating-related routines, to the detriment of self-care, social life, and meaningful engagement (Godfrey 2013, St-Pierre et al. 2023). Ultimately, DEAB reshapes occupational balance and reinforces cycles of dysfunction (Lock and Pépin 2019, Elliot 2012). In summary, the interaction between body perceptual disturbances, DEAB, and environmental contexts creates a complex occupational landscape. These factors, compounded by family dynamics, societal ideals, and cognitive distortions, significantly impact daily functioning and participation in eating-related occupations.

1.2 The dark side of eating-related occupations

The concept of the "dark side of occupation" refers to occupations that may be harmful, socially unacceptable, or stigmatized, yet remain meaningful and purposeful for those involved (Twinley 2021). In the context of DEAB, this concept offers valuable insights into behaviours that many pathologize, yet individuals integrate into their daily routines and psychological coping mechanisms. Cowan and Sørlie (2021) examine how individuals with DEAB not only experience this dark side of occupations but also how therapists can incorporate it into occupational therapy interventions. Similarly, Elliott (2012) challenges the traditional view that occupations are inherently health-promoting by framing actions such as eating restriction, bingeing, and purging as occupations in their own right—intentional, structured, and meaningful within the individual's lived experience.

Overinvestment in body image and weight often occurs at the expense of other meaningful occupations (Cash and Pruzinsky 1990, Lock and Pépin 2019, St-Pierre et al. 2022). Obsessive thoughts about eating and body shape significantly influence daily routines, with an increasing amount of time and energy dedicated to behaviours such as binge eating, self-induced vomiting, excessive exercise, or prolonged fasting (Tchanturia et al. 2012, Cowan and Sorlie 2019). The darker side of occupations often acts as a maladaptive coping strategy, providing individuals with a fleeting sense of control or emotional regulation in response to psychological distress, and gradually developing into highly structured and time-consuming occupational patterns (Cowan and Sorlie 2019, St-Pierre et al. 2023). Although often triggered by a desire to lose weight or prevent weight gain, these behaviours are incorporated into daily routines with regularity and purpose (Pettersen et al. 2013, Morris 2012, Vansteelandt et al. 2007). For example, physical activity or more specifically, excessive exercise might be undertaken not for health or enjoyment, but as a compensatory act, reinforcing disordered patterns (Campbell et al. 2025)

Some occupations arise indirectly from DEAB-related routines, such as purchasing specific products (e.g., laxatives, slimming aids), carefully monitoring one's appearance, or managing financial costs associated with these items (Morris 2012). These tasks further disrupt daily rhythms and reinforce symptom-driven occupational patterns. This gives rise to the concept of "symptom-occupations" behaviours rooted in psychopathological symptoms but operating as meaningful, structured occupations in daily life. These include not only eating-related behaviours but also the cognitive and emotional investments associated with them (St-Pierre et al. 2022). Symptom-occupations are daily occupations grounded in psychopathological behaviours like excessive exercise, binge eating, and restriction. Over time, they can replace leisure, social, and productive roles, worsening psychosocial dysfunction (Morris 2012, St-Pierre et al. 2022). Behaviours such as purchasing laxatives or obsessively managing appearance disrupt routines and incur substantial time and financial costs. Therefore, analyzing daily routines in detail can reveal how over- and under-investment in various occupations, particularly those related to eating, contribute to the psychosocial difficulties experienced by individuals with DEAB (St-Pierre et al. 2022). This perspective encourages occupational therapists to recognize the ambivalent nature of meaning in occupation and to support clients in rebuilding healthier and more balanced occupational identities.

1.3 Occupational investment continuum in dysfunctional eating attitudes and behaviours

A recent scoping review highlights that an excessive focus on eating-related occupations can lead to insufficient or no engagement in other areas of life, particularly those involving social interaction, where individuals are exposed to others' perceptions (St-Pierre et al. 2022). For example, individuals might neglect work or academic duties because their preoccupation with eating or body image dominates their ability to participate productively. Conversely, under-engagement in eating-related occupations may lead to over-engagement in other occupations, often as a way to avoid food or drink intake. Such imbalances in occupational engagement, whether through avoidance or over-involvement, are frequently linked to distorted body perceptions. This results in variable participation in meaningful occupations, shaped by the person's lived experience. Under-investment may manifest as avoiding specific occupations or settings. For instance, someone might steer clear of dining out or joining group sports because these heighten concerns about body image or eating. Conversely, over-investment may involve excessive dedication to specific occupations, such as compulsive exercise used to compensate for food or drink intake or to lessen fears of weight gain.

The individual's self-perception and their belief about how others perceive them significantly influence their level of investment in any occupation involving body exposure. In this regard, relational difficulties often arise, leading to social withdrawal (Clark and Nayar 2012). Studies show that social and leisure occupations are usually the first to be abandoned by individuals with disordered eating (Quiles-Cestari and Ribeiro 2012), contributing to widespread imbalance across social roles. Moreover, self-care occupations are also affected, often burdened by negative self-perceptions (Lock and Pépin 2019). For example, body image concerns and discomfort with being seen may limit participation in clothing-related occupations such as shopping or trying on clothes (Morris 2012), while hygiene routines may be either over-performed or entirely avoided (Clark and Nayar 2012). Eating-related occupations exert a disruptive influence on overall occupational routines (Clark and Nayar 2012). DEAB frequently results in occupational imbalance, significantly impacting the ability to fulfil social roles (Gardiner and Brown 2012, Lock and Pépin 2019). Individuals may choose solitary occupations over social interaction. Although DEAB is most visible during bingeing or restriction episodes, its impact extends beyond eating to surrounding occupations. Grocery shopping, for instance, becomes emotionally charged and rigidly structured, marked by calorie obsession, eating rules, and ritualized behaviours (Clark and Nayar 2012). Meal preparation is similarly affected, with duration and frequency fluctuating based on dysfunctional beliefs (Morris 2012). Some individuals may eat during food or drink preparation to justify not eating later. According to Singlehurst et al. (2007), preoccupation with eating can become so dominant that it reduces opportunities for other occupations and damages interpersonal relationships. Avoidant behaviours may include eating alone, feigning illness to avoid eating with others, declining eating-related work occupations, or using other occupations to distract during eating crises. Additionally, rigid eating rituals, such as strict control over eating and body weight, obsessive calorie counting, frequent weighing, excessive exercise, and compensatory behaviours, further contribute to occupational disruption (Clark and Nayar 2012, Gardiner and Brown 2012, Pettersen et al. 2013).

Ultimately, body perceptual disturbances closely influence the presence of DEAB and play a central role in the occupational dysfunction that affected individuals experience, particularly in eating-related occupations.

2. Empirical and clinical support

2.1 Occupational analysis

Therapeutic and meaningful occupations are central to occupational therapy practice, valued both as tools to achieve therapeutic goals and as desired outcomes of intervention (Hinojosa et al. 2017). A meaningful occupation provides personal purpose and contributes to a sense of self or satisfaction (Ikiugu et al. 2015). To evaluate meaningfulness, practitioners consider occupational roles, culture, age, gender, interests, and the cognitive, emotional, and physical dimensions of

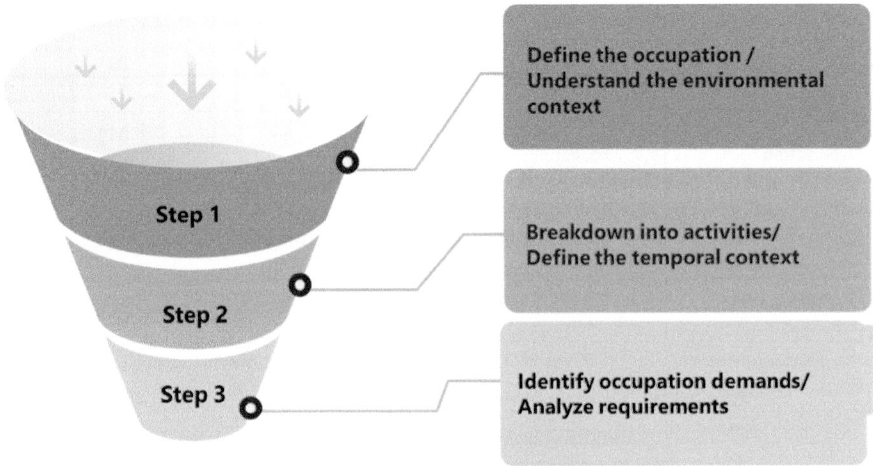

Figure 1. 3-Steps of occupational analysis.

the person's life. Occupational analysis is a structured process that examines the interaction between the occupation (the key to meaning and participation), the person or group (the lock that must align with the occupation), and the context (the keystone that shapes opportunities and constraints). This approach helps uncover how occupations influence health, well-being, and participation while identifying supports and barriers in the individual's complex environment (Gillen and Ramugondo 2024, Mackenzie et al. 2020, Thomas 2024). Used in both assessment and intervention planning (Thomas 2024), occupational analysis reveals strengths and challenges in daily performance, guiding the development of personalized strategies to promote engagement in meaningful occupations.

The three steps of occupational analysis offer a systematic and detailed approach. The steps outlined in this chapter represent a consolidated method based on well-established processes in the academic literature, with particular emphasis on the work of Thomas (2024). It describes each step and illustrates them in Figure 1.

Step One: Define the occupation and understand the environmental context. Analyzing an occupation starts with identifying the occupation and understanding its personal significance, as this meaning defines its role in the individual's life. Key characteristics to outline include the type and purpose of the occupation, required tools or resources, and the environmental context in which it occurs. Table 1 summarizes these key components.

Several authors (Christiansen et al. 2024, Hasselkus and Dickie 2024) emphasize that understanding an occupation requires considering its subjective and contextual meanings. This involves exploring how the person perceives the occupation, shaped by their experiences, preferences, and cultural background, to support their better engagement and performance.

Table 1. Categories and details of Step 1—Define the occupation and understand the environmental context.

Categories	**Details**
Type and Purpose of Occupation	**Self-care**: Occupations related to personal health and well-being (e.g., hygiene, eating, rest and sleep) **Productivity**: Occupations that are useful or necessary (e.g., work, education, household tasks) **Leisure**: Occupations enjoyed for pleasure or relaxation (e.g., hobbies, sports, play, outings)
Relevance and importance	Who is performing the occupation? The individual's abilities, interests, and motivations
Required equipment or resources and environment/context	**Place**: Where is the occupation taking place (e.g., at home, in a restaurant)? **Time**: When (e.g., time of day, season, life stage, duration)? **Tools and materials used** **Physical/social environment** **Cultural/institutional/virtual context**

Step Two: Break down into smaller, sequential activities and define the temporal context. This facilitates a detailed understanding of the demands, resources, and challenges at each stage, whether the occupation is complex or straightforward. For example, "going for a walk" can be separated into preparation, initiation, execution, completion, and recovery, each involving specific motor, cognitive, and emotional processes. This breakdown also clarifies the actions needed for full participation and uncovers often implicit elements of daily occupations. Simultaneously, analyzing the temporal context, such as life stage, time of day or year, duration, frequency, and regularity, adds a dynamic dimension. Understanding when and how often an occupation takes place helps to situate it within a person's routine and indicates whether it remains stable or varies over time.

Step three: Identify occupation demands and analyze requirements. At this stage, the focus is on examining the various demands of the occupation, particularly in relation to bodily functions, structures, and performance skills (Thomas 2024). This helps to understand the specific demands of the occupation and how they correspond with the individual's skills. First, identifying the necessary body functions is often the most detailed and comprehensive part of the analysis. According to the World Health Organisation (2001), body functions refer to the "physiological functions of body systems," encompassing not only physical aspects such as joint mobility and muscle power, but also sensory, cognitive, and emotional functions. Understanding these requirements clarifies what the occupation demands from the client in terms of mental, physical, and emotional involvement. Next, the analysis includes identifying the required body structures, which are the anatomical parts essential to performing the occupation. These go beyond basic life-sustaining structures and focus on those specifically involved in performing the occupation. Finally, it is essential to identify the required actions and performance skills—the observable abilities and movements that the client must demonstrate to engage successfully in the occupation. By analyzing these components in detail, practitioners gain a clearer understanding of the occupation's complexity and how it aligns with the individual's abilities and therapeutic objectives.

Identifying and analyzing these requirements facilitates supporting participation in meaningful occupations. In the final stages of occupational analysis, practitioners must identify all barriers that prevent the person from performing the occupation. Occupational science understands optimal performance as occurring when the person, the occupation, and the environment align. Disruptions or imbalances among these elements can hinder successful engagement in everyday occupations (Bass et al. 2024). The Person-Environment-Occupation-Performance (PEOP) model conceptualizes this dynamic interplay, emphasizing that occupational performance emerges from the continuous and reciprocal interaction among three core components (Christiansen et al. 2024).

3. Applications to the sociocultural context

This section examines occupational analysis within the context of eating-related occupations, aiming to define their structure and the influence of their context in daily life and cultural context.

Define the occupation and understand the environmental context of DEAB (step 1). Both the surrounding context and the individual's abilities, interests, and motivations influence decision-making and actions (Dickie et al. 2006). In the case of eating-related occupations, an individual's choice to engage in or continue a particular occupation depends on how they perceive the context as supporting or hindering it. For individuals with DEAB, negative perceptual filters such as guilt about eating or anxiety over body image or contextual filters like societal pressure to conform to beauty ideals shape their view of eating-related occupations. These filters determine whether individuals see eating as a source of nourishment or as an emotionally distressing activity. Together, these factors shape how individuals experience, understand, and carry out eating-related occupations. Furthermore, clinicians and researchers should avoid simply classifying eating-related occupations as self-care or nutrition. Instead, they should be understood in terms of their significance and personal fulfilment, reflecting the individual's overall sense of experience. This perspective emphasizes that eating-related occupations play a vital role in shaping one's identity, social interactions, and emotional well-being, rather than merely satisfying basic physical needs (Eklund and Argentzell 2016, Hammell 2015). Table 2 provides a detailed explanation of each context, offering a clear understanding of how they influence the way eating-related occupations occur.

Breakdown into activities and define the temporal context (step 2). This section provides a detailed breakdown of the occupation into its component subtasks or activities, placing each within its proper temporal context. To ensure this step was effectively completed, a structured method grounded on focused discussions with experts in occupational analysis allowed for a deeper understanding of eating-related occupations. The initial model, developed by the principal author of this chapter and presented in a book on healthy eating, was considered to enhance the occupational

Table 2. Environmental Contexts Influencing Occupations.

Context	Elements	Details
Physical Environment	Lighting	Proper lighting enhances visibility, reduces the risk of accidents, and fosters a pleasant atmosphere.
	Space	Size and layout of the space (kitchen, dining area) influence how easily individuals can carry out eating-related tasks.
	Tools	Availability and suitability of kitchen tools (knives, cutting boards, adaptive utensils).
	Accessibility	Easy access to food storage, preparation areas, and dining spaces is essential for independence, especially for individuals with mobility impairments.
Social Environment	Presence of Others	Eating with family/friends/colleagues improves communication, emotional bonds, and social interaction experience.
	Social Expectations or Norms	Social norms regarding dining (table manners, mealtimes, etiquette) shape how eating is experienced and foster a sense of belonging.
Cultural Context	Cultural Beliefs and Practices	Cultural factors influence what is eaten, how it is prepared, and how it is served, as well as dietary restrictions shaped by religious or cultural beliefs.
	Specific Eating Rituals	Rituals surrounding mealtimes, such as prayers, greetings, or specific ways of serving and eating, shape the social dynamics of meals.
	Culinary Preferences	Cultural preferences influence food and drink choices, cooking techniques, and meal structures (e.g., communal vs. individual servings).
	Meaning of the Occupation	The cultural importance of eating-related occupations can vary, with eating playing a central role in social bonding in some cultures, while others see it as more functional.
Institutional Context	Workplace Rules	Rules in workplace settings regarding mealtimes, food and drink consumption, and designated eating areas.
	Healthcare Protocols	Dietary guidelines, meal schedules, and rules governing food and drink consumption in healthcare settings, particularly for individuals with specific health conditions.
Virtual Context	Digital Tools	Online recipe websites, cooking apps, virtual grocery shopping, meal delivery services, and digital health trackers.
	Online Social Interaction	Virtual eating-related experiences (online dinners or cooking events) add a layer of social engagement when physical interaction is not possible.

perspective (Monthuy-Blanc et al. 2025). Categorizing eating-related occupations into three phases (1) PRE-intake, (2) PER-intake, and (3) POST-intake provided a clear framework for their definition. This sequential model, which reached consensus and is illustrated in Figure 2, conceptualizes food and drink intake as an occupational sequence structured around these distinct yet interconnected stages.

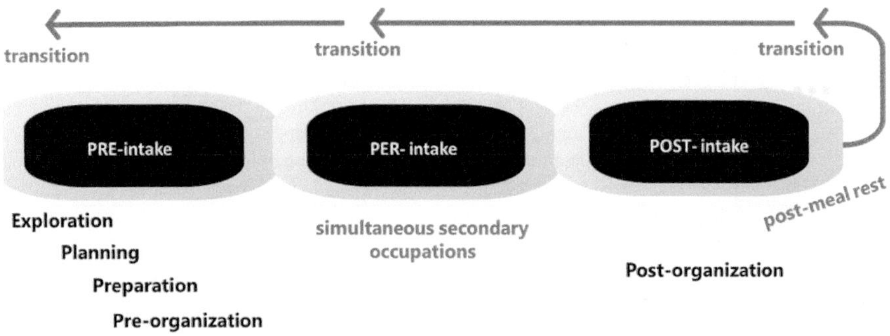

Figure 2. Time sequence of eating-related occupations.

- The **PRE-intake** phase includes four key stages: exploration, planning, preparation, and pre-organization. Each stage plays a crucial role in setting the foundation for an efficient and enjoyable eating experience.
- The **PER-intake** phase involves the tasks and interactions that occur during the actual act of eating. This includes not only the physical process of consuming food or drink but also potential elements of social participation.
- The **POST-intake** phase focuses on occupations that occur after eating. These are essential for maintaining physical well-being and ensuring a clean, organized environment (restore). This phase comprises one main stage: post-organization, which enhances the overall eating experience by fostering comfort, relaxation, and readiness for future meals.

Although not formally classified as a post-intake subtask, the post-meal rest period holds cultural and occupational significance. This phase supports physical digestion and emotional decompression, especially after socially engaging meals. Across cultures, resting after eating, whether lying down, sitting quietly, or engaging in light conversation, reflects a valued moment of integration, allowing the body and mind to process not only the food but also the shared experience that accompanies it. Eating and resting together contribute meaningfully to well-being and deserve acknowledgment within occupational analysis.

A transition dynamic is underway, driven by an active and constantly evolving process that reflects how eating-related occupations adapt and respond to individual and contextual changes. Refer to Table 3 for a comprehensive breakdown of each sub-task and a detailed analysis of the occupations involved at each stage.

The temporal context of eating-related occupations encompasses various aspects that help to understand how this activity integrates into a person's daily routine, including culturally shaped rhythms. Eating usually occurs multiple times a day at regular intervals such as in the morning, at midday, and in the evening making it a routine, daily, and often cyclical occupation. The duration required to prepare, eat, and clean up after meals can vary (e.g., a quick breakfast versus a more elaborate dinner), and occupations tend to follow predictable patterns. A fast-paced lifestyle may result in quicker meals, while others may have more time to enjoy them. Throughout the lifespan, eating habits may evolve depending on the stage of

Table 3. Occupational sequence of eating-related occupations: PRE-, PER-, and POST- intake phases.

Phase	Stage	Description	Examples of Occupations/Tasks
PRE-intake	Exploration	The initial stage involves gathering ideas and information for food and drink.	Looking up recipes Watching food/drink videos Reading nutrition labels
	Planning	Organizing what to eat and how to get it.	Making a shopping list Choosing meals for the week Grocery shopping (in-store or online) Washing and cutting vegetables
	Preparation	Actions taken to prepare ingredients and begin cooking.	Marinating meat Pre-cooking steps (boiling, blanching) Collecting utensils and cookware
	Pre-Organization	Setting up the environment for eating.	Setting the table Cleaning kitchen surfaces Preparing condiments
PER-intake	Eating Setup	Preparing oneself and the environment for eating.	Sitting at the table or another eating space Adjusting the seating for comfort and accessibility
	Handling Food	Managing tools and interacting with the food.	Choosing appropriate cutlery Cutting, spreading, and picking up food
	Chewing and Swallowing	Physical process of consuming food/drink.	Chewing food Swallowing safely
	Social Participation	Engaging with others during the meal (if applicable).	Conversing with family or friends Sharing mealtime traditions
POST-intake	Post-Organization	Cleaning and organizing the eating environment.	Washing dishes Storing leftovers Wiping tables and counters Disposing of food waste and packaging properly

life. A child, an adolescent, an adult, or an older adult may have different nutritional requirements and routines. Seasonal variations can impact both the timing and type of food or drink consumed—for example, differences between summer and winter meals—as well as specific events or traditions, such as festive gatherings or religious fasting. Additionally, daily routines such as eating-related occupations depend on the time of day (e.g., breakfast, lunch, dinner), personal or family schedules, and cultural customs. Appreciating this temporal context offers a richer, more dynamic understanding of eating-related occupations, their stability, regularity, and role in structuring daily life, thereby deepening the analysis and relevance of occupational practices.

Identify occupation demands/analyze requirements (step 3). The multidimensionality of eating-related occupations emphasizes the complexity of sub-tasks or activities that

Table 4. Overview of demands/requirements for eating-related occupations.

Categories	Demands/requirements/Details
Physical skills and effort.	**Movements involved:** Hand-eye coordination, fine and gross motor skills and posture control. **Physical Demands:** Strength and physical endurance.
Mental processes cognitive processing, emotional and social dimension	**Planning and organization:** Cognitive skills are required to structure the sequence of tasks **Memory:** Remembering recipe steps, ingredients, and portions **Problem-solving:** Cognitive flexibility and decision-making are crucial for adapting to unexpected challenges that arise during meal preparation. **Emotional:** Comfort, pleasure, or the satisfaction of a shared meal. Emotional hunger can contribute to the development of dysfunctional eating when eating becomes the primary means of relieving emotions. **Motivation:** The motivation to prepare and consume food or drink is often influenced by personal preferences, habits, and mental or emotional states. **Interaction:** Eating with others can enhance the enjoyment of the meal and strengthen social bonds. Additionally, conforming to social norms is often part of the eating experience.
Sensory components Sensory experiences are central to eating-related occupations, making them highly engaging and enjoyable for many people.	**Taste, smell, and texture of food and drink:** The five basic senses contribute significantly to the overall eating experience. Becoming fully aware of them allows an increased perceived palatability, improves the enjoyment of a meal, and improves eating satisfaction. **Sensitivity to stimuli:** Other environmental sensory stimuli, such as kitchen noise (from blenders and timers), lighting, or even the temperature of the kitchen, can influence the food and drink preparation process.

occur before, during, and after food or drink intake. Understanding the full spectrum of demands and requirements, including the tasks and skills involved, enables a more comprehensive occupational analysis and helps identify areas where support may be needed to improve an individual's ability to perform and find satisfaction in eating-related occupations. At this stage of the analysis, it is essential to examine each of these dimensions to gain a comprehensive understanding of how individuals carry out eating-related occupations and to anticipate potential challenges (Thomas 2024). Table 4 offers a structured overview of these requirements, serving as a practical tool to guide this in-depth assessment and support personalized intervention planning.

3.1 Application to a clinical case from the Canadian cultural landscape

To illustrate a holistic view of eating-related occupation, we will present a clinical example that highlights the multifaceted nature of meal preparation within a family context. Clara, a mother of two, used to gather her family around a home-cooked meal every Sunday evening. This time was not simply a routine, but a significant occupation that impacted many aspects of their lives (Mack et al. 2024). Within the Canadian cultural landscape, families often ritualize the Sunday evening meal as a tradition that fosters intergenerational ties and maintains a sense of familial continuity and social cohesion. To better understand Clara's meal preparation, practitioners can break down the occupation into sequential activities. This enables detailed analysis and helps identify challenges or resources that affect her participation, particularly in the context of DEAB.

Clara begins her Sunday by planning the evening meal. What was once an enjoyable task now presents significant cognitive and emotional challenges. As she tries to select a menu that suits her family's tastes and nutritional needs, intrusive thoughts related to calorie content, fear of weight gain, and a need for control often dominate her decision-making process. This internal conflict is further compounded by the "weight" of cultural and familial expectations associated with traditional practices, making it difficult for her to prioritize her family's preferences over her own restrictive eating patterns. With her list in hand, Clara heads to the market to shop for ingredients. She can navigate the space and select fresh, high-quality ingredients, drawing on her knowledge of nutrition, food, and drink preparation. However, the act of choosing food and drink is not neutral. She feels overwhelmed by concerns about what is "healthy" or "unhealthy," and the emotional weight of these decisions can slow her down and increase her stress. Once home, Clara prepares the ingredients. She completes physical tasks such as washing, chopping, and organizing with skill and efficiency. Still, body image concerns disrupt Clara's concentration—she may pause to check her appearance or engage in rituals that provide a sense of control, but that interfere with the flow of the activity. These behaviours not only reduce her engagement in the task but also add to her mental fatigue. Cooking the meal involves a combination of physical and cognitive demands. Clara must coordinate the timing, adjust the seasoning, and ensure that the food and drink are prepared safely. While she is capable of multitasking and adapting recipes, anxiety often intensifies at this stage. She may be preoccupied with the caloric content of the meal, double-check portions, or over-monitor the preparation process, which detracts from her confidence and enjoyment. As the meal nears completion, Clara turns to setting the table. This task, although relatively simple, involves a social and cultural dimension, honouring family traditions, creating a welcoming environment, and attending to presentation details. However, her relationship with the act of eating and body image can interfere here as well, making her overly concerned about how the meal will be perceived, or how much food and drink the hosts are serving. During the meal, Clara serves each family member and joins them at the table. Despite the opportunity for social connection, this moment often brings heightened emotional tension. Fear of eating, anxiety over portion sizes, and difficulty being present due to body perceptual disturbances may prevent her from fully participating or enjoying the experience. She may limit her intake or focus on others rather than herself, maintaining a distance from the food on her plate. After the meal, Clara is responsible for cleaning up. She completes the tasks: washing dishes, putting away leftovers, and tidying the kitchen. But by this point, the cumulative physical and mental demands of the day become evident. The emotional strain of managing eating-related thoughts and behaviours throughout the process leaves her feeling exhausted. This example illustrates how a seemingly routine family occupation can become deeply affected by the cognitive, emotional, and behavioral impacts of disordered eating. Clara retains many functional skills and values the meaning of shared meals, yet her ability to engage fully is compromised.

By breaking the occupation into sequential steps, we gain a clearer understanding of the barriers and supports that influence her occupational performance in the context of DEAB.

Clara's relationships with her family, cultural traditions, and even her own body would become strained as the influence of DEAB permeated every aspect of this once cherished family ritual. For Clara to participate effectively in this occupation, it is essential to consider her personal beliefs. It struggles around food, drink, and body image, as well as the environmental and social factors that might either obstruct or support her involvement. Recognizing where Clara encounters difficulties in the process allows for a more customized approach in therapy or intervention to help her regain a sense of control and satisfaction in performing this meaningful occupation.

Conclusion

This chapter reveals the complexity of eating-related occupations through occupational analysis, showing how body perceptual disturbances can turn nourishment into distress. These occupations are deeply personal, shaped by physical, emotional, social, and cultural factors. By identifying specific challenges in the eating process, tailored interventions can support agency and well-being. Ultimately, eating is not just a routine; it is a meaningful experience shaped by the dynamic interplay between person, environment, and occupation.

Acknowledgments

We wish to express our sincere gratitude to all the occupational analysis experts who were consulted for their valuable insights, which significantly contributed to the writing of this chapter.

References

Alleva, J.M. and T.L. Tylka. 2021. Body functionality: a review of the literature. Body Image 36: 149–171.

Aparicio-Martinez, P., A.J. Perea-Moreno, M.P. Martinez-Jimenez, M.D. Redel-Macías, C. Pagliari and M. Vaquero-Abellan. 2019. Social media, thin-ideal, body dissatisfaction and disordered eating attitudes: an exploratory analysis. Int. J. Environ. Res. Public Health 16(21): 4177.

Bass, J.D., J.K. Marchant, S.L. de Sam Lazaro and C.M. Baum. 2024. Application of the Person–Environment–Occupation–Performance model: a scoping review. OTJR: Occup. Ther. J. Res. 44(3): 521–540.

Campbell, C., X. Greig, J. Griffiths, D. Hashman, T. Sottile, M. Isobe et al. 2025. The prevalence of excessive exercise in eating disorders: a systematic review and meta-analysis. Eur. Eat. Disord. Rev.

Cash, T.F. and T. Pruzinsky. 1990. Body Image: Development, Deviation and Change. Guilford Press, New York, USA.

Cash, T.F. 2002. Cognitive-behavioral perspectives on body image. pp. 38–46. *In*: Cash, T.F. and T. Pruzinsky (eds.). Body Image: A Handbook of Theory, Research, and Clinical Practice. Guilford Press, New York, USA.

Christiansen, C.H., J. Bass and C.M. Baum. 2024. Occupational Therapy: Performance, Participation, and Well-being. Taylor and Francis.

Clark, M. and S. Nayar. 2012. Recovery from eating disorders: a role for occupational therapy. N. Z. J. Occup. Ther. 59(1): 13–17.

Cowan, M. and C. Sørlie. 2021. The dark side of occupation in an eating disorder intensive day service. pp. 114–121. *In*: Twinley, R. (ed.). Illuminating the Dark Side of Occupation: International Perspectives from Occupational Therapy and Occupational Science. Routledge, Abingdon, UK.

Crouch, R. and V. Alers. 2014. The treatment of eating disorders in occupational therapy (chap. 25). *In*: Crouch, R. and V. Alers (eds.). Psychiatry and Mental Health. 5th ed. John Wiley and Sons, Ltd., Toronto, Canada.

Dickie, V., M.P. Cutchin and R. Humphry. 2006. Occupation as transactional experience: a critique of individualism in occupational science. J. Occup. Sci. 13(1): 83–93.

Eklund, M. and E. Argentzell. 2016. Perception of occupational balance by people with mental illness: a new methodology. Scand. J. Occup. Ther. 23(4): 304–313.

Elliot, M.L. 2012. Figured world of eating disorders: occupations of illness. Can. J. Occup. Ther. 79(1): 15–22.

Espeset, E.M.S., K.S. Gulliksen, R.H.S. Nordbo, F. Skarderud and A. Holte. 2012. The link between negative emotions and eating disorder behavior in patients with anorexia nervosa. Eur. Eat. Disord. Rev. 20: 451–460.

Farooq, F. and S. Zareef. 2025. Role of social media use and socio-cultural attitude towards appearance in eating problems among adults. Res. Med. Sci. Rev. 3(2): 376–397.

Gardiner, C. and N. Brown. 2010. Is there a role for occupational therapy within a specialist child and adolescent mental health eating disorder service? Br. J. Occup. Ther. 73(1): 38–43.

Gardner, R.M. 2001. Assessment of body image disturbance in children and adolescents. Body Image: 193–213.

Gillen, G., C. Brown and E. Ramugondo. 2024. Willard and Spackman's Occupational Therapy. 14th ed. Wolters Kluwer, Philadelphia, USA.

Glashouwer, K.A., I. Masselman and P.J. de Jong. 2019. Reducing body dissatisfaction by means of an evaluative conditioning procedure in undergraduate women: a replication study. Behav. Res. Ther. 121.

Godfrey, N. 2013. Occupational impact of anorexia nervosa: occupational meaning, motivation and engagement. Br. J. Occup. Ther. 76: 42–42.

Hammell, K.W. 2015. Occupational rights and critical occupational therapy: rising to the challenge. Aust. Occup. Ther. J. 62(6): 449–451.

Hasselkus, B.R. and V. Dickie. 2024. The Meaning of Everyday Occupation. Routledge, Abingdon, UK.

Hinojosa, J., P. Kramer and C. Brasic Royeen. 2017. The complexity of occupation. pp. 1–22. *In*: Hinojosa, J., P. Kramer and C. Brasic Royeen (eds.). Perspectives on Human Occupation: Theory Underlying Practice. 2nd ed. F.A. Davis Company, Philadelphia, USA.

Ikiugu, M.N., A.K. Hoyme, B. Mueller and R.R. Reinke. 2015. Difference between meaningful and psychologically rewarding occupations: findings from two pilot studies. J. Occup. Sci. 23(2): 266–277.

Jiotsa, B., B. Naccache, M. Duval, B. Rocher and M. Grall-Bronnec. 2021. Social media use and body image disorders: association between frequency of comparing one's own physical appearance to that of people being followed on social media and body dissatisfaction and drive for thinness. Int. J. Environ. Res. Public Health 18(6): 2880.

Lock, L.C. and G. Pépin. 2019. Eating disorders. pp. 154–168. *In*: Brown, C., V. Stoffel and J.P. Muñoz (eds.). Occupational Therapy in Mental Health: A Vision for Participation. 2nd ed. F.A. Davis Company, Philadelphia, USA.

Mack, R.A., C.E. Stanton and M.R. Carney. 2023. The importance of including occupational therapists as part of the multidisciplinary team in the management of eating disorders: a narrative review incorporating lived experience. J. Eat. Disord. 11: 37.

Mack, R.A., K. Kelleher, J. Bhattarai and T. Spence. 2024. Individuals with eating disorders' perspectives on a meal preparation intervention. Occup. Ther. Ment. Health 40(4): 371–390.

Mackenzie, L., G. O'Toole and C. James. 2020. Core business: activity, task and occupational analysis. pp. 215–226. *In*: Occupational Therapy in Australia. Routledge, Abingdon, UK.

Merino, M., J.F. Tornero-Aguilera, A. Rubio-Zarapuz, C.V. Villanueva-Tobaldo, A. Martín-Rodríguez and V.J. Clemente-Suárez. 2024. Body perceptions and psychological well-being: a review of the impact

of social media and physical measurements on self-esteem and mental health with a focus on body image satisfaction and its relationship with cultural and gender factors. Healthcare 12: 1396.
Monthuy Blanc, J., É. Therrien and J. Harnois. 2025. Santé, boire & manger : l'alimentation en transdisciplinarité selon les perceptions. Éditions JFD, Québec, Canada.
Morris, R. 2012. Assessment of occupation and social performance. pp. 61–74. *In*: Fox, J. and K. Goss (eds.). Eating and Its Disorders. Wiley Blackwell, Oxford, UK.
Pawaskar, M., E.A. Witt, D. Supina, B.K. Herman and T.A. Wadden. 2017. Impact of binge eating disorder on functional impairment and work productivity in an adult community sample in the United States. Int. J. Clin. Pract. 71(7).
Pettersen, G., K.-B. Thune-Larsen, R. Wynn and J.H. Rosenvinge. 2013. Eating disorders: challenges in the later phases of the recovery process. A qualitative study of patients' experiences. Scand. J. Caring Sci. 27(1): 92–98.
Pollan, M. 2009. In Defense of Food: An Eater's Manifesto. Penguin, New York, USA.
Quiles-Cestari, L.M. and R.P. Ribeiro. 2012. The occupational roles of women with anorexia nervosa. Rev. Latino-Am. Enfermagem. 20: 1–2.
Roy, M. and F. Forest. 2007. Assessment of body image distortion in eating and weight disorders: the validation of a computer-based tool (Q-BID). Eat. Weight Disord. 12: 1–11.
Singlehurst, H., S. Corr, S. Griffiths and K. Beaulieu. 2007. The impact of binge eating disorder on occupation: a pilot study. Br. J. Occup. Ther. 70: 493–501.
Sørlie, C., M. Cowan, J. Chacksfield, E. Vaughan and K.E. Atler. 2020. Occupation-focused assessment in eating disorders: preliminary utility. Occup. Ther. Ment. Health 36: 145–161.
St-Pierre, M.-J., P.-Y. Therriault, S. Béliveau and J. Monthuy-Blanc. 2022. Le sous- et sur-investissement de l'occupation, une porte ouverte vers la compréhension des troubles du comportement alimentaire: étude de portée. Rev. Francoph. Rech. Ergothérapie 8: 13–46.
St-Pierre, M.-J., P.-Y. Therriault, U. Faghihi and J. Monthuy-Blanc. 2023. Eating disorders: when food "eats" time. Appetite 185: 106509.
Taylor, R.R. (ed.). 2017. Kielhofner's Model of Human Occupation: Theory and Application. 5th ed. Wolters Kluwer, Philadelphia, USA.
Thomas, H. 2024. Occupational and Activity Analysis. Taylor & Francis, Abingdon, UK.
Tchanturia, K., H. Davies, A. Harrison, J.R.E. Fox, J. Treasure and U. Schmidt. 2012. Altered social hedonic processing in eating disorders. Int. J. Eat. Disord. 45: 962–969.
Townsend, E., H.J. Polatajko, N. Cantin and Association canadienne des ergothérapeutes. 2013. Habiliter à l'occupation: faire avancer la perspective ergothérapique de la santé, du bien-être et de la justice par l'occupation. 2e éd. CAOT Publications ACE, Ottawa, Canada.
Twinley, R. (ed.). 2021. Illuminating the Dark Side of Occupation: International Perspectives from Occupational Therapy and Occupational Science. (Routledge Advances in Occupational Science and Occupational Therapy Series). Routledge, Abingdon, UK.
Vansteelandt, K., F. Rijmen, G. Pieters, M. Probst and J. Vanderlinden. 2007. Drive for thinness, affect regulation and physical activity in eating disorders: a daily life study. Behav. Res. Ther. 45: 1717–1734.
World Health Organization (WHO). 2001. International Classification of Functioning, Disability and Health. WHO, Geneva, Switzerland.

Chapter 11

Challenges and Perspectives for Informal Caregivers in Dysfunctional Eating Attitudes and Behaviors

French Insights

Elisabetta Scanferla[1,2,3,*] and *Romain Rey*[4,5,6]

INTRODUCTION

Informal caregivers play a pivotal role in supporting individuals with severe or long-term mental health disorders, including dysfunctional eating attitude and behaviors (DEAB), with eating disorders representing the most severe forms of DEAB. Scientific literature worldwide highlights the vital contribution of families and friends in assisting individuals with mental health disorders to cope and overcome challenges (Bremmers et al. 2022, del Castillo 2024).

[1] Université Paris Cité, CRPMS (EA 3522), IHSS, Paris, France.
[2] GHU Paris Psychiatrie et Neurosciences, CMME, Hôpital Sainte-Anne, Paris, France.
[3] Unité de Recherche Loricorps, Centre de Recherche de l'Institut Universitaire en Santé Mentale de Montréal, (CR-IUSMM), 7331, Rue Hochelaga, Montreal, QC H1N 3V2, Canada.
[4] Centre Lyonnais des Aidants en Psychiatrie (CLAP), Le Vinatier-Psychiatrie Universitaire Lyon Métropole, Bron, France.
[5] Fondation FondaMental, Créteil, France.
[6] INSERM, U1028; CNRS, UMR5292; Université Lyon 1; Centre de Recherche en Neurosciences de Lyon, équipe PsyR2, Lyon, France.
Email: romain.rey@ch-le-vinatier.fr
* Corresponding author: e.scanferla@ghu-paris.fr

DOI: 10.1201/9781032718125-13

Caregivers often provide their loved one with vital financial, practical and emotional support throughout their care and recovery process (Andrade et al. 2022). The assistance of family and friends can take different forms, not mutually exclusive, including: facilitating the access to care, providing logistical support, motivating the person to engage in treatment, coordinating the care sequences, participating in therapeutic decision-making (McDaid and Park 2022). The impact of this support is significant, extending beyond clinical and functional outcomes, influencing the quality of life both for the individual and their family. For healthcare professionals and other stakeholders involved in the care process, collaborating with informal caregivers is crucial, and there is an increase in interest among them with regard to this role (Hengelaar et al. 2018).

This chapter will firstly delineate the main issues related to the role of informal caregivers and their needs. It will then explore the essential support they require, along with various types of interventions available in the context of DEAB and conclude by introducing a novel promising early psychoeducational intervention.

1. Conceptual framework

1.1 The long-term impact of caring responsibilities on caregivers' mental and physical health

Caring responsibilities in the context of mental health disorders frequently come with a significant burden, encompassing physical, psychological, social, and financial long-term consequences (Gupta et al. 2015). The mental health toll on caregivers may be profound, with many exhibiting symptoms of clinical depression and anxiety (Bremmers et al. 2022). As compared to the general population, they are at a greater risk of experiencing social isolation, limiting time for personal relationships and leisure activities, reduced quality of life, and altered mental health (Bremmers et al. 2024). Caregivers often endure elevated stress levels, pervasive feelings of hopelessness, and chronic emotional exhaustion (Mittendorfer-Rutz et al. 2019).

The physical health impacts of caregiving are equally concerning (Phillips et al. 2023). Chronic stress associated with caregiving has been linked to a range of physical health issues, including weakened immune function, and increased susceptibility to chronic illnesses (Lindt et al. 2020). Sleep deprivation, poor dietary habits, and a lack of physical activity are common consequences, which further contribute to an altered physical health. The caregivers' burden often manifests as a state of emotional and physical exhaustion (George et al. 2020). Additionally, caregiving responsibilities often impose significant financial and social strains. Caregivers may need to reduce their work hours or leave employment to accommodate caregiving duties. This loss of income compounds the financial burden associated with treatment costs, further straining caregivers' burden (Surgenor et al. 2022). Available research highlights a cyclical relationship where a decline in the caregiver's well-being negatively affects their ability to provide effective care, which in turn further impacts their well-being. If these combined mental and physical challenges remain unaddressed, the capacity of caregivers to provide effective support is also compromised, which is crucial for their loved ones to achieve recovery (Applebaum and Sannes 2025).

Although caregivers in the context of DEAB may have distinctive requirements and expectations, they also exhibit commonalities with caregiving experience in other mental disorders. Providing care for a loved one facing such challenges necessitates constant vigilance, navigating intricate healthcare systems, and coping with the emotional burden of witnessing someone grappling with a life-threatening condition (Zabala et al. 2009). Because of their demanding responsibilities, caregivers often experience significant psychological distress. They also report elevated levels of expressed emotion, including feelings of helplessness, guilt, and strained family dynamics (Pehlivan et al. 2024). The process of attempting to adapt to the situation often reshapes family relationships, creating a dynamic interplay of tension and support. Caregivers often struggle to find the right balance between providing adequate support and avoiding actions that may be perceived as intrusive or counterproductive, insidiously exacerbating the symptoms of DEAB (Kumar et al. 2024). Additionally, the lived experience of caregivers is frequently characterized by alterations to their worldview, relationships, and sense of identity (Highet et al. 2005). Societal misconceptions about dysfunctional eating attitudes and behaviors, coupled with a dearth of comprehension regarding their etiology and treatment, further foster feelings of isolation and blame among caregivers (Treasure and Schmidt 2013). Furthermore, a significant number of caregivers report feelings of being marginalized within the care process and a lack of guidance from professionals (Determeijer et al. 2024). Organizational obstacles, including fragmented care delivery, lack of coordination between services, and inadequate training of healthcare providers on engaging with caregivers, may impede effective collaboration. This is a regrettable circumstance, given that available research highlights caregivers' participation may alleviate some of the pressure on healthcare systems bridging gaps in care (Stephenson et al. 2022).

1.2 Identifying and addressing caregivers' needs

Although caregivers may have distinctive requirements and expectations, they also exhibit commonalities. This encompasses the necessity for transparent and detailed information regarding the disorder in question, including its underlying causes, symptoms, potential progression, and treatment options (Lin et al. 2018). Beyond receiving information, caregivers benefit from acquiring practical skills such as effective communication with their loved ones and healthcare providers, techniques for managing crises, and strategies to promote treatment adherence. Additionally, caregivers require assistance in navigating the healthcare system and accessing available resources. In particular, caregivers need to feel listened to and acknowledged. Furthermore, they aspire to establish trusting relationships with healthcare providers and to play an active role in the care process for their loved ones (Cree et al. 2015). To provide effective long-term assistance for their loved ones, caregivers need to reassess and adjust beliefs and expectations about the loved one, to recognize and accept their limitations, while valuing their strengths and resources (Izal 2005). Furthermore, caregivers have to recognize and change unrealistic expectations one may have about one's own abilities to care for and solve all problems.

Caregivers also need social and emotional support. Therefore, they need to work on building a support network. Such a network has to be strong enough to allow them to cope with ongoing stress, feelings of isolation, negative emotions related to guilt, and moral exhaustion, as well as catastrophic thoughts and self-stigmatization, which further aggravates isolation. As early as possible, caregivers should be given the opportunity to meet and work with other families in a similar situation. Joining a support group, participating in a psychoeducational program or in a training with other caregivers allow them to meet others going through similar challenges and offer a place to feel understood and less lonely. The relationships built on such occasions are often strong and lasting and help structure the caregivers' network. Furthermore, engaging with family associations is a way to meet volunteers, who have previously benefited from support themselves. Volunteers inspire hope and encourage caregivers to engage in a lasting support process.

Eventually, it is important for them to achieve a balance between caregiving responsibilities and the maintenance of their own well-being. This process involves cultivating healthy coping mechanisms, seeking professional assistance to manage stressful situations and negative emotions (Bighelli et al. 2021). By learning to take care of oneself, caregivers not only do something beneficial for themselves, they also ensure their ability to provide lasting support to their loved one. However, few caregivers initially grant themselves this freedom: they always prioritize supporting their loved one and consider their own well-being as secondary. Their natural tendency is to consider that they don't have time to devote to their own well-being. Without appropriate support, most of the caregivers are not aware that taking care of themselves is also beneficial to the support they provide to their loved one.

2. Empirical and clinical support

2.1 A model for structuring comprehensive clinical support for caregivers

International and national guidelines and recommendations advocate for early, systematic and sustainable support for caregivers (MacCourt 2013, NICE 2020). Strategically, support interventions should be designed to address the dynamic needs and evolving expectations of caregivers while providing sustainable solutions. Services should thus be conceptualized as a continuous support pathway, ensuring ongoing assistance tailored to caregivers' changing circumstances. The "Family care pyramid", developed in Australia in 2005, is consistent with these requirements and provides a template on which healthcare professionals can base their everyday practice with caregivers (Mottaghipour and Bickerton 2005) (Figure 1).

The *Family Care Pyramid* provides a structured, integrated and flexible framework to organize caregiver support through five levels of interventions, ranging from foundational to highly specialized. It may be adapted to the specificities of diverse healthcare settings (Selick et al. 2017). The first two levels of the pyramid are *Connection and assessment* (level 1) and *General education* (level 2). They serve as the cornerstone of the support system and are universally applicable to all caregivers. These foundational interventions aim to ensure broad access to essential resources and are often implemented collaboratively by healthcare professionals and

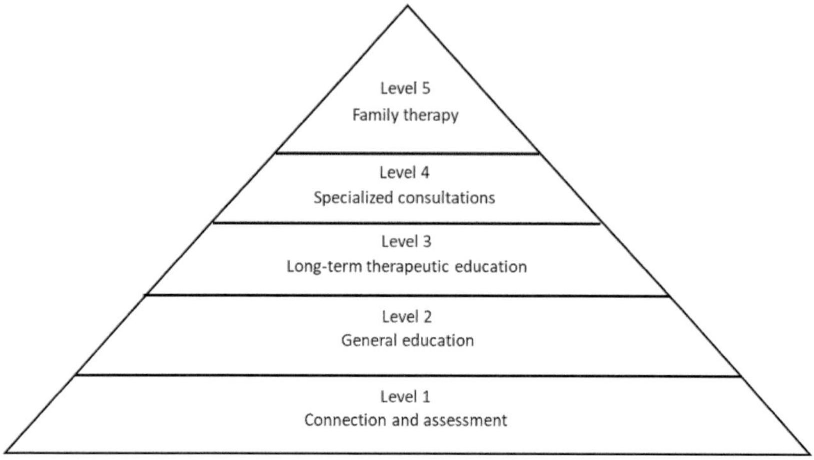

Figure 1. The *Family care pyramid* adapted from Mottaghipour and Bickerton 2005.

family associations. At level 1, interventions focus on welcoming families, actively listening to their concerns, assessing their needs, providing them basic knowledge and skills and connecting them with appropriate resources. Level 2 provides general education on caregiving, offering caregivers a broad understanding of mental health challenges and coping strategies. These foundational levels establish a strong base, allowing caregivers to engage more effectively with advanced interventions. As levels 1 and 2 require minimal training for healthcare professionals and members of family associations, they are the most generalizable interventions and, as such, should be systematically provided to all caregivers. Once the minimum level of support has been provided, caregivers with additional demands may benefit from the three higher levels, if relevant. These higher-level interventions include *long-format therapeutic education*, or psychoeducation (level 3). Advanced psychoeducational programs provide deeper, thematic training for caregivers. These programs typically focus on enhancing communication skills and fostering caregivers' resilience. The *Specialist consultations* level (level 4) address unmet needs through personalized consultations and might involve referrals to other services or practitioners. The *Family therapies* level (level 5) is the pinnacle of the pyramid. These interventions are particularly targeted for families with complex needs requiring multidisciplinary support. They often focus on reshaping family dynamics, improving interactions, and contribute to the integration of caregivers into the treatment process. Notably, advanced interventions (levels 3 to 5) are longer than the initial interventions and more intensive. They are more complex to implement than that of the first two levels and require highly trained facilitators necessitating the investment of a significant amount of time. The successful deployment of caregiver support interventions relies on enhancing healthcare providers' awareness to caregivers needs and critical role, and increasing their competencies to support them.

The availability of support interventions varies significantly depending on the healthcare context of each country. Some countries prioritizing patient- and family-centered care models, such as those in Northern Europe, the United States, Canada, and Australia, have taken the lead in implementing well-structured caregiver support systems (Kokorelias et al. 2019).

2.2 Caregivers support pathways in the context of DEAB

In the context of dysfunctional eating behaviors and attitudes, the need for specialized and consistent support and training for caregivers has become increasingly acknowledged as crucial (Hibbs et al. 2015). Consistently with the *Family Care Pyramid* model, interventions developed to support those caregivers include initial steps focused on welcoming and assessment, as well as more advanced and complex resources, such as advanced psychoeducational interventions, specialized consultations and family-based treatments (Crone et al. 2023). For adolescents living with DEAB, family and multifamily therapies, level 5 interventions, have historically constituted the recommended approach (NICE 2017, Dodge et al. 2024). Such interventions not only address the emotional impact of caregiving but also emphasize active parental involvement in restoring healthy eating behaviors and challenging disordered thoughts (Fisher et al. 2019). The efficacy of these treatments in reducing symptoms, improving treatment adherence and preventing relapse in adolescents with DEAB has been consistently demonstrated (Baudinet and Eisler 2024). A significant strength of family-based treatments is their capacity to establish secure environments for open dialogue, thereby facilitating emotional validation for caregivers and alleviating their burden. Considering the lasting impact of family relationships far beyond adolescence, family and multifamily therapies have been recently adapted and recommended for young adults and their families with DEAB. In case of DEAB, the extension of family-based treatments to young adults acknowledges the ongoing importance of familial relationships during transitional life stages (Dodge et al. 2024). Adapting family therapy principles allows these interventions to address developmental needs and thereby ensuring the intervention's efficacy across different life stages (Dimitropoulos et al. 2015).

The main aims of advanced psychoeducation for caregivers in the context of DEAB are as follows:

- To provide caregivers with a foundational understanding of DEAB, including their causes, symptoms, and potential complications. Such knowledge allows caregivers to gain a deeper comprehension of their loved one's predicament, thereby reducing the distress and burden associated with caregiving, as well as to collaborate with healthcare professionals in a more informed manner (Sadeh-Sharvit et al. 2020).
- To equip caregivers with practical tools for the management of challenging behaviors. This includes strategies for the de-escalation of conflict, the promotion of adherence to treatment and the addressing of triggers for disordered eating behaviors and attitudes. Training interventions may also focus on communication strategies, assisting caregivers in negotiating delicate conversations (e.g., about food restrictions, or body appearance) and cultivating a supportive and non-judgmental environment (Langley et al. 2018).

- To help caregivers recognize the vital importance of self-care and resilience in preventing burnout and sustaining their ability to provide long-term support. Peer-led training programs, which incorporate the lived experiences of caregivers, have demonstrated efficacy in enhancing these competences (Lewis and Foye 2021).

2.3 Potential areas of innovation

Lived experience support in intervention for informal caregivers. Peer mentoring has been shown to inspire hope, promote resilience, and foster recovery through the shared experiences of peers who have navigated similar challenges (Grennan et al. 2022). It can take various forms, such as online support groups, in-person support meetings, chat or mentorship programs (Lewis and Foye 2021). Lived experience support contributes to the creation of a community based on shared understanding, enabling collective advocacy and caregiver empowerment within healthcare systems (Joo et al. 2022). This approach appears to be promising in the context of DEAB (Lefkovits et al. 2024, LaMarre et al. 2024). Recent literature suggests that virtual peer-led support groups help parents feel less isolated and relieved of shame related to their loved ones' condition, while also providing effective coping strategies emotional validation, and informational support for families (Murray et al. 2025). Online support groups also may help build capacity, increase knowledge about DEAB and reduce the caregiver burden. This intervention could be recommended as an adjunctive resource for parents either waiting for professionally-led interventions or following them (Nicula et al. 2023). This type of support complements professional healthcare interventions, particularly in emotionally demanding contexts such as mental health care or chronic illness management. Adequate training, supervision, and ongoing psychological support are essential to protect peer mentors well-being and ensure the sustainability and effectiveness of mentoring programs (Lewis and Foye 2022).

Digital resources and online interventions. Digital tools have become essential in providing support both for users and caregivers, revolutionizing the way assistance and resources are delivered, and enhancing progress towards the implementation of international guidelines regarding support to caregivers. These tools offer accessible, scalable, and customizable support, catering to the diverse and evolving needs of caregivers, thus breaking down barriers of time, geography, and access to resources (Siddiqui et al. 2023). Online e-learning platforms provide accessible, evidence-based information and training programs. National health organizations and services host dedicated websites providing caregivers with essential user-friendly information and guidance materials. Mobile applications, such as *eBREF* in France, further expand the reach of digital support by fostering connectivity between caregivers and accessible dedicated resources, especially family associations, thereby promoting peer-to-peer interaction, seeking advice and building a sense of community among caregivers. As digital tools continue to evolve, they are now playing an increasingly significant role in supporting caregivers. The integration of emerging technologies, such as interactive modules and Artificial Intelligence-driven tools, into existing platforms offers a range of benefits, including personalized feedback, real-time monitoring and predictive insights (Sun and Zhou 2023). As these technologies evolve, they hold significant promise for enhancing both the caregiving experience and the outcomes for those who provide support (Borna et al. 2024).

The integration of in-person and digital strategies allows for the provision of a comprehensive, tailored assistance that is responsive to the diverse needs and profiles of caregivers (Siddiqui et al. 2023).

3. Adaptations to the sociocultural context

3.1 The gradual structuring of support for caregivers in France

In France, support pathways for caregivers in mental health are being progressively structured, integrating resources from healthcare professionals and family associations to create a comprehensive framework. Consistently with the *Family care pyramid*, this framework includes a sequence of increasingly specific and complementary interventions. Currently, foundational and general education support (levels 1 and 2) are not widely available in France, necessitating flexibility in the model. Many caregivers begin at level 3 (long-format therapeutic education or psychoeducation) or level 5 (family therapy). Indeed, specialized, complex interventions have been prioritized in healthcare systems, while users and family associations have focused on addressing immediate family needs.

Most of the general education interventions (level 2) are provided by family associations in France, such as Unafam, the national association of families and friends of individuals living with mental disorders. Training opportunities include general training programs, which feature support groups and workshops led by trained volunteers, sometimes in partnership with healthcare professionals. Topics covered include mental healthcare, legal frameworks, and family rights, giving caregivers a comprehensive understanding of the caregiving landscape. The *Prospect* program, a peer-to-peer empowerment and recovery program developed by Eufami, the federation of European family associations, fosters collaboration, shared learning among caregivers, and mutual comprehension within the mental health ecosystem (EUFAMI). Noteworthily, in addition to the training pathways for caregivers, the *Prospect* program offers a specific pathway for individuals with lived experience, and another one for mental health and social care professionals.

Several level 3, advanced psychoeducational programs addressing the specific and varied needs of caregivers and encouraging mutual support among participants are available, such as *Léo,* a comprehensive toolkit for caregivers of individuals with severe mental health conditions, irrespective of the diagnosis (Lespine et al. 2024), *Profamille,* designed for those supporting individuals with psychotic disorders (Hode et al. 2024), and *Family Connections*, for those who care for individuals with borderline personality (Hoffman et al. 2005). They are delivered in a variety of formats, including in-person workshops, support groups and digital platforms, thereby ensuring accessibility and inclusivity.

In the specific context of DEAB, both national health authorities and the national federation of healthcare professionals in eating disorders (FFAB) advocate for actively involving families in the care pathway of individuals with eating disorders (FFAB-DGOS 2019). Altogether, international and national recommendations converge on a holistic management model, recognizing that supporting families is crucial to achieve lasting recovery (Austin et al. 2023).

While efforts to integrate caregivers into treatment frameworks, and to offer them tailored resources are increasing, much more progress is required to address these challenges in a systematic and sustainable way (Hénaut et al. 2017). Implementing short, early, and cost-effective interventions could be a game-changer, offering a scalable and systematic way to enhance support for caregivers.

3.2 Focus on the BREF-ED Program: An early, short, psychoeducational intervention

In order to facilitate access to support without delays the BREF program was created in 2016 to address the dearth of level 1 interventions to caregivers. BREF was developed through participatory research by the Lyon Center for Caregivers in Psychiatry (CLAP) and the peer-family association *Unafam*, the French national association for families of individual living with mental disorders. The BREF program is an early, individualized and structured support program that serves as an effective initial approach to support caregivers and to guide them through their caregiving journey (Rey 2023). BREF was designed as a short, single-family intervention. It includes three one-hour sessions, facilitated by two healthcare professionals, that address key issues for caregivers, such as information on their loved-one condition, navigation in the healthcare system, and acknowledgment of their role. A trained Unafam volunteer co-facilitates the final session, enriching discussions and fostering peer-to-peer connections. A follow-up three months after the program evaluates participants' progress and encourages ongoing engagement with support systems. By connecting caregivers to family associations and other resources, the program establishes a strong foundation for ongoing support while also improving the coordination and integration of local resources and services, thereby fostering a structured and cohesive caregiver pathway. The BREF program has been adapted to the needs of caregivers of individuals with DEAB, referred as the *BREF-Eating Disorders* (BREF-ED) program (Scanferla et al. 2024). The objective of this program is to facilitate an open environment in which specific concerns about the loved one's dysfunctional eating behaviors and attitudes can be shared. Caregivers' representations regarding DEAB and the healthcare system are explored, thereby facilitating the personalization of support. Practical strategies are introduced with the objective of managing challenging behaviors and supporting the recovery process...

The program adaptation process exemplifies a participatory approach to intervention design, in which input from caregivers, individuals with lived experience of dysfunctional eating, and specialists shaped the program's development. Through this participative process, key topics of interest for caregivers were identified and selected. These topics were used to inform the design of the illustrated cards used during the program to facilitate meaningful exchanges with caregivers. The twenty-eight identified topics were divided into two decks. Deck 1 covers challenges caregivers face directly related to their loved one's symptoms, attitudes and care. In this deck, the cards most frequently selected by caregivers are, in descending order: the relative's fear and anxiety; false-self functioning; ambivalence towards care; body dysmorphia; food restrictions; hyperactivity; denial of symptoms; perfectionism; and consequences of the nutritional deficiencies. Deck 2 focuses on issues affecting the caregivers' own lives and well-being, and the most frequently selected cards are, in descending order: social withdrawal; difficulty navigating the care system; fatigue/helplessness; disruption to family life; guilt; fear for their loved one's future; the relative's fragility; lack of understanding of available care options; and care-related costs. The program's content is structured around these themes, thereby ensuring that it directly addresses the most pressing concerns of those in a caring role. The incorporation of peer support, i.e., people who have lived experience of the disorder, either through personal experience or as caregivers supporting someone living with this disorder, is a distinctive aspect of the BREF-ED program. Indeed, in addition to the volunteer from a family association co-facilitating the last session, one of the two healthcare professionals facilitating each session of the BREF-ED can be a certified peer support worker.

The preliminary outcomes of the BREF-ED program are promising. In a recent study (Scanferla et al. 2025), caregivers attending the program reported notable improvements by the end of the third session and at the three-month follow-up: a significant reduction in depressive symptoms was observed, accompanied by a significant decrease in the emotional burden typically felt by caregivers. In terms of qualitative assessment, participants valued particularly its individualized approach, addressing relevant needs of participants, and its dual emphasis on professional expertise and peer insights. Overall, the BREF-ED program key strengths include:

- *Accessibility*: resource-efficient format, compatible with health services with limited human and financial resources, this program can be widely offered;
- *Customization*: the program can be easily tailored to the specific caregiving dynamics within each family;
- *Peer support integration*: this provides hope, reassurance and a supportive network on the long term.

These strengths position the BREF-ED program as an innovative model that effectively addresses key barriers in supporting caregivers early and systematically, particularly given that traditional family psychoeducation models are often lengthy and resource-intensive. As the demand for effective, scalable, time- and resource-efficient interventions for caregivers grows, BREF-ED's innovative model offers a blueprint for addressing these needs and represents a valuable addition to the existing mental health frameworks, in France and beyond.

Conclusion

Informal caregivers play a crucial role in supporting individuals with dysfunctional eating attitudes and behaviors. While indispensable, this role often entails considerable emotional, physical, and financial strain. Tailored interventions—such as the

BREF-ED, an early, brief, psychoeducational program—help alleviate caregiver distress, enhance resilience, and connect caregivers to a structured, coherent and sustainable pathway. Incorporating peer support from individuals with lived experience adds depth to these interventions by fostering hope, empowerment, and a shared sense of understanding within supportive networks. To amplify their reach, future efforts should prioritize broader access to caregiver support, promote the integration of digital tools, and encourage collaboration among healthcare professionals, caregivers, and family associations.

A holistic approach to caregiver support is vital for cultivating environments where families feel equipped and confident throughout the care journey. Meaningful assistance not only strengthens caregivers' ability to provide sustained support but also empowers them to advocate for systemic improvements. This advocacy can drive policy change, expand available resources, and advance a more inclusive, responsive, and comprehensive model of care.

Acknowledgments

The authors warmly thank UNAFAM, the French national association of families and friends of individuals living with mental disorders, for contributing their time and experiences to the development of the BREF program and for their continued support.

References

Andrade, C., M. Tavares, H. Soares, F. Coelho and C. Tomás. 2022. Positive mental health and mental health literacy of informal caregivers: a scoping review. Int. J. Environ. Res. Public Health 19: 15276.

Applebaum, A.J. and T.S. Sannes. 2025. The importance of honoring family caregiver burden: challenges in mental health care delivery. J. Clin. Psychol. Med. Settings 32: 193–201.

Austin, A., U.D. Silva, C. Ilesanmi, T. Likitabhorn, I. Miller, M. da L.S Fialho et al. 2023. International consensus on patient-centred outcomes in eating disorders. Lancet Psychiatry 10: 966–973.

Baudinet, J. and I. Eisler. 2024. Multi-family therapy for eating disorders across the lifespan. Curr. Psychiatry Rep. 26: 323–329.

Bighelli, I., A. Rodolico, H. García-Mieres, G. Pitschel-Walz, W.-P. Hansen, J. Schneider-Thomas et al. 2021. Psychosocial and psychological interventions for relapse prevention in schizophrenia: a systematic review and network meta-analysis. Lancet Psychiatry 8: 969–980.

Borna, S., M.J. Maniaci, C.R. Haider, C.A. Gomez-Cabello, S.M. Pressman, S.A. Haider et al. 2024. Artificial intelligence support for informal patient caregivers: a systematic review. Bioengineering 11: 483.

Bremmers, L.G.M., I.N. Fabbricotti, E.S. Gräler, C.A. Uyl-de Groot and L. Hakkaart-van Roijen. 2022. Assessing the impact of caregiving on informal caregivers of adults with a mental disorder in OECD countries: A systematic literature review of concepts and their respective questionnaires. Plos One 17.

Bremmers, L.G.M., I.N. Fabbricotti, E.S. Gräler, C.A. Uyl-de Groot and L. Hakkaart-van Roijen. 2024. The impact of informal care provision on the quality of life of adults caring for persons with mental health problems: A cross-sectional assessment of caregiver quality of life. Health Psychol. Open. 11: 20551029241262883.

Del Castillo, F.A. 2024. Valuing informal care and recognizing care as foundational. J. Public Health. 46: e344–e345.

Cree, L., H.L. Brooks, K. Berzins, C. Fraser, K. Lovell and P. Bee. 2015. Carers' experiences of involvement in care planning: a qualitative exploration of the facilitators and barriers to engagement with mental health services. BMC Psychiatry 15: 208.

Crone, C., L.J. Fochtmann, E. Attia, R. Boland, J. Escobar, V. Fornari et al. 2023. The American Psychiatric association practice guideline for the treatment of patients with eating disorders. Am. J. Psychiatry 180: 167–171.

Determeijer, J.J., J.D. van Waard, S.J. Leopold, R. Spijker, C. Agyemang and M. van Vugt. 2024. The barriers and facilitators family caregivers experience when participating in resource-limited hospital care: a qualitative systematic review. BMJ Glob. Health. 9: e015956.

Dimitropoulos, G., A. Toulany, J. Herschman, A. Kovacs, C. Steinegger, J. Bardsley et al. 2015. A qualitative study on the experiences of young adults with eating disorders transferring from pediatric to adult care. Eat. Disord. 23: 144–162.

Dodge, E., J. Baudinet, A. Austin, I. Eisler, D. Le Grange and G. Dimitropoulos. 2024. Family therapy for emerging adults with anorexia nervosa: Expert opinion on evidence, practice considerations, and future directions. Eur. Eat. Disord. Rev. 1–11

EUFAMI. EUFAMI's Prospect Training (unpublished data).

Fisher, C.A., S. Skocic, S. Rutherford and S.E. Hetrick. 2019. Family therapy approaches for anorexia nervosa. Cochrane Database Syst. Rev. 5: CD004780.

George, E.S., M. Kecmanovic, T. Meade and G.S. Kolt. 2020. Psychological distress among carers and the moderating effects of social support. BMC Psychiatry 20: 154.

Grennan, L., M. Nicula, D. Pellegrini, K. Giuliani, E. Crews, C. Webb et al. 2022. "I'm not alone": a qualitative report of experiences among parents of children with eating disorders attending virtual parent-led peer support groups. J. Eat. Disord. 10: 195.

Gupta, S., G. Isherwood, K. Jones and K. van Impe. 2015. Assessing health status in informal schizophrenia caregivers compared with health status in non-caregivers and caregivers of other conditions. BMC Psychiatry 15: 162.

Hénaut, L., J.-C. Sardas and S. Gand. 2017. Aider les proches aidants: Comprendre les besoins et organiser les services sur les territoires. Presses des Mines via OpenEdition.

Hengelaar, A.H., M. van Hartingsveldt, Y. Wittenberg, F. van Etten-Jamaludin, R. Kwekkeboom and T. Satink. 2018. Exploring the collaboration between formal and informal care from the professional perspective—A thematic synthesis. Health Soc. Care Community 26: 474–485.

Hibbs, R., N. Magill, E. Goddard, C. Rhind, S. Raenker, P. Macdonald et al. 2015. Clinical effectiveness of a skills training intervention for caregivers in improving patient and caregiver health following in-patient treatment for severe anorexia nervosa: pragmatic randomised controlled trial. B.J. Psych. Open. 1: 56–66.

Highet, N., M. Thompson and R.M. King. 2005. The experience of living with a person with an eating disorder: the impact on the carers. Eat. Disord. 13: 327–344.

Hode, Y., R. Padovani, W. Hikmat, N. Guillard-Bouhet, J. Attal, M.-C. Bralet et al. 2024. Family psychoeducation in schizophrenia and schizophrenia related disorder, treatment compliance, and suicidal risk reduction: questions about their relationship from a naturalistic observation. Front. Psychiatry 15.

Hoffman, P.D., A.E. Fruzzetti, E. Buteau, E.R. Neiditch, D. Penney, M.L. Bruce et al. 2005. Family connections: a program for relatives of persons with borderline personality disorder. Fam. Process. 44: 217–225.

Izal, M., I. Montorio, M. Marquez and A. Losada. 2005. Caregivers' expectations and care receivers' competence: Lawton's ecological model of adaptation and aging revisited. Arch. Gerontol. Geriatr. 41: 129–140.

Joo, J.H., L. Bone, J. Forte, E. Kirley, T. Lynch and H. Aboumatar. 2022. The benefits and challenges of established peer support programmes for patients, informal caregivers, and healthcare providers. Fam. Pract. 39: 903–912.

Kokorelias, K.M., M.A.M. Gignac, G. Naglie and J.L. Cameron. 2019. Towards a universal model of family centered care: a scoping review. BMC Health Serv. Res. 19: 564.

Kumar, A., H. Himmerich, J.L. Keeler and J. Treasure. 2024. A systematic scoping review of carer accommodation in eating disorders. J. Eat. Disord. 12: 143.

LaMarre, A., J. Couturier, G. Dimitropoulos, S. Jones, S. Kumar, N. Obeid et al. 2024. Peer support for eating disorders in Canada: program user perspectives. J. Eat. Disord. 12: 133.

Langley, J., J. Treasure and G. Todd. 2018. Caring for a Loved One with an Eating Disorder: The New Maudsley Skills-Based Training Manual. Routledge, London.

Lefkovits, A.M., G. Pepin, A. Phillipou, S. Giles, J. Rowan and I. Krug. 2024. Striving to support the supporters: A mixed methods evaluation of the strive support groups for caregivers of individuals with an eating disorder. Eur. Eat. Disord. Rev. 32: 880–897.

Lespine, L.-F., B. de Martène, B. Zeltner, B. Chenu, C.D. Berbey and R. Rey. 2024. Leo program, a short multi-family skill-based psychoeducational program for caregivers of relatives living with a severe mental disorder: a retrospective pilot study. Front Psychiatry 15: 1374540.

Lewis, H.K. and U. Foye. 2022. From prevention to peer support: a systematic review exploring the involvement of lived-experience in eating disorder interventions. Ment. Health Rev. J. 27: 1–17.

Lin, E., J. Durbin, D. Guerriere, T. Volpe, A. Selick, J. Kennedy et al. 2018. Assessing care-giving demands, resources and costs of family/friend caregivers for persons with mental health disorders: A scoping review. Health Soc. Care Community 26: 613–634.

Lindt, N., J. van Berkel and B.C. Mulder. 2020. Determinants of overburdening among informal carers: a systematic review. BMC Geriatr. 20: 304.

MacCourt, P. 2013. National guidelines for a comprehensive service system to support family caregivers of adults with mental health problems and illnesses: Directives pancanadiennes en faveur d'un système de prestation de services pour les proches aidants d'adultes ayant une maladie mentale.

McDaid, D. and A.-L. Park. 2022. Understanding the economic value and impacts on informal carers of people living with mental health conditions. Int. J. Environ. Res. Public Health. 19: 2858.

Mittendorfer-Rutz, E., S. Rahman, A. Tanskanen, M. Majak, J. Mehtälä, F. Hoti et al. 2019. Burden for parents of patients with schizophrenia-a nationwide comparative study of parents of offspring with rheumatoid arthritis, multiple sclerosis, epilepsy, and healthy controls. Schizophr. Bull. 45: 794–803.

Mottaghipour, Y. and A. Bickerton. 2005. The Pyramid of Family Care: A framework for family involvement with adult mental health services. Aust. E.J. Adv. Ment. Health. 4: 210–217.

Murray, M.F., J.S. Kandel, R. Rifkin, J. Hendelman, J. Tsen and A.A. Haedt-Matt. 2025. Initial examination of virtual support groups as a resource for caregivers of individuals with eating disorders. Eat. Disord. 1–17.

Eating disorders: recognition and treatment (Nice guideline NG69). 2020. London: National Institute for Health and Care Excellence (NICE).

Supporting adult carers (Nice guidelines 150). 2020. London: National Institute for Health and Care Excellence (NICE).

Nicula, M., L. Grennan, T. Loewen, E. Crews, K. Giuliani, C. Webb et al. 2023. Virtual parent-led peer support groups for parents of children with eating disorders: A mixed methods feasibility study. Int. J. Eat. Disord. 56: 2107–2119.

Pehlivan, M.J., B. Rodgers, J. Schlage, S. Maguire and J. Miskovic-Wheatley. 2024. Characteristics, correlates of burden and support service use of a help-seeking carers of loved ones with an eating disorder. Eur. Eat. Disord. Rev. 32: 458–475.

Phillips, R., M. Durkin, H. Engward, G. Cable and M. Iancu. 2023. The impact of caring for family members with mental illnesses on the caregiver: a scoping review. Health Promot. Int. 38.

Rey, R. 2023. A further step towards early and systematic psychoeducation for caregivers with the BREF program. Eur. Psychiatry 66.

Sadeh-Sharvit, S., M.R. Sacks, C.D. Runfola, C.M. Bulik and J.D. Lock. 2020. Interventions to empower adults with eating disorders and their partners around the transition to parenthood. Fam. Process. 59: 1407–1422.

Scanferla, E., J. de Salle, J. Monthuy-Blanc, R.L. Mancusi, L-F. Lespine, R. Rey et al. 2025. Short-term impact of BREF-ED, an early, single-family psychoeducational programme for caregivers of individuals with eating disorders: A retrospective pilot study. Eur. Psychiatry 68: 1–9.

Scanferla, E., J. de Salle and P. Gorwood. 2024. Adaptation of the brief psychoeducational intervention programme (BREF) for carers of patients with eating disorders. Eur. Psychiatry 67.

Selick, A., J. Durbin, N. Vu, K. O'Connor, T. Volpe and E. Lin. 2017. Barriers and facilitators to implementing family support and education in Early Psychosis Intervention programmes: A systematic review. Early Interv. Psychiatry 11: 365–374.

Siddiqui, F., D. Varghese, P. Singh, S.B. Bayyavarapu, S. Lindsay, D. Chandrasekara et al. 2023. Exploring the digital support needs of caregivers of people with serious mental illness. Proc. 2023 CHI Conference on Human Factors in Computing Systems, 2023. ACM, Hamburg, Germany. 1–16.

Stephenson, A.L., M. Raj, S.C. Thomas, E.E. Sulliva, M.J. DePuccio, B. Fleuren et al. 2022. Reconceptualizing family caregivers as part of the health care team. J. Hosp. Manag. Health Policy. 6.

Sun, G. and Y.-H. Zhou. 2023. AI in healthcare: navigating opportunities and challenges in digital communication. Front. Digit. Health. 5: 1291132.

Surgenor, L.J., S. Dhakal, R. Watterson, B. Lim, M. Kennedy, C. Bulik et al. 2022. Psychosocial and financial impacts for carers of those with eating disorders in New Zealand. J. Eat. Disord. 10: 37.

Treasure, J. and U. Schmidt. 2013. The cognitive-interpersonal maintenance model of anorexia nervosa revisited: a summary of the evidence for cognitive, socio-emotional and interpersonal predisposing and perpetuating factors. J. Eat. Disord. 1: 13.

Zabala, M.J., P. Macdonald and J. Treasure. 2009. Appraisal of caregiving burden expressed emotion and psychological distress in families of people with eating disorders: A systematic review. Eur. Eat. Disord. Rev. 17: 338–349.

Chapter 12

Patient Partner in DEAB Intervention

Experiential Knowledge of the Body

Liette St-Pierre

INTRODUCTION

Anyone living with a health problem acquires experience and becomes something of an expert in their own situation. In addition to having to learn to live *with* their illness, they also have to make decisions that very often have a direct effect on their quality of life. Healthcare professionals must therefore attach importance to the patient, and encourage their participation in the care and services offered. This is where the patient-partner (PP) approach takes on its full meaning and becomes a must in the healthcare field. The experience of members of the eLoriCorps team, a research group working with patients with dysfunctional eating attitudes behaviours (DEAB), is presented in this chapter. The chapter begins with a brief review of the fundamental concepts of the PP approach and an explanation of how the philosophy was implemented within the team. This is followed by concrete examples of PP's involvement in care, to conclude with the importance of supporting such an approach to improve care and services.

1. Conceptual framework

At the turn of the 1980s, the so-called "paternalistic" conception of healthcare frequently used by healthcare professionals was replaced by more patient-centered

Research Unity Loricorps, Montreal Mental Health University Institute Research Center, 7401, rue Hochelaga, H1N 3MG, Montréal, QC, Canada.
Chaire IRISS (chaire interdisciplinaire de recherche et d'intervention dans les services de santé), Université du Québec à Trois-Rivières, Trois-Rivières, QC, Canada.
Email: liette.st-pierre@uqtr.ca

DOI: 10.1201/9781032718125-14

approaches and even migrated towards an approach integrating the patient into the care team (Karazivan et al. 2015, Pomey et al. 2015). The importance given to patients in their care, the efforts made to integrate them into the team as well as their involvement at all levels of the healthcare system are based on a premise that aims to improve, among other things, the health of the population and the quality of care and services offered in the healthcare system (Pomey et al. 2015). At the turn of the 21st century, the health partnership approach opened the door to collaboration between healthcare professionals and patients. Patients were finally able to express their needs and expectations in relation to their health condition, and thus modify the services offered to them. In Quebec, this paradigm shift was made possible by the increase in chronic health problems, the importance attached by the government to mobilizing citizens in the development of health policies, and the democratization of access to information. The recognition of patients' experiential knowledge was a major advance at the time, and opened the door to the possibility of patients being seen as full members of the care team (Abelson et al. 2022, Bird et al. 2020, Goulet et al. 2015, MSSS 2018). Patients, in collaboration with healthcare professionals, are increasingly seen as the people best able to make the best decisions in relation to their life choices based on their health condition (Ibarra 2006, Légaré et al. 2008). The philosophy of care is thus evolving, moving from "doing for" the patient, to "being with" the patient (Stewart 2003). In 2010, a team of researchers at the Université of Montréal developed a model of care that includes the patient as partner (PP). Since then, the Montreal model (Pomey et al. 2015a, b) has been the subject of several clinical and research projects and is now used in several countries. The PP approach recognizes, among other things, that the patient's experiential knowledge is just as important as the professionals' clinical knowledge; that collaboration between professionals and patients is essential to finding solutions that meet the patient's expressed needs; and that an openness to discussion between the different partners enables a better understanding of the issues and challenges of the healthcare system in which clinicians and PPs work, leading to more effective and sustainable solutions. Collaboration and the concept of co (working together) as co-construction, co-management are important elements of the model, and relationships between professionals and PPs need to be dynamic as they evolve over the course of teamwork. The experiential knowledge of the PP (Goulet et al. 2015) in relation to the health problems they experience on a daily basis and throughout their trajectory of care and services represents an important asset for the researchers who developed the Montreal model (Goulet et al. 2015). This concept of the central role that the PP should have throughout the continuum of care, and the philosophy of engaging the PP in their health care process, explains why the members of the eLoriCorps program team chose this model. This model offers an integrated care structure where the PP's experiential knowledge, needs, concerns and life project are recognized, and their care skills developed with the help of team members (Flora et al. 2016, Pomey et al. 2015a, b, Richards et al. 2013).

2. Empirical and clinical support

Since 2011, a team of researchers at the Université du Québec à Trois-Rivières has been developing an outpatient program for DEAB clients. This transdisciplinary team is made up of health and education professionals from various disciplines, including nursing, occupational therapy, health education, psycho-education, psychology and medicine. In order to facilitate the work of each team member, one member takes on the role of "disciplinary facilitator", a person whose mandate is to oversee the team's transdisciplinary work, while ensuring that the reserved acts specific to each professional are respected (Monthuy-Blanc et al. 2022). Co-construction with the PP and all professionals is an essential part of the eLoriCorps program philosophy. Objectives, evaluation methods and interventions, although guided by the same vision, can sometimes differ according to the needs of the PP and the team (Monthuy-Blanc et al. 2022) precisely "reserve" the intervention of disciplines for situations that require it. The intervention team is no longer made up of professionals from the health, humanities or social sciences sectors, but rather of a case manager who is responsible for making appointments and following up with the PP, and who works in close collaboration with the other professionals. Naturally, in certain situations, the needs of the PP may require care and services corresponding to a specific discipline (for example, a doctor or nurse practitioner when a prescription for medication is required), but the vast majority of the PP's follow-up is carried out by the members of the team, regardless of profession. Practitioners thus transcend the "simple" expression of their identity and disciplinary culture (psychologist, physician, etc.) and express or play a role co-constructed according to the needs of the team and the PP, which corresponds to transdisciplinary work (Monthuy-Blanc et al. 2022). Little is known on implemented transdisciplinary work, but it is particularly recommended in the treatment of so-called holistic and complex mental health disorders such as body perception disturbance (BPD) (Golan 2013, Ozier and Henry 2011), so the clientele of the eLoriCorps program is one that fits these criteria. BPD (APA 2013), including specified disorders such as anorexia nervosa, bulimia nervosa, binge eating disorder are defined by persistent and pervasive disturbances in attitudes and behaviors related to eating, weight control and body image (Fairburn 2008, APA 2013). Knowing that recovery is long for the majority of DEAB individuals and that around 50% of people still present BPDs 10 to 20 years after interventions (Fichter et al. 2008) including the PP in the team can be a guarantee of success. It is also important to understand that the act of eating and drinking is part of every human being's daily life, which makes DEAB omnipresent, like a chronicity that sticks to the skin of people who, for the most part, hate their body envelope. The PP's participation in the team is therefore essential, and their knowledge and experience are considered a major source of expertise for the team. The transdisciplinary eLoriCorps program, which lasts approximately 20 weeks, is offered on an outpatient basis to people with a continuum of mild to moderate subclinical and clinical BPDs, referred to by our team as DEAB. With a dimensional focus on the continuum of care (promotion, prevention, screening and treatment), this program offers, among other things, a psychosocial intake/general services for DEAB patients with situational problems generating temporary adjustment difficulties; a privileged self-management service for DEAB patients able to mobilize their strengths and motivate change; and a specific follow-up consultation service, both individual and group, for DEAB patients. The main objective is the holistic recovery of the PP through their power to act, focusing in particular on perceptual and bodily disorders, in order to move towards the living environment and balanced eating. More specifically, this program targets four elements, referred to as active transdisciplinary ingredients: perceptions, relationships, occupations and sensations relating to eating attitudes and behaviors. Briefly, perceptions refer to the way a person perceives their body image. Relationship refers to relationships with others, i.e., how the PP socializes in interactions with family, peers and work colleagues, among others. Occupations are defined by everything the person does in its daily life that gives meaning to their existence. Sensation represents the recognition of bodily sensations such as hunger and satiety signals, body movements and the presence of bodily pain.

By respecting the PP's wishes, they are actively involved in the process of receiving care or services and is always invited to participate in decisions relating to their health. The following paragraphs will attempt to demonstrate the practical application of this approach. Adhering to a model of care in which the PP is the expert in their own situation may seem trivial to some healthcare professionals, but more often than not it comes with its own set of challenges. In fact, before the 2010s, very few university programs presented or promoted the PP approach to future healthcare professionals. Even today, there are still programs that barely touch on this approach. Of course, the place of the resource user is increasingly established in the healthcare field in Quebec (MSSS 2018), yet its integration into daily clinical practice is not acquired by all healthcare professionals. This observation was also made by the eLoriCorps team. It was therefore necessary to think about ways of implementing the PP approach in a concerted way in the program, so that it could occupy its rightful place in the care and services offered.

Awareness of the PP approach was therefore raised and training was designed so that program stakeholders could understand, integrate and adhere to this common aim. The Montreal model (Pomey et al. 2015) was chosen as a basis for reflection and as a foundation to guide choices in connection with the implementation of the PP approach. Naturally, healthcare professionals must adhere to the fundamental values that guide the PP approach in order to subsequently present an interest in working with PP. The importance and added value of PP were never questioned by team members. However, a paradigm shift had to be made, mainly with regard to the PP's leading and decision-making role throughout the program. A number of challenges had to be overcome, including the fact of having to accept that the PP could decide on the objectives to be achieved during the process. The usual schedule set by professionals was disrupted by the need to modulate clinical meetings to take into account the needs of the PP. Some of the more rigid and corporatist professionals had to work on their openness to the PP's place in the team; this approach was sometimes seen as intrusive in their professional practice. Some professionals have even preferred to leave the team, unable to recognize the added value that the PP brings to their journey and recovery. Professionals who have decided to embark on the PP inclusion experience have received educational support to guide them in this new clinical practice. Although acceptance of the new PP role is largely harmonious, there are still daily challenges for those in charge of the program, who have to remind, emphasize and ensure that the PP's voice is always heard, that their opinions are known and that decisions are made with respect for their choices. The qualities required for successful integration of this approach include open-mindedness, good adaptability and an acceptance of not always being the person who guarantees the PP's progress, since they are entitled to take detours, difficult paths and even slow down the pace, before arriving at their goal. They are entitled to explore other avenues even if, in the professional's experience, the path taken presents a risk. You have to be willing to see and do things differently, because there are many paths that can lead to a situation that is acceptable to the PP. The repercussions of the approach for the PP are so positive that the choice naturally appears to be the best way of working with the client. Naturally, regular discussions were held with the team to decide on the deployment of the approach and the strategies to be used to promote the integration of the PP throughout the program. In addition, a consensus was also reached to ensure that the essential activities to be carried out with PP were respected by all healthcare professionals. Indeed, in addition to the philosophy of accompaniment, which calls for PP to be part of the solution to the health problems with which it has to contend, healthcare professionals must also ensure that they encourage the active participation of the people involved in the program. To do this, team members have decided on the team meetings where the PP's presence was essential, and on the activities that would encourage their active involvement.

2.1 PP tools

More than a dozen tools have been developed by the eLoriCorps team to promote the inclusion of PP in the program. Three of these tools are presented in the following pages.

The integrated concept map. The concept map is a visual map designed to present, on one page, a global picture of the problem experienced by the PP and the impact of this problem on their life (the map is used at the beginning and at the end of the program to assess PP progress). Each PP is paired with a healthcare professional - the "case manager" - who becomes responsible for the person's continuum of care and services throughout the program. The PP is invited to take part in a few meetings with the team, and to co-construct a conceptual map covering the program's four active ingredients: perceptions, relationships, sensations, occupations, and in relation to their experience of the BPD. After several meetings, the case manager draws up a precise visual and schematic portrait of the person. The concept map is discussed with the PP and other team members, to ensure a shared understanding of the illustrated concepts and support the approach. A concept map helps to prioritize the information gathered and reflect the patient's authentic overall experience. The discrepancies between the healthcare team's perception and the PP's actual experience open up the discussion, enabling the different points of view to be exchanged, and form the basis for a solid collaboration that takes into account the needs expressed by the PP. At the "concept map presentation" meeting, several team members join the case manager to symbolize the transdisciplinary contribution of the entire team in supporting and accompanying the PP at every stage of the program. The benefits of using the concept map include nuancing the information gathered, reflecting the PP's real-life experience, and identifying additional protective and risk factors. It's an activity that PPs really appreciate because it represents a "high point" for them, as they are able to visualize the extent to which their health problems affect their daily lives. One PP reports "...it's quite impressive to see this image of Me...made by a team......it's as if, for the first time in my life, I can have a picture in front of me that shows my journey, my life, and all the pain and shame I go through every day.....it's not easy to look at....but ...it's Me"

Educational capsules. The eLoriCorps team has also developed a series of educational capsules to illustrate each of the program's active ingredients. This ambitious project drew on the expertise and experience of the PPs and team members. Attractive, visual educational vignettes were created to provide a teaching aid that could be used at any time by PPs. In addition to the visual media available, explanatory and descriptive leaflets can also be consulted by PPs. In a world where the use of technology is of interest to many people, these vignettes make it possible to respond to requests made by PPs regarding the accompanying material available as support throughout their journey, thus facilitating a degree of autonomous management of their health problem. What's more, these educational capsules can be reconsulted when PPs leave the program. The pooling of knowledge advocated in the philosophy of applied and integrated research that values the use of new technologies in health propels the principles of self-care through the development of skills and knowledge to act on one's own health (Gomes Chaves et al. 2021, Huang et al. 2021). The implementation of the content of each capsule mobilizes the experiential knowledge of some PPs who have completed follow-up to support the recovery of other PPs who continue their journey through the program. For example, the practice of breathing techniques can be suggested and demonstrated in a video capsule by a PP. In practical terms, the informative content is delivered by various experts, of which the PPs are an integral part.

The therapeutic letter. The final tool presented in this chapter is the therapeutic letter (Mitchell et al. 2014, Pyle 2006). Team members chose to use this writing strategy, which takes place in the final weeks of the program. This activity is suggested on a voluntary basis, but adherence to this writing exercise was noted for all PPs. Two letters are written, one by the PP and the other by the care team. Some PPs prefer to use art or handicrafts to illustrate the emotions, feelings and sensations they want to share with the team, and this is naturally allowed. With a view to inclusion, pictorial representation is an alternative form of presentation that can sometimes overcome literacy difficulties. Real "works" by way of pictorial or literary representation have captured the attention and emotion of team members. Even if some PPs find it more difficult to write, they agree to share their text, even if it's short and unimaginative, but so representative of their experiences. The power of words, and the choice of words used, are a clear indication of the PPs' investment in and commitment to their life journey within the program. The therapeutic letter written by the PP is given to the team, and it is the PP who decides whether they prefer to read it or simply leave it for the members to read later. The instructions are the same for the PP, who has the choice of when they wish to read the contents of the letter written for him or her. In fact, the case manager signs the letter, but there is always a team discussion to ensure that the content to be addressed to the PP is properly targeted, and that nothing is forgotten about the progress and efforts made by him or her. In the eLoriCorps program, this strategy consolidates the activities carried out in connection with the concept map, and promotes the consolidation of acquired knowledge. The outcomes of this activity are positive for the PP, but even more so for the team members. First of all, it provides meaningful feedback to the PP, sharing and reminding him or her of the highlights of their journey, and acknowledging their skills and experiential knowledge. For team members, receiving the letter written by the PP encourages a pause in which to welcome and accept comments on the entirety of the PP's progress through the different phases of the program. It's as if, for a moment, the team gave itself permission to receive a balm to savor together, courtesy of the PP's journey and their generosity in sharing it. It was also an opportunity to listen to suggestions for improvement based on the PP's experience. The decision to integrate the therapeutic letter into the program gave rise to a great deal of discussion. In fact, some team members and PPs were worried about not knowing what to write in their letter, or how to react when it was handed in. So we had to take the time and be open to discussion, explaining and convincing them to try to do the exercise as simply as possible, without having any precise expectations or putting any pressure on them. The hard work and generosity of the first PPs who took up the "challenge" are to be thanked, as they were immediately enchanted by the strength and power of this medium. Sharing their feelings, emotions and experiences along the way is now an essential part of the program.

2.2 Reflections regarding the PP approach

The PP approach requires everyone's involvement and time to facilitate co-development between the PP and team members. Throughout the program and progressively, the person is accompanied by the team in the development of their PP skills, and is always invited to share their opinion with the various professionals, and to make choices regarding the objectives, activities and meetings suggested to them. In addition, the program provides for voluntary co-development meetings with other PPs, so that they can exchange views with team members and share their comments on the continuum of care and services offered by eLoriCorps. Meetings can be held as a group or individually, depending on the PP's preference. Feedback is shared as a team, with a view to continuous improvement of the program and the continuum of care and services to be offered to the PP. The outcomes and benefits of the PP approach are numerous, both for the PPs and for the healthcare professionals involved in the eLoriCorps program. Comments gathered from PPs illustrate in part the interest and motivation they have in the activities and in the program. For many, this is their first experience in a program where the emphasis is on their interests, opinions and values, as the following comments illustrate: "I was stressed at first because you were always asking me what I am thinking, if I had anything to say... then there was the conceptual map, then I could change the size of the circles and the color...then everyone was okay with it....then I understood that it wasn't like the other times..."; '...it seems that here I don't have to pretend...I can always tell the truth, I'm not judged...'. PPs also say they realize that the suggestions they make can make a difference to other patients in the program. They feel that a concept of value is being created, and these comments echo those of the healthcare professionals. In fact, they mention that the opportunity to work closely with the PP and to adhere to the approach fosters the creation of values in care. In addition, team members point out that working in partnership with PPs promotes an important value for the program: continuous improvement. Much more than just a fashionable concept, continuous improvement is a must for team members, who focus on the most optimal continuum of care and services possible for the PP, and make sure to modify the approaches or activities used if necessary. This integration of the PP into the care team symbolizes the concerted efforts made by the team to offer care and services that meet the needs of the PP. For their part, the comments of professionals are also evocative of the power of this approach in health care: "...it's done...I don't practice the way I did before....I'm now 'tinted' by the approach....and that's so much better!"; "I love the work we do as a team, the exchanges are so rich and authentic, it's even emotional sometimes ...". What's more, the strength of the PP approach also makes it possible to organize the care and services offered to patients with a view to quality, and the positive points that emerge concur with those mentioned by various authors (Flora 2013, Lecocq et al. 2017, MSSS 2018, Ortiz et al. 2020, Pomey et al. 2015a, b, Saraga 2018). These elements include the need to make sense of what they are doing in treatment (both for healthcare professionals and for the PP), to highlight the limits of the intervention and find solutions to improve them, to increase the PP's motivation in the face of treatment and to find solutions to enable a pleasant day-to-day life.

3. Applications to the sociocultural context

The Quebec healthcare system is a public system that provides free services to the population. It is governed by the Ministère de la Santé et des Services sociaux (MSSS), and its mission is to provide quality, safe and accessible care and services to the Quebec population, in order to maintain, restore and improve people's health and well-being. Care and services are offered in a variety of healthcare facilities, ranging from outpatient services (outpatient health clinics: family medicine group, home care: 1st line) to integrated health and social services centers (general hospitals; 2nd line) and university hospital centers (specialized and superspecialized hospitals, e.g., traumatology, forensic psychiatry; 3rd line). The continuity of care of a patient using the healthcare system presents its share of challenges. This is illustrated in the following paragraphs. The first paragraph presents the trajectory in the Quebec healthcare system, followed by the one set up by the eLoriCorps team.

Healthcare trajectory in Quebec. When a patient consults a healthcare professional, they can move through the different levels of service offered, depending on the episode of care. Taking the example of a DEAB patient, it may therefore be possible to meet the patient for an initial assessment in a medical clinic (1st line) where a DEAB diagnosis could be made. A few months after diagnosis, and despite follow-up, the patient may develop a more severe eating disorder requiring an emergency consultation (2nd line). Following a brief hospitalization, the patient may again be monitored in 1st line for some time. After a few months, the patient may develop a more serious, health-threatening problem requiring hospitalization in a specialized or super-specialized setting (3rd line). Throughout this process, the patient remains the same person, but requires different care and services as their health problems evolve. In order to ensure that the follow-up offered to this patient corresponds to their needs, and that the interventions chosen are as appropriate as possible, communications (oral or written) and the availability of the patient record must be accessible and available to all those involved, and they should be able to work collaboratively. However, we have to admit that it is often very complicated for people working in different sectors to take the time to collaborate on a particular case. Heavy workloads and the organization of care and services make inter-sectoral and interdisciplinary work sometimes very complex, forcing some healthcare professionals to work in silos.

The eLoricorps care and service follow-up model. Building on several years of research into care and service trajectories, the IRISSS chair researchers teamed up with researchers from the eLoricorps group to develop a care and service follow-up model for people with a DEAB. The work done by the transdisciplinary team was developed in collaboration with the various team members, while leaving room for the PP, who is the focal point of their own trajectory. eLoriCorps care and services are provided exclusively on an outpatient basis. Initial meetings are used to carry out a summative evaluation of the DEAB person, to explain the program and to decide with the PP whether they wish to integrate and actively participate in the eLoriCorps program. The program usually lasts 18 to 20 weeks, with one meeting per week. In this way, an "ideal" pathway through the program has been devised.

This continuum of care includes the main stages of the program, with "suggested" timeframes for a "normal" pathway. To ensure that the caregivers and the PP had an overall view of the program, it was decided to post the care trajectory on a wall in the clinic, in a locked, confidential room. This trajectory served as a discussion tool and enabled exchanges between team members with a view to assessing the patient's progress as part of their follow-up. A patient identification card is installed on the care trajectory. This card is removable and is moved as the patient progresses through recovery. At the weekly team meeting, a color code is used to illustrate and evaluate each patient's progress. The code is simple: a green circle indicates that everything is going well in the PP's pathway and that they are progressing adequately in the program. A yellow circle is used when the pathway raises questions for the caregiver or the PP. For example, the PP may have been absent for no reason for several weeks and then decide to return. Team members can then discuss the problem with the PP to find solutions to ensure that absences are reduced or no longer occur. Naturally, frank and open discussions are held to understand the issues that led to the absences. Under no circumstances are PPs obliged to finish the program if motivation is no longer there. However, we do need to talk to patients and be ready to adapt solutions as a team to adjust the care and services offered, with the aim of restoring health. Usually, the case manager is the one who puts a yellow circle on the PP's chart, and the team members must then discuss ways of resolving the problem. It's important to understand that this visual method makes it possible to quickly identify the priorities to be addressed in a patient's caseload. So, if there are several yellow circles on the care trajectory, the team meeting leader will manage the time to resolve the issues. Sometimes, PPs are unable to attend team meetings, but it's important to understand that the solutions proposed by the team are presented to the patient so that they can decide with him or her what will be put in place to ensure a better care path. The PP is the one who has the most power over the decision, since it's their journey that is important. It's worth mentioning that the PPs involved in the eLoriCorps program are, for the most part, always very interested in the discussions and suggestions that come from the program's team members. As one PP puts it: "What I really liked about this approach was that you could talk to the people involved even if you didn't agree with them, and that they listened and respected our decisions if we wanted to do things a little differently.... and, in fact, we often realize that maybe they were right... but I....wasn't there yet....so, I needed more time to get there, and I took another route that was more similar to what I am".

Finally, a red code is affixed to the identification card when there is a major problem with the PP's progress. This problem must be referred to the team as quickly as possible. The main cases that have come to our team are hospitalizations for worsening symptoms and program dropouts. Naturally, in the event of hospitalization, the program is paused, but the PP is informed that when they are ready, the eLoriCorps team will be happy to welcome him or her back into the program. It is possible and desirable for a professional member of the care team where the PP is hospitalized to contact a member of the eLoriCorps program. While respecting codes of ethics and data confidentiality, discussions can take place between health system partners and program staff to ensure that the PP's progress is as smooth as possible, and that the care team is aware of the patient's involvement in their care throughout the program. These exchanges take place with a view to publicizing all the recovery work done by the PP and highlighting the efforts, steps and strategies put in place to resolve the health problem.

Continuity of care is a priority for eLoriCorps program staff, and team meetings have always aimed to prioritize interventions that meet the needs of PPs. The care trajectory is therefore a tool for keeping a perspective on the PP's progress towards recovery. It should also be noted that the program is managed by a transdisciplinary team that has appointed a program manager. The program manager manages the administrative side of the program (number of patients monitored, up-to-date patient files, management of caregivers, etc.). This manager represents the strategic side of program planning, development and deployment. With regard to the care trajectory, the program manager ensures that the PP' pathway is properly followed, and that team members address any program management issues to her. The trajectory's color codes enable the manager to ensure that the program is running smoothly and that performance indicators are being met (waiting time, length of sessions, number of drop-outs, reasons for dropping out, PP satisfaction). The issues that need to be addressed at the strategic level relate to the program's mission, vision and values, as well as to the political issues of program deployment and operation. When trajectory issues are dealt with at the strategic level, they usually involve issues that need to be dealt with between different healthcare facilities, or with healthcare professionals who want to obtain information about PP followed in the program. Clinical facilitators are also full members of the eLoriCorps program, and may be involved in PP care, but their main role is that of clinical leader. They act at the tactical level of the trajectory, ensuring that decisions taken at the strategic level can be applied at the operational level. They are also responsible for monitoring the performance indicators used to measure the results of PP interventions.

Conclusion

The active and dynamic involvement of the PP in the intervention among people living with DEAB can have a positive effect on many dimensions during treatment, including improving the level of motivation and involvement in treatment; increasing the sense of empowerment and self-determination; strengthening the therapeutic alliance; facilitating the identification of patients' needs; and identifying possible solutions to treatment problems, limitations and challenges.

Despite the fact that the PP approach is becoming increasingly well known in the healthcare field, it would be wrong to claim that all professionals want to integrate this approach into their practice. Moreover, it must also be understood that the health and social services network in Quebec does not always offer optimal conditions for deploying the PP approach in its services, which sometimes makes it more difficult for care teams to collaborate with PPs (MSSS 2018). Efforts are being made in this direction, but there is still a long way to go and healthcare professionals must capitalize on this approach and take the time to properly integrate these concepts in order to defend the rights of PPs in their continuum of care and services, promote their integration into care teams and thus succeed in offering optimal services for PPs.

For the members of the eLoriCorps team, the initial investment required to understand the foundations of the PP approach is not very costly compared to the positive effects of integrating such an approach into their practice. The time invested in ensuring that each professional understands the central role that the PP plays in their health care pathway is a guarantee of success for the subsequent involvement of the PP in the care and services offered to him or her. Sharing the expertise of PP and healthcare professionals, as well as the collaboration between them, enriches their daily lives, enabling them to co-construct new experiences together, and to become even more attentive to each other. Professionals accept that health is a personal commitment that each person chooses, embodying the priorities they value in their lives. Each person gives meaning to their experiences and co-constructs the steps to be taken in order to live fully, despite the problems that stand in the way. The individual is the sole owner of their own health, and listening to him or her and letting him or her make their own decisions becomes a mark of respect, facilitating support throughout the process and ensuring the success of the approach implemented jointly with him or her. It has become unthinkable to see the patient as anything other than a person whose involvement is commensurate with their importance in daily life. In this way, the strength of the team is increased tenfold by the investment the PP makes in the continuum of care and services. It's worth mentioning, of course, that when the PP joins a team, the team can say without a shadow of a doubt that 1 + 1 = 3, or even that 1 + 1 = 1 when integration is complete.

Acknowledgments

A thank you to all the patient partners with whom I had the chance to share and learn and who helped me grow.

References

Abelson, J., C. Canfield, M. Leslie, M.A. Levasseur, P. Rowland, L. Tripp et al. 2022. Understanding patient partnership in health systems: lessons from the Canadian patient partner survey. BMJ Open 12: e061465.

American Psychiatric Association. 2013. DSM-5: Diagnostic and statistical manual of mental disorders 5e ed. Washington, DC: American Psychiatric Association.

Black, D. and J. Black. 2009. A review of the urban development and transport impacts on public health with particular reference to australia: trans-disciplinary research teams and some research gaps. Int. J. Environ. Res. Public Health 6: 1557–1596.

Bird, M., C. Ouellette, C. Whitmore, L. Li, K. Nair, M.H. McGillion et al. 2020. Preparing for patient partnership: A scoping review of patient partner engagement and evaluation in research. Health Expect. 23: 523–539.

Fairburn, C.G. 2008. Cognitive Behavior Therapy and Eating Disorders. Guilford Press.

Flora, L., A. Berkesse, A. Payot, V. Dumez and P. Karazivan. 2016. L'application d'un modèle intégré de partenariat dans la formation des professionnels de la santé : vers un nouveau paradigme humaniste et éthique de coconstruction des savoirs en santé. J. Int. Bioéthique 27: 59–72.

Flora, L. 2013. Savoirs expérientiels des malades, pratiques collaboratives avec les professionnels de santé : état des lieux. Éducation permanente. 195: 59–72.

Golan, M. 2013. The journey from opposition to recovery from eating disorders: Multidisciplinary model integrating narrative counseling and motivational interviewing in traditional approaches. J. Eat. Disord. 1: 1–8.

Gomes Chaves, B., C. Briand and K. Bouadida. 2021. Innovation in healthcare organizations: concepts and challenges to consider. Int. J. Health Res. Innov. 9: 1–14.

Huang, H., D. Leone, A. Caporuscio and S. Kraus. 2021. Managing intellectual capital in healthcare organizations. a conceptual proposal to promote innovation. J. Intellect. Cap. 22: 290–310.

Ibarra, A. 2006. L'élaboration du projet de vie chez les jeunes adultes, Université de Fribourg.

Karazivan P., V. Dumez, L. Flora, M-P. Pomey, C. Del Grande, D.P. Ghadiri et al. 2015. The patient-as-partner approach in health care: a conceptual framework for a necessary transition. Acad. Med. J. Assoc. Am. Med. Coll. 90: 437–41.

Lecocq, D., H. Lefebvre and A. Néron. 2017. Le patient partenaire. Un modèle pour améliorer l'adhésion aux traitements, la qualité des soins et réduire les coûts. Soins et système de soins. 4: 44–54.

Légaré, F., S. Ratté, K. Gravel and I.D. Graham. 2008. Barriers and facilitators to implementing shared decision-making in clinical practice: update of a systematic review of health professionals' perceptions. Pat. Educ. Couns. 73: 526–535.

Ministère de la Santé et des Services Sociaux. 2018. Cadre de référence de l'approche de partenariat entre les usagers, leurs proches et les acteurs en santé et en services sociaux. Québec : Bibliothèque et Archives nationales du Québec.

Ortiz, H.I., B. Scholtes, B. Voz, N. Gillain, N. Durieux, A. Odero et al. 2020. "Patient participation" and related concepts: A scoping review on their dimensional composition. Patient Educ. Couns. 103: 5–14.

Ozier, A.D. and B.W. Henry. 2011. Position of the American Dietetic Association nutrition intervention in the treatment of eating disorders. J. Am. Diet. Assoc. 111: 1236–1241.

Mitchell, P., P. Rhodes, A. Wallis and V. Wilson. 2014. A comparison of two systemic family therapy reflecting team interventions. J. Fam. Ther. 36: 237–254.

Monthuy-Blanc, J., M-J. St-Pierre, J. Ménard and L. St-Pierre. 2022. La transdisciplinarité en santé, la puissance plutôt que l'absence des disciplines. Ann. Méd. Psychol. 180: 350–359.

Pomey, M-P., L. Flora, P. Karazivan, V. Dumez, P. Lebel, M-C. Vanier et al. 2015a. Le «Montreal model» : enjeux du partenariat relationnel entre patients et professionnels de la santé. SP. 1: 41–50.

Pomey, M.-P., H. Hihat, M. Khalifa, P. Lebel, A. Néron and V. Dumez. 2015b. Patient partnership in quality improvement of healthcare services: Patients' inputs and challenges faced. Patient Exp. J. 2: 29–42.

Pyle, N.R. 2006. Therapeutic letters in counselling practice: client and counsellor experiences. Can. J. Couns. 40: 1, 17–31.

Richards, T., V.M. Montori, F. Godlee, P. Lapsley and D. Paul. 2013. Let the patient revolution begin. BMJ 346: f2614.

Saraga, M. 2018. Transparence, transfert et patient partenaire. Psycho-Oncol. 12: 24–28.

Stewart, M. 2003. Patient-Centered Medicine: Transforming the Clinical Method, Abingdon, Radcliffe Medical.

Chapter 13

Bodies in Context

How Gender and Sexuality Shape Body Perception Disturbances and Dysfunctional Eating Attitudes and Behaviors

Georg Halbeisen and *Georgios Paslakis**

INTRODUCTION

Body perception disturbances (BPD) are considered core symptoms underlying the development and maintenance of dysfunctional eating attitudes and behaviors (DEAB) (American Psychiatric Association 2013). The over-evaluation of body weight and shape, and the preoccupation with controlling them, can lead to extreme body shaping and dieting behaviors, including severe dietary restraint, excessive exercising, purging, laxative abuse, and loss-of-control (binge) eating (Fairburn et al. 2003). Historically, BPD and DEAB have been conceptualized in reference to a thin body ideal, i.e., a slender figure coupled with low body fat and a toned physique, which especially heterosexual women in Western countries continue to internalize through exposure to media portrayals and social media use (Paterna et al. 2021). However, there is an increasing recognition that the preeminence of the thin ideal could delay the detection of DEAB in Sexual and Gender Minority

University Clinic for Psychosomatic Medicine and Psychotherapy, Medical Faculty, Campus East-Westphalia, Ruhr-University Bochum, Virchowstr. 65, 32312 Luebbecke, Germany.
Email: georg.halbeisen@rub.de
* Corresponding author: georgios.paslakis@rub.de

DOI: 10.1201/9781032718125-15

(SGM) populations and that diverse body ideals and concerns are increasingly prevalent across different social groups (Halbeisen et al. 2022). In fact, past research consistently shows that adults and adolescents in SGM populations, e.g., people that identify as lesbian, gay, bisexual, trans*, queer, and intersex, tend to be at greater risk for DEAB when compared to their heterosexual and cisgender counterparts (Parker and Harriger 2020). DEAB incidence has also increased in recent years among men, older adults, underrepresented ethnic groups, and adults with intellectual disabilities (Halbeisen et al. 2022). These socio-demographical shifts, among other things, point to a critical role of gender and sexuality in DEAB etiology and to potential opportunities and challenges in DEAB care.

This chapter focusses on the roles of gender and sexuality in BPD and DEAB presentation. The first part outlines prominent theoretical models that link gender and sexuality in SGM populations to qualitative differences in BPD and to the increased prevalence rates of DEAB. We argue that these models offer a conceptual framework for advancing our understanding of DEAB presentation beyond SGM populations. The second part reviews empirical evidence that investigated the roles of gender and sexuality in DEAB presentation, comorbidities, and overarching contextual factors that attenuate or aggravate sexuality- and gender-based differences. Finally, in the third part, we turn our attention toward gender and sexuality in DEAB treatment in Germany and discuss the emerging challenges for improving medical education and care.

1. Conceptual framework

1.1 The minority stress model

How do gender and sexuality link to variations in BPD and DEAB? One prominent idea is that increased levels of stigma-related stress experienced among SGM populations increase the risk for mental health problems. Specifically, the minority stress model assumes that stress can originate from experiencing prejudice and discrimination based on one's socio-economic status, race, ethnicity, gender, or sexuality (Frost and Meyer 2023). Unlike everyday stress (e.g., when needing to meet a deadline), minority stress is considered unique in that it is experienced by stigmatized groups in addition to everyday stress, and in that it is more enduring (chronic) due to the social structures that perpetuate stigmatization (Frost and Meyer 2023). Individuals from SGM populations may experience stress "distally" from discriminatory policies or institutions (e.g., transgender people needing to undergo psychiatric evaluations to change their name and gender status), and from being discriminated against overtly or covertly (e.g., a physician not taking DEAB symptoms seriously based on the "looks" of a patient). Moreover, SGM populations experience stress "proximally" from anxiously expecting negative reactions and social rejection (Rood et al. 2016), from internalizing socially perpetuated prejudicial attitudes (e.g., "homonegativity") (Berg et al. 2016), or from needing to conceal one's (non-conforming) gender identity or sexual orientation (Rood et al. 2017). The psychological consequences of these stressors, such as increased rumination tendencies and feelings of hopelessness, are assumed to directly increase the risk of developing psychopathologies (Hatzenbuehler

2009) and to aggravate existing psychopathologies by interfering with help-seeking behaviors (Spengler et al. 2023).

The minority stress model has been influential in understanding health disparities in SGM compared to cisgender and heterosexual populations (Frost and Meyer 2023). To the extent that minority stress explicitly relates to body image and eating behaviors, it also provides a plausible model for increased prevalence rates of BPD and DEAB among SGM populations and their overrepresentation in clinical settings (see Chapter 5).

However, although minority stress is frequently associated with overall reduced mental health in SGM populations and elevated DEAB psychopathology (Parker and Harriger 2020, Santoniccolo and Rollè 2024), it has limited implications for addressing the diversity in BPD and DEAB presentation. The minority stress model does not address why different groups present with different body image concerns and that not all body concerns are created equal. For example, men tend to be less concerned with thinness and seek to increase body mass and muscularity (Lavender et al. 2017). In contrast, trans* women have been found to report higher femininity concerns compared to cisgender women (Mofradidoost and Abolghasemi 2020). By definition, the minority stress model also cannot explain the increasing prevalence rates of BPD and DEAB among cultural majority groups (e.g., among cisgender men and older individuals), although individuals from these groups may experience other forms of discrimination in specific contexts (e.g., cisgender men with disordered eating in health care settings; Richardson and Paslakis 2021). Thus, understanding the diversity in BPD and DEAB presentation requires further considerations.

1.2 The tripartite influence model

The tripartite influence model has been proposed to address how sociocultural factors associated with gender and sexuality can lead to qualitative differences in BPD and DEAB (Thompson et al. 1999). Specifically, the model and later extensions propose that different body ideals are internalized due to the constant appearance-related pressures encountered by peers, family members, and the media (Tylka 2011). For heterosexual women in Western cultures, having a thin and slender body remains the dominant body ideal (Mingoia et al. 2017). In contrast, heterosexual men in Western cultures tend to internalize a lean, albeit muscular, and athletic body ideal (Paterna et al. 2021). Due to the often unrealistic or extreme nature of appearance ideals, internalization, in turn, increases the chances for unfavorable comparisons and dissatisfaction with body fat or muscularity, which then leads to disordered eating and other forms of body-shaping behaviors (Schaefer et al. 2015).

Consistent with the historical research focus, the tripartite influence model has been extensively explored and validated among girls and young women (Rodgers et al. 2011). However, because appearance pressures are assumed to vary with peer, media, and family influences, and because peer, media, and family influences differ by gender and sexuality (Lanzieri and Cook 2013), it is also a suitable model for addressing qualitative differences in BPD and DEAB in groups other than (cisgender) women. Studies with SGM populations show that, among heterosexual and gay adult men, both thinness- and muscularity-oriented appearance processes contribute to DEAB (Tylka and Andorka 2012, Schaefer et al. 2021). Links between peer pressures and body dissatisfaction are pronounced in lesbian and bisexual women, suggesting that some SGM communities could be more prone to reinforcing societal expectations around ideal body types; however, the structure of processes remains similar (i.e., internalization processes mediate between appearance pressures and disordered eating symptoms; Hazzard et al. 2019).

One US-based study recently corroborated that, on average, thin-ideal internalization and media pressures are particularly pronounced in people seeking men as partners (heterosexual women and gay men), showing the importance of male partner pressures and possibly self-objectification (Fredrickson and Roberts 1997). In comparison, muscular-ideal internalization is pronounced in heterosexual men, and Black men especially (Frederick et al. 2022). The latter observation hints at the importance of also considering intersecting identities for understanding BPD, as the endorsement of prototypically male body ideals could be a way of asserting a fragile masculine gender identity that is threatened, for example, by experiencing ethnicity-based prejudice and discrimination (Frederick et al. 2017).

1.3 Towards a social-ecological framework

Taken together, the evidence favoring the minority stress model and the tripartite influence model suggests that sexual and gendered social ecologies in which people live are important determinants of BPD and DEAB. The minority stress model highlights how overarching, contextual factors interact with gender and sexuality to create adverse conditions that favor the development of BPD and DEAB (Frost and Meyer 2023). That is, the gender and sexuality of people interact with population structures, healthcare policies, and cultural beliefs that lie largely outside of an individual´s control, which predisposes for discriminatory experiences. In comparisons, the tripartite influence model focuses prominently on the more active roles of sexuality and gender in shaping immediate social interactions and comparisons on an interpersonal level; that is, gender and sexuality affect which media people consume, their family interactions, which peers and partners they engage with, and which body ideals they internalize. Thus, both the context in which people's bodies are put in, and the interactions their bodies create are important factors for how gender and sexuality shape BPD and DEAB.

Interestingly, and highlighting the utility of an integrative perspective (see also Barnhart et al. 2022), processes related to contextual and interpersonal levels appear to reinforce each other in SGM populations. For example, although engagement with SGM peer communities can be understood as an adaptive response to coping with stress due to heterosexist discrimination, engagement with peer communities among SGM populations has been, at times, found to increase rather than buffer against appearance-related comparison pressures (Convertino et al. 2021). In other words, engaging with peer communities can provide support and affirmation but also contribute to BPD and DEAB, potentially creating a vicious cycle in which minority discrimination and peer pressures converge (Nagata et al. 2024).

However, we would argue that processes described within an integrative perspective also offer a conceptual framework for advancing our understanding of BPD and DEAB presentation beyond SGM populations. As addressed earlier, DEAB incidence also increases among men, older adults, and underrepresented ethnic groups (Halbeisen et al. 2022). Thus, there may be challenges for DEAB detection and access to care in other populations that have also rarely been considered in previous research. Moreover, although SGM populations may experience minority stress, both SGM and cisgender populations face overarching adversities that could interact with gender and sexuality to create or aggravate mental health conditions (e.g., climate change, global pandemics, and loneliness). Thus, in exploring the role of gender and sexuality in disordered eating, it could be fruitful to consider a broader range of contextual factors.

In the next part of this chapter, we review empirical evidence that investigated the role of gender and sexuality in DEAB presentation and comorbidities, and that considered further contextual factors that attenuate or aggravate sexuality- and gender-based differences.

2. Empirical and clinical support

2.1 Gender and sexuality in DEAB presentation

It is crucial to advance our understanding of the diverse forms of DEAB presentation to improve clinical assessments and people's access to care. There is concern among healthcare professionals that DEAB symptoms could often go unnoticed due to differences in presentation across diverse gender and sexuality groups (Matsumoto and Rodgers 2020). Indeed, most standard psychopathology assessments and diagnostic criteria were developed based on DEAB presentation in girls and young women and usually do not assess symptoms potentially more relevant in other populations, including SGM. Factor analyses have confirmed these validity concerns among standard disordered eating assessments for men and SGM populations (Laskowski et al. 2023, Nagata et al. 2024), highlighting the need to consider a broader range of symptoms.

One increasingly popular approach for analyzing DEAB presentation is network analysis (Tomei et al. 2022). Network analyses visualize specific symptoms (e.g., body dissatisfaction, driven exercise, binge eating) and their associations. The arrangement of symptoms can be evaluated to detect clusters of highly associated symptoms, similar to factors in factor analyses, and to quantify how strongly individual symptoms (such as body dissatisfaction) "activate" other disordered eating cognitions and behaviors.

A systematic review of 25 network analyses among women with diagnosed eating disorders found overvaluation of body shape and weight and cognitive restraint to be most influential (i.e., associated with other symptoms), consistent with diagnostic criteria, together with feelings of ineffectiveness, lower interoceptive awareness, and emotional regulation difficulties (Monteleone and Cascino 2021). Network analyses with men are rare, but their findings point to a more central role of muscularity concerns, consistent with predominant cultural ideals (Paterna et al.

2021). For example, among men, the guilt associated with missed training sessions and the use of supplements were closely associated with core DEAB symptoms, such as weight and shape overvaluation and the fear of losing control over eating (Forrest et al. 2019). Similarly, muscularity-related attitudes and behaviors emerged as central next to weight and shape overvaluation and leanness concerns in male and female adolescent symptom networks (Prnjak et al. 2021).

We recently expanded upon these findings by analyzing associations with disordered eating symptoms beyond stereotypically male and female presentations (Eschrich et al. 2024, Jürgensen et al. 2025). Specifically, we further included symptoms regarding the obsessive preoccupation with healthy eating (Orthorexia Nervosa) as well as symptoms of Avoidant/Restrictive Food Intake Disorder (ARFID), which are independent of specific body image concerns. The results showed that muscularity concerns still emerged as central in men's and women's disordered eating networks. However, we also found a symptom cluster of body shaping and rule-based dieting behaviors beyond muscularity-related manifestations in men (i.e., related to healthy eating), separate from "thin ideal" dieting and weight-control behaviors such as counting calories or restricting food intake. These findings suggest that DEAB presentation could be more heterogeneous than previously assumed and that it is not limited to conforming to either just thin or muscular body ideals.

The literature thus far has been predominantly concerned with exploring gender-based differences in DEAB presentation, and we are not aware of similar systematic comparisons of symptom structures based on sexuality or other identity features. Nonetheless, several disordered eating assessments have been developed that focus on attitudes and behaviors toward increasing muscle size and definition (Eschrich et al. 2024), and norms for popular eating disorders symptom scales are also available for SGM populations (Nagata et al. 2024), providing a solution until more specific and inclusive disordered eating assessments have been developed.

2.2 Gender and sexuality in DEAB comorbidities

Psychiatric comorbidities are common in individuals with eating disorders (Ulfvebrand et al. 2015), with some differences based on sexuality and gender. For example, DEAB has been frequently associated with autistic traits and autism spectrum disorders, especially among women (Barnett et al. 2021), although it is currently unclear if these effects are genuine or due to gendered assessment biases (see above). Autism and autistic traits are also more frequent among SGM compared to cisgender populations (Warrier et al. 2020), suggesting a potential for interconnections between gender and sexuality in autistic comorbidity. Similarly, individuals with borderline personality disorder, display higher rates of "sexual identity disturbances" (Frías et al. 2016), and the comorbidity with eating disorders is found more often in women compared with men (Qian et al. 2022). We again cannot exclude diagnostic biases, but the available evidence nevertheless points towards the potential of exploring the interconnections between gender, sexuality, disordered eating, and borderline personality disorder more closely.

Recent studies further show associations between sexuality, gender, and general psychopathology in patients with eating disorders. One retrospective chart review among sexual minority adolescents and young adults found higher rates of depression, anxiety, post-traumatic stress disorder, and self-injury behaviors compared to their heterosexual counterparts (Chaphekar et al. 2023). Similar patterns were observed when comparing transgender youths to cisgender boys and girls with eating disorders (Baker et al. 2024). Another study showed that depressive symptoms were associated with increases in caloric restriction, diet pill use, purging, laxatives, and binge eating, suggesting a critical role of general psychopathology and comorbidities in disordered eating development in SGM youths (Roberts et al. 2022).

Because young men and women appear increasingly concerned with body muscularity, we recently explored gender differences in the link between body image disturbances, disordered eating, and the use of anabolic androgenic steroids (Zaiser et al. 2024). These compounds contain derivatives of testosterone and are predominantly utilized within sports contexts to augment muscle size and definition, as well as to improve athletic performance. The synthesis of 22 studies showed that men were more likely to use anabolic steroids and that non-heterosexual men reported higher lifetime use compared to heterosexual men. DEAB risk increased in individuals using anabolic steroids. Only one study compared associations between anabolic steroids use and DEAB by gender, finding comparable detrimental effects across men and women. Studies that investigated the effects of anabolic steroids use thus far did not distinguish between cisgender and SGM populations. However, given the increased usage rates of other (legal) appearance and performance-enhancing supplements among transgender men, gender-expansive people, and transgender women (Nagata et al. 2022), we might expect at least similar associations with body image disturbances and disordered eating.

2.3 The interplay of gender and sexuality with overarching adversities

Both SGM and cisgender populations face overarching challenges that could interact with gender and sexuality to create or aggravate mental health conditions, including BPD and DEAB. For example, the COVID-19 pandemic has led to food shortages, increased food prices, and loss of income, i.e., food insecurity, which has been linked to predisposing or exacerbating disordered eating in children and adolescents (Paslakis et al. 2021). Households headed by women are particularly vulnerable to food insecurity (Jung et al. 2017). Thus, gender disparities in DEAB may have increased during the COVID-19 pandemic.

In a recent systematic review conducted during the first half of the pandemic, we found large increases in the number of hospitalizations and DEAB symptoms, anxiety, and depression in people with eating disorders during the COVID-19 pandemic (Devoe et al. 2023). Qualitative studies attributed this deterioration to decreased access to care and treatment, changes in routines and loss of structure, a negative influence by the media, and social isolation. Unfortunately, there was a lack of diversity in terms of sexualities and genders in the samples of the included studies, calling for further research on the impact of the COVID-19 pandemic as a contextual factor on gender- and sexual orientation-related disparities in disordered eating. Still, according to another synthesis of systematic reviews of our group (Laskowski et al. 2024), women and SGM populations, although overall underrepresented in COVID-19-related research, experienced increased mental health problems during the COVID-19 pandemic compared to cisgender men and the general population, respectively. Another systematic review specifically reported increased DEAB symptoms in SGM populations, which could be attributed to increased exposure to interpersonal pressures, such as weight stigmatization in social media messaging, and non-acceptance of one's sexual identity by family members (Datta and Mukherjee 2023).

In two upcoming reviews with extended databases (Laskowski et al. 2024, 2025), we examined gender differences in DEAB in the general adult population during the COVID-19 pandemic, and gender differences in BPD, respectively. The first review found SGM populations to display highest disordered eating symptom scores when compared to cisgender men and women, and that elevated levels of pandemic-related stress in SGM individuals could be linked to DEAB, corroborating the potentially crucial role of overarching factors in explaining gender- and sexuality-related disordered eating disparities. The second review also found higher levels of weight and body shame in SGM groups and women when compared to (cisgender) men, consistent with the assumed roles of minority stress and societal pressures.

Loneliness following social isolation has also been suspected to be a key variable for explaining the adverse effects of the COVID-19 pandemic, while at the same time, loneliness itself (i.e., independent from pandemic-associated public health measures) has been recognized as a growing public health problem, especially among older adults, including those from SGM populations (Freedman and Nicolle 2020). We recently explored gender differences in patients with eating disorders based on sociodemographic patterns, including potential markers of loneliness such as relationship status and living circumstances (Traut et al. 2023). Using a latent class analysis, we found that men with eating disorders had significantly higher odds than women to belong to a "single-childfree-working" class. Moreover, while there were few overall differences in DEAB-related symptoms and general psychopathology between men and women, single-childfree-working men presented with higher general psychopathology symptoms than men in the other classes. Although the study did not assess loneliness directly, a lack of social support and loneliness might pose a particular vulnerability for DEAB in men. However, the overall evidence seems thus far inconclusive (Meneguzzo et al. 2024), suggesting that more research is needed on the interplay of gender, sexuality, loneliness, and DEAB.

3. Applications to the sociocultural context

The emerging evidence for gender- and sexuality-related disparities in DEAB prevalence and presentation indicates a need to improve current disordered eating assessment and care. There is concern that the overrepresentation of cisgender women in research may have inadvertently facilitated the development of treatment settings geared toward that population, including in Germany (Halbeisen et al. 2022). Although first examples of gender- and SGM-based comparisons suggest overall equality in treatment outcomes, we know that discrimination by healthcare providers is a common experience for trans* individuals and that even cisgender men, otherwise in the majority, face unique challenges accessing or during treatment, often struggling to be understood by therapists, feeling unwanted in the treatment environment, or that their experiences are not taken into account (Richardson and Paslakis 2021). Thus, there is a continuing need to advance our current models of care and its access.

At the interpersonal level, interventions can be designed to help empower individuals to cope with disordered eating and when facing discriminatory experiences (Roberts et al. 2022). At the contextual level, it is crucial to address sources of stigmatization in health care and to improve access to care. Perceiving stigmatization can be a potent barrier to seeking help for disordered eating (Lehe et al. 2024), which health care professionals can (unwittingly) communicate through implicit and explicit biases. Although some biases might be attitudinal, our research suggests that a lack of knowledge on variations in disordered eating presentation may be the most common source of stigmatization among health care professionals.

3.1 The state of German medical education

We recently conducted a first nationwide online survey on SGM healthcare and education among 670 medical students from 33 German universities (Brandt et al. 2022b). Overall, most respondents reported low confidence regarding their medical training sufficiently preparing them for SGM patients, stating that SGM themes were not covered during training and agreeing that the inclusion of such themes is urgently needed. A review of our group on existing SGM-related medical trainings yielded important conclusions on how to design such interventions (Brandt et al. 2022a); even a single-hour lecture can increase students' knowledge. Lectures can be an effective means of imparting knowledge on SGM-related healthcare; nevertheless, to promote attitude change, direct or indirect contact with lived experiences of SGM individuals is essential. For example, this kind of contact can take place as discussion groups with former patients.

3.2 Combatting stigmatization through professional training

It is also important to combat the stigmatization of people with eating disorders among practicing health care professionals. A particularly important group are general practitioners (GPs), who in Germany serve as gatekeepers and entry points to advanced and mental health care. As a starting point, we recently developed an intervention to improve disordered eating assessment and care for men (https://maennermitessstoerung.rub.de). The aim of the intervention was to reduce eating disorder stigma by raising awareness of the existence of eating disorders in men and improving GPs' knowledge in terms of assessment, treatment, and communication with patients of different genders and sexual orientations (Lehe et al. 2026).

Of course, it will be essential to incorporate experiences related to gender and sexuality directly into disordered eating care. Unique experiences of discrimination and social pressures can be core components of exacerbated feelings of body dissatisfaction in SGM and other populations. Focusing solely on treating symptoms without addressing the underlying causes, such as stigma, would be an incomplete approach.

Conclusion

This chapter focused on the roles of gender and sexuality in BPD and DEAB presentation. We argued that existing theoretical models that link gender and sexuality to qualitative differences in BPD and to the increased prevalence rates of DEAB offer a conceptual framework for advancing our understanding of DEAB presentation beyond SGM populations. We corroborated this perspective based on our review of variations in BPD and DEAB symptom presentation, patterns of co-morbidities, and the interplay of gender and sexuality with overarching adversities such as the COVID-19 pandemic, food insecurity, and loneliness. We thus believe it is essential to address gender- and sexuality-related disparities in disordered eating assessment and care on both interpersonal and contextual levels, which, in Germany, could be pursued through improving medical education and offering targeted professional training.

References

American Psychiatric Association. 2013. Diagnostic and Statistical Manual of Mental Disorders (5th ed.). Washington, DC: American Psychiatric Publishing.

Baker, J.H., D. Freestone, K. Cai, S. Silverstein, B. Urban and D. Steinberg. 2024. Eating disorder clinical presentation and treatment outcomes by gender identity among children, adolescents, and young adults. J. Adolesc. Heal. 75: 254–260.

Barnett, A., K. Edwards, R. Harper, E. Evans, D. Alexander, M. Choudhary et al. 2021. The association between autistic traits and disordered eating is moderated by sex/gender and independent of anxiety and depression. J. Autism Dev. Disord. 51: 1866.

Barnhart, W.R., H. Sun, Z. Lin, C. Lu, X. Han and J. He. 2022. Integrating the tripartite influence, minority stress, and social comparison theories to explain body image and disordered eating in Chinese sexual minority men and women. Body Image 43: 95–106.

Berg, R.C., H.M. Munthe-Kaas and M.W. Ross 2016. Internalized homonegativity: a systematic mapping review of empirical research. J. Homosex. 63: 541.

Brandt, G., L. Prüll and G. Paslakis. 2022a. LGBTIQ + Related healthcare aspects in medical education in Germany. PPmP Psychother. Psychosom. Medizinische Psychol. 72: 397–409.

Brandt, G., J. Stobrawe, S. Korte, L. Prüll, N.M. Laskowski, G. Halbeisen et al. 2022b. Medical students' perspectives on LGBTQI+ healthcare and education in Germany: results of a nationwide online survey. Int. J. Environ. Res. Public Health 19: 10010.

Chaphekar, A.V., A. Downey, A.K. Garber, M. Kuykendall, P. Bojorquez-Ramirez, K.T. Ganson et al. 2023. Eating disorders in sexual minority adolescents and young adults: examining clinical characteristics and psychiatric co-morbidities in an inpatient medical setting. J. Eat. Disord. 11: 32.

Convertino, A.D., J.L. Helm, J.L. Pennesi, M. Gonzales and A.J. Blashill. 2021. Integrating minority stress theory and the tripartite influence model: A model of eating disordered behavior in sexual minority young adults. Appetite 163: 105204.

Datta, S. and T. Mukherjee. 2023. Impact of COVID-19 stress on the psychological health of sexual & gender minority individuals: A systematic review. Front. Glob. Women's Heal. 4: 1132768.

Devoe, D.J., A. Han, A. Anderson, D.K. Katzman, S.B. Patten, A. Soumbasis et al. 2023. The impact of the COVID-19 pandemic on eating disorders: A systematic review. Int. J. Eat. Disord. 56: 5–25.

Eschrich, R.L., G. Halbeisen, S. Steins-Loeber, N. Timmesfeld and G. Paslakis. 2024. Investigating the structure of disordered eating symptoms in adult men: A network analysis. Eur. Eat. Disord. Rev. 33: 80–94.

Fairburn, C.G., Z. Cooper and R. Shafran. 2003. Cognitive behaviour therapy for eating disorders: a "transdiagnostic" theory and treatment. Behav. Res. Ther. 4: 509–528.

Forrest, L.N., N.M. Perkins, J.M. Lavender and A.R. Smith. 2019. Using network analysis to identify central eating disorder symptoms among men. Int. J. Eat. Disord. 52: 871–884.

Frederick, D.A., L.M. Shapiro, T.R. Williams, C.M. Seoane, R.T. McIntosh and E.W. Fischer. 2017. Precarious manhood and muscularity: Effects of threatening men's masculinity on reported strength and muscle dissatisfaction. Body Image 22: 156–165.

Frederick, D.A., E. Pila, V.L. Malcarne, E.J. Compte, J.M. Nagata, C.R. Best et al. 2022. Demographic predictors of objectification theory and tripartite influence model constructs: The U.S. Body Project I. Body Image 40: 182–199.

Fredrickson, B.L. and T.A. Roberts. 1997. Toward understanding women's lived experiences and mental health risks. Psychol. Women Q. 21: 173–206.

Freedman, A. and J. Nicolle. 2020. Social isolation and loneliness: The new geriatric giants Approach for primary care. Can. Fam. Physician 66: 176–182.

Frías, Á., C. Palma, N. Farriols and L. González. 2016. Sexuality-related issues in borderline personality disorder: A comprehensive review. Personal Ment. Health 10: 216–231.

Frost, D.M. and I.H. Meyer. 2023. Minority stress theory: Application, critique, and continued relevance. Curr. Opin. Psychol. 51: 101579.

Halbeisen, G., G. Brandt and G. Paslakis. 2022. A plea for diversity in eating disorders research. Front. Psychiatry 13: 145.

Hatzenbuehler, M.L. 2009. How does sexual minority stigma "get under the skin"? A psychological mediation framework. Psychol. Bull. 135: 707–730.

Hazzard, V.M., L.M. Schaefer, K. Schaumberg, A.M. Bardone-Cone, D.A. Frederick, K.L. Klump et al. 2019. Testing the Tripartite Influence Model among heterosexual, bisexual, and lesbian women. Body Image 30: 145–149.

Jung, N.M., F.S. De Bairros, M.P. Pattussi, S. Pauli and M.B. Neutzling. 2017. Gender differences in the prevalence of household food insecurity: A systematic review and meta-analysis. Public Health Nutr. 20: 902–916.

Jürgensen, V., G. Halbeisen, M.S. Lehe and G. Paslakis. 2025. Muscularity concerns and disordered eating symptoms in adult women: a network analysis. Eur. Eat. Disord. Rev.

Lanzieri, N. and B.J. Cook. 2013. Examination of muscularity and body fat depictions in magazines that target heterosexual and gay men. Body Image 10: 251–254.

Laskowski, N.M., G. Halbeisen, K. Braks, T.J. Huber and G. Paslakis. 2023. Exploratory graph analysis (EGA) of the dimensional structure of the eating disorder examination-questionnaire (EDE-Q) in women with eating disorders. J. Psychiatr. Res. 163: 254–261.

Laskowski, N.M., G. Brandt and G. Paslakis. 2024. Gender Inequalities of the COVID-19 Pandemic: A synthesis of systematic reviews with a focus on sexual and gender minorities. PPmP Psychother. Psychosom. Medizinische Psychol. 74: 57–69.

Laskowski, N.M., G. Brandt, C.B. Reque, L. Sabel, M. Pahlenkemper, C. Zaiser et al. 2025. The collateral effects of the COVID-19 pandemic: A gender-specific systematic review of disordered eating behaviour in the general population. Eur. Eat. Disord. Rev. 33: 254–288.

Lavender, J.M., T.A. Brown and S.B. Murray. 2017. Men, muscles, and eating disorders: an overview of traditional and muscularity-oriented disordered eating. Curr. Psychiatry Rep. 19: 32.

Lehe, M.S., G. Halbeisen, S. Steins-Loeber and G. Paslakis. 2024. Invisible walls? Stigma-related perceptions are associated with reduced help-seeking intentions for disordered eating in men. J. Eat. Disord. 12: 200.

Lehe, M.S., G. Halbeisen, S. Steins-Loeber and G. Paslakis. 2026. Efficacy of the intervention against the stigmatization of men with eating disorders in primary healthcare (iSMEsH): Results from a randomized waitlist-controlled study. Int. J. Eat. Disord. 2026 Mar 9. doi: 10.1002/eat.70080. Epub ahead of print. PMID: 41804178.

Matsumoto, A. and R.F. Rodgers. 2020. A review and integrated theoretical model of the development of body image and eating disorders among midlife and aging men. Clin. Psychol. Rev. 81: 101903.

Meneguzzo, P., S. Terlizzi, L. Maggi and P. Todisco. 2024. The loneliness factor in eating disorders: Implications for psychopathology and biological signatures. Compr. Psychiatry 132: 152493.

Mingoia, J., A.D. Hutchinson, C. Wilson and D.H. Gleaves. 2017. The relationship between social networking site use and the internalization of a thin ideal in females: A meta-analytic review. Front. Psychol. 8: 239871.

Mofradidoost, R. and A. Abolghasemi. 2020. Body image concern and gender identities between transgender and cisgender persons from Iran. J. Sex Marital. Ther. 46: 260–268.

Monteleone, A.M. and G. Cascino. 2021. A systematic review of network analysis studies in eating disorders: Is time to broaden the core psychopathology to non specific symptoms. Eur. Eat. Disord. Rev. 29: 531–547.

Nagata, J.M., F.H. McGuire, J.M. Lavender, T.A. Brown, S.B. Murray, R.E. Greene et al. 2022. Appearance and performance-enhancing drugs and supplements, eating disorders, and muscle dysmorphia among gender minority people. Int. J. Eat. Disord. 55: 678–687.

Nagata, J.M., E. Stuart, J.O. Hur, S. Panchal, P. Low, A.V. Chaphekar et al. 2024. Eating disorders in sexual and gender minority adolescents. Curr. Psychiatry Rep. 26: 340–350.

Parker, L.L. and J.A. Harriger. 2020. Eating disorders and disordered eating behaviors in the LGBT population: a review of the literature. J. Eat. Disord. 8: 1–20.

Paslakis, G., G. Dimitropoulos and D.K. Katzman. 2021. A call to action to address COVID-19-induced global food insecurity to prevent hunger, malnutrition, and eating pathology. Nutr. Rev. 79: 114–116.

Paterna, A., M. Alcaraz-Ibáñez, M. Fuller-Tyszkiewicz and Á. Sicilia. 2021. Internalization of body shape ideals and body dissatisfaction: A systematic review and meta-analysis. Int. J. Eat. Disord. 54: 1575–1600.

Prnjak, K., E. Fried, J. Mond, P. Hay, K. Bussey, S. Griffiths et al. 2021. Identifying components of drive for muscularity and leanness associated with core body image disturbance: a network analysis. Psychol. Assess. 34: 353–366.

Qian, X., M.L. Townsend, W.J. Tan and B.F.S. Grenyer. 2022. Sex differences in borderline personality disorder: A scoping review. PLoS One 17: e0279015.

Richardson, C. and G. Paslakis. 2021. Men's experiences of eating disorder treatment: A qualitative systematic review of men-only studies. J. Psychiatr. Ment. Health Nurs. 28: 237–250.

Roberts, S.R., A.J. Maheux, R.J. Watson, R.M. Puhl and S. Choukas-Bradley. 2022. Sexual and gender minority (SGM) adolescents' disordered eating: Exploring general and SGM-specific factors. Int. J. Eat. Disord. 55: 933–946.

Rodgers, R.F., H. Chabrol and S.J. Paxton. 2011. An exploration of the tripartite influence model of body dissatisfaction and disordered eating among Australian and French college women. Body Image 8: 208–215.

Rood, B.A., S.L. Reisner, F.I. Surace, J.A. Puckett, M.R. Maroney and D.W. Pantalone. 2016. Expecting rejection: understanding the minority stress experiences of transgender and gender-nonconforming individuals. Transgender Heal. 1: 151–164.

Rood, B.A., M.R. Maroney, J.A. Puckett, A.K. Berman, S.L. Reisner and D.W. Pantalone. 2017. Identity concealment in transgender adults: A qualitative assessment of minority stress and gender affirmation. Am. J. Orthopsychiatry 87: 704–713.

Santoniccolo, F. and L. Rollè. 2024. The role of minority stress in disordered eating: a systematic review of the literature. Eat. Weight Disord. 29: 1–11.

Schaefer, L.M., N.L. Burke, J.K. Thompson, R.F. Dedrick, L.J. Heinberg, R.M. Calogero et al. 2015. Development and validation of the sociocultural attitudes towards appearance questionnaire-4 (SATAQ-4). Psychol. Assess. 27: 54–67.

Schaefer, L.M., R.F. Rodgers, J.K. Thompson and S. Griffiths. 2021. A test of the tripartite influence model of disordered eating among men. Body Image 36: 172–179.

Spengler, E.S., D. Tierney, L.C. Elledge and P.R. Grzanka. 2023. Beyond the individual: sexual minority help-seeking and the consequences of structural barriers. J. Couns. Psychol. 70: 133–145.

Thompson, J.K., L.J. Heinberg, M. Altabe and S. Tantleff-Dunn. 1999. Exacting Beauty: Theory, Assessment, and Treatment of Body Image Disturbance. American Psychological Association, Washington, DC.

Tomei, G., M.F. Pieroni and E. Tomba. 2022. Network analysis studies in patients with eating disorders: A systematic review and methodological quality assessment. Int. J. Eat. Disord. 55: 1641–1669.

Traut, P., G. Halbeisen, K. Braks, T.J. Huber and G. Paslakis. 2023. Sociodemographic and clinical features of men and women with eating disorders: a diagnosis-matched, retrospective comparison among inpatients. Front. Psychiatry 14: 1192693.

Tylka, T.L. 2011. Refinement of the tripartite influence model for men: Dual body image pathways to body change behaviors. Body Image 8: 199–207.

Tylka, T.L. and M.J. Andorka. 2012. Support for an expanded tripartite influence model with gay men. Body Image 9: 57–67.

Ulfvebrand, S., A. Birgegård, C. Norring, L. Högdahl and Y. von Hausswolff-Juhlin. 2015. Psychiatric comorbidity in women and men with eating disorders results from a large clinical database. Psychiatry Res. 230: 294–299.

Warrier, V., D.M. Greenberg, E. Weir, C. Buckingham, P. Smith, M.C. Lai et al. 2020. Elevated rates of autism, other neurodevelopmental and psychiatric diagnoses, and autistic traits in transgender and gender-diverse individuals. Nat. Commun. 11: 3959.

Zaiser, C., N.M. Laskowski, R. Müller, K. Abdulla, L. Sabel, C. Ballero Reque et al. 2024. The relationship between anabolic androgenic steroid use and body image, eating behavior, and physical activity by gender: A systematic review. Neurosci. Biobehav. Rev. 163: 105772.

Chapter 14

Body Image and Embodied Cognition in Eating Disorders

Clinical and Therapeutic Perspectives

Amandine Turcq[1,*] and *Pierre Dechelotte*[2]

INTRODUCTION

Eating disorders (EDs) are traditionally associated with altered body image perception, or body dysmorphic disorder, characterized by an allocentric perception of the self (Monthuy-Blanc et al. 2020). This perception is strongly influenced by the ideal of thinness and the culture of performance promoted by Western society, both recognized as significant risk factors in EDs development (Striegel-Moore and Bulik 2007).

Body image occupies a predominant place in Western culture, a phenomenon amplified by globalization and the rise of social media. This evolution has had significant repercussions on individuals' identity construction and self-esteem. Several studies have highlighted an increase in the prevalence of EDs in countries and cultures previously less affected (Caqueo-Urízar et al. 2011, Gerbasi et al. 2014, Xu et al. 2010). The COVID-19 pandemic accentuated this phenomenon, with a dramatic increase in screen time observed, accompanied by increased body dissatisfaction. In

[1] Department of Nutrition Hospital Croix-Rouge Française, 459 Chemin de la Breteque 76230 Bois Guillaume.

[2] Department of Nutrition Hospital CHU Rouen, 37 bd Gambetta, 76000 Rouen.
Email: pierre.dechelotte@chu-rouen.fr

* Corresponding author: amandine.turcq@croix-rouge.fr

DOI: 10.1201/9781032718125-16

the months following the pandemic's onset, a generalized resurgence of EDs was observed in most countries (Devoe et al. 2023, Monthuy-Blanc et al. 2023, Tavolacci et al. 2021). These observations underscore the profound impact of sociocultural and environmental factors on body image perception and ED development. However, body perception is not limited to this allocentric dimension; it also encompasses an egocentric dimension, involving sensory, emotional, and motor experiences lived through the body. This less-studied perspective deserves attention.

1. Conceptual framework

Allocentric body perception refers to a third-person perspective in which the body is perceived as an object integrated into the surrounding physical environment. This perspective corresponds to how we see others' bodies or our own body in a mirror, involving an external representation of the body based on visual and spatial landmarks. According to Riva et al. (2018), allocentric perception shapes "body memory" and includes knowledge, beliefs, and attitudes related to one's own body.

Egocentric body perception refers to the first-person, embodied perspective of one's own body as experienced from the viewpoint of the perceiver. It involves an internal body representation based on proprioceptive, interoceptive, and kinesthetic sensations. According to Riva et al. (2018), the egocentric perspective originates from somatoperceptions—the neural processes by which the brain constructs real-time representations of the body's current state through the integration of tactile, proprioceptive, and interoceptive signals from multiple sensory receptors. These two perspectives differ in their nature and function. Allocentric perception relies on external visual cues to represent the body's position in space, while egocentric perception integrates internal sensory signals (proprioceptive, interoceptive, vestibular) to construct first-person bodily experience. The former enables environmental spatial awareness, whereas the latter generates the subjective sense of embodied selfhood.

According to Corno et al. (2018), allocentric perspective processing may be more strongly associated with body perception disturbances, whereas egocentric perspective processing appears less influenced by these factors. The "allocentric lock" theory developed by Riva posits that patients with EDs may become "locked" into negative mental representations of their body that are no longer updated by current perceptual information, even following significant changes in body shape and size (Riva et al. 2018).

1.1 The somesthetic model and embodied cognition

The Exteroception-Interoception-Proprioception model provides a conceptual framework for understanding how the brain integrates different sources of sensory information to construct a coherent experience of the self and the environment (Figure 1). Exteroception involves the perception of external stimuli through the traditional senses (vision, hearing, smell, taste, and touch), playing a crucial role in environmental perception and interaction. Through multisensory integration processes, exteroceptive inputs contribute to forming a coherent perception of the

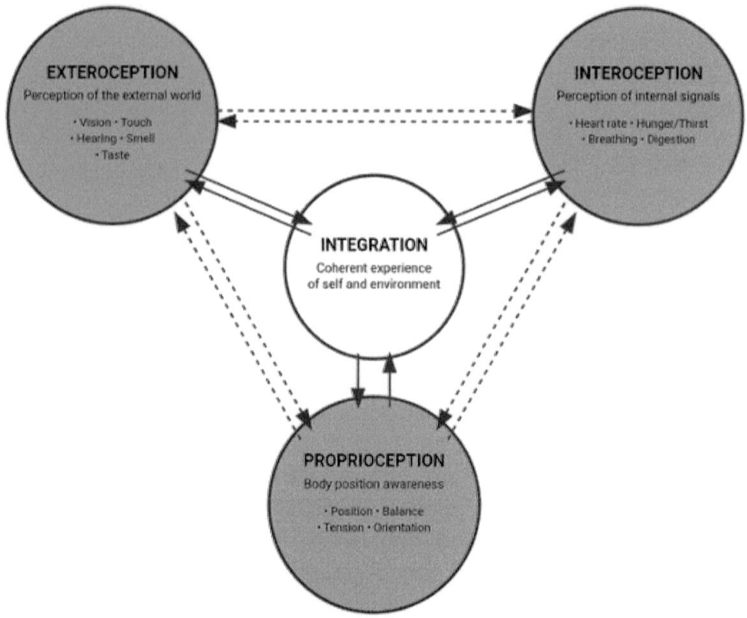

Figure 1. Exteroception-Interoception-Proprioception Model based on works by Craig (2002), Blanke (2012), Proske and Gandevia (2012) and Khalsa et al. (2018).

external world, which is essential for complex functions such as body awareness and spatial orientation (Blanke 2012).

Interoception relates to the perception of internal bodily signals (heartbeats, digestive sensations, respiratory changes) via receptors located in blood vessel walls, lungs, intestinal tract, and other internal organs. These signals are transmitted through afferent pathways, primarily the vagus nerve and spinal cord, to brain structures including the brainstem, thalamus, insula, and somatosensory cortex (Craig 2002). Proprioception involves the awareness of body position and movement (Khalsa et al. 2018) through receptors located in skin, muscles, and joints. Proprioception enables awareness of limb and body position and movement in space, even without visual feedback (Proske and Gandevia 2012). While these three systems are presented distinctly for clarity, their boundaries are not clearly delineated in practice. Recent studies emphasize the importance of interactions between these systems in providing a unified perception of bodily state. For example, Aspell et al. (2013) demonstrated that manipulation of interoceptive signals can influence exteroceptive body perception.

Interactions between these systems in body image formation. The somatosensory system, encompassing exteroception, interoception, and proprioception, plays a fundamental role in the formation and maintenance of body image. Exteroception, which processes cutaneous stimuli, contributes to delimiting body boundaries (Serino and Haggard 2010). Interoception, involving the perception of internal signals, influences awareness of physiological states and affects global body perception

(Craig 2003). Proprioception, essential for perceiving body position and movement, is crucial for precise spatial body representation (Proske and Gandevia 2012). Body and facial perception results from continuous integration of multisensory inputs (visual, tactile, proprioceptive, and interoceptive) (Riva 2017, Riva et al. 2018). These systems interact continuously, creating a dynamic and multidimensional body image. Tsakiris et al. (2011) demonstrated that interoceptive sensitivity predicts the malleability of body representations. During movement, proprioception provides information about limb position, exteroception about the environment, while interoception signals physiological changes related to effort (Kilteni et al. 2015).

The concept of embodiment, also known as embodied cognition, which emerged from cognitive psychology, is increasingly appearing in the literature on psychiatric and psychological disorders. This concept proposes that mental processes, emotional states, and behaviors are deeply rooted in physical and bodily experiences. In other words, embodiment suggests that cognitive, affective, and behavioral processes are intimately linked to how the body interacts with its environment and the sensations it experiences.

Link between sensory processing deficits and EDs. EDs are increasingly recognized as involving sensory processing deficits, particularly interoceptive dysfunction. Several studies have highlighted these associations. For example, Zucker et al. (2013) and Jacquemot et al. (2020) demonstrated that individuals with anorexia nervosa present altered interoceptive sensitivity. Jacquemot et al. (2020) examine the role of interoception in anorexia nervosa pathogenesis and treatment, highlighting reduced interoceptive sensitivity and disturbed interoceptive awareness. These deficits are associated with several aspects of anorexia nervosa, including altered perception of hunger and satiety, body schema prediction errors, emotional awareness difficulties, and body dysmorphia. Altered interoceptive sensitivity in EDs may be linked to autonomic nervous system dysfunction, particularly involving the vagus nerve, which plays a crucial role in bidirectional brain-gut communication (Faris et al. 2000). Mazurak et al. (2011) demonstrates reduced heart rate variability, while Jenkins et al. (2021) show increased parasympathetic activity and decreased sympathetic activity in subjects with anorexia nervosa, suggesting autonomic dysregulation.

1.2 Comorbidity of ED with autism spectrum disorders (ASD)

It should be noted that findings supporting the predominance of allocentric perspective processing appear relevant primarily for neurotypical populations. However, among autistic individuals, who represent a significant subgroup within EDs populations, allocentric perspective processing alone may be insufficient to fully account for EDs onset and maintenance. Indeed, Gesi et al. (2020) demonstrate that patients with anorexia nervosa, bulimia nervosa, and binge eating disorder exhibit significantly elevated autistic traits compared to neurotypical controls. Symptoms associated with autism spectrum disorders are overrepresented in emergency services, particularly among anorexia nervosa. Studies indicate that 4% to 52.5% of hospitalized patients with anorexia nervosa score above the clinical threshold for autism spectrum disorder on standardized assessment tools (Westwood et al. 2017). Moreover, autistic individuals appear less concerned with the social (allocentric) perception of their body. Brede et al. (2020) emphasize that concerns about weight and physical appearance are not primary motivations for autistic females with anorexia nervosa. Similarly, autistic males with obesity appear less concerned about social perception of their body, which, according to Must et al. (2017), may explain the lower frequency of weight reduction attempts during adolescence or adulthood.

1.3 The embodied cognition approach in ED with ASD comorbidity

In the context of EDs, the embodied cognition approach offers an innovative perspective. This approach suggests that altered body perceptions, dysfunctional eating behaviors, and associated emotional states form an interconnected system with bidirectional influences (Riva 2018). Interoceptive sensations triggered by eating can generate discomfort, negative emotions, and anxiety, while bodily changes modify proprioceptive experiences and, consequently, self-image (Monteleone and Maj 2013).

Particularly illuminating is the model developed by Crespi and colleagues (2019), which conceptualizes autism and psychotic-affective disorders as situated at opposite poles of an embodiment continuum. According to this model, autism is characterized by increased interoceptive precision and more rigid self-boundaries, while psychotic disorders present reduced interoceptive precision and more permeable self-boundaries. This latter configuration predisposes individuals to EDs, such as anorexia nervosa, thus providing a potential explanation for the frequent comorbidities observed between these disorders (Westwood et al. 2017). This conceptualization of EDs as embodiment disorders enables better understanding of patients' lived bodily experience beyond manifest symptoms, considering both neurobiological and phenomenological foundations of embodied experience.

2. Empirical and clinical support

2.1 New treatment approaches based on integrative approach

Embodiment-based interventions aim to provide treatment by targeting not only cognitions and behaviors but also bodily and sensory experiences, offering a more integrative therapeutic approach. Given the proposed embodiment spectrum ranging from autism to schizophrenia (Crespi 2019), a personalized approach that considers each individual's position on this continuum is essential for optimizing therapeutic intervention effectiveness. For autism, this would involve therapies aimed at expanding self-boundaries through sensory integration training and mindfulness-based interventions to enhance metacognitive awareness. For EDs, which are situated on this spectrum, several authors demonstrate the relevance of therapies targeting empathy, self-reflexivity, and psycho-affective cognition (Adamson et al. 2018, Dandil et al. 2020, Saure et al. 2022).

2.2 The role of oxytocin in body perception regulation and ED with ASD comorbidity

The investigation of neurobiological mechanisms underlying eating disorders (EDs) provides valuable insights into their pathophysiology and treatment potential, particularly in the context of comorbidity with autism spectrum disorder (ASD) (Romano et al. 2016, Adams et al. 2024). Oxytocin (OT) has emerged as a promising therapeutic candidate due to its documented involvement in social behavior, feeding regulation, and sensory processing.

Neuroimaging and attentional mechanisms. Yao et al. (2018) conducted a pharmaco-fMRI study involving 83 participants, demonstrating that intranasal OT can shift attentional allocation from interoceptive signals toward socially relevant external stimuli. Specifically, OT administration reduced interoceptive precision during heartbeat detection when participants were concurrently exposed to emotional faces, enhanced right anterior insula activation, and increased functional connectivity between the right anterior and left posterior insula. These findings suggest that OT may rebalance the weighting of bodily versus social cues—a mechanism relevant to both EDs and ASD.

Plemeniti Tololeski et al. (2021), in a narrative clinical review on ASD–anorexia nervosa comorbidity, highlighted the frequent co-occurrence of alexithymia, insular hypoactivation reported in previous neuroimaging studies, and lower endogenous OT levels in these populations. They proposed this constellation as a potential shared mechanism contributing to both social–emotional difficulties and disturbed body awareness. However, this remains a conceptual framework rather than an empirically validated causal model.

Genetic, epigenetic, and behavioral correlates. Several studies indicate that variability in the oxytocin receptor gene (OXTR) may influence susceptibility to EDs phenotypes. Burmester et al. (2021) reviewed evidence that OXTR polymorphisms—particularly rs53576 and rs2254298—are associated with eating behavior patterns, with the A allele of rs2254298 linked to restrictive behaviors and the G allele of rs53576 associated with binge-type behaviors. Given heterogeneity across studies, these associations should be interpreted cautiously.

On the behavioral level, Kim et al. (2014) employed a double-blind, placebo-controlled, within-subject crossover design with 31 anorexia nervosa patients and 33 healthy controls. Using a visual probe detection task, they found that OT reduced attentional bias toward negative food- and body-related stimuli and attenuated vigilance toward disgust expressions in both groups, while shifting avoidance of angry faces toward vigilance in anorexia patients. These results indicate that OT may modulate both body-related and socio-emotional processing.

Emerging epigenetic data further suggest sex-specific[1] regulation of the OXTR gene. Adams et al. (2024) hypothesised that similar methylation alterations in EDs and ASD could represent a shared biological mechanism underlying their

[1] 'Sex' here refers to biological sex as defined in genetic studies, which do not take gender into account.

frequent co-occurrence. Supporting this view, Giel et al. (2022) observed OXTR hypomethylation in men with binge eating disorder, whereas Thaler et al. (2020) reported OXTR hypermethylation in women with active anorexia nervosa. These differences may contribute to the higher prevalence of obesity in autistic males and the overrepresentation of females in ASD–anorexia comorbidity, though longitudinal confirmation is needed.

Clinical trial evidence. Translation of mechanistic findings into therapeutic applications has yielded mixed results. In anorexia nervosa, Russell et al. (2018) reported limited positive signals on eating behaviors in females following intranasal OT, but effect sizes were modest and require replication. More recently, a large multicenter RCT failed to confirm benefits on weight restoration or core psychopathology (Maguire et al. 2024).

In ASD, the large-scale NEJM trial by Sikich et al. (2021; n=290) found no significant improvement in primary social outcome measures compared to placebo, although exploratory analyses did not exclude potential benefit in specific subgroups. Baseline OT levels may be one such moderator: Parker et al. (2017) found that autistic children with lower endogenous OT responded more strongly to intranasal OT treatment, suggesting a possible biomarker-guided approach. This is consistent with meta-analytic evidence (John and Jaeggi 2021) showing reduced baseline OT in autistic children, though not consistently in adults.

Integrative framework. Taken together, neuroimaging, behavioral, genetic, and clinical findings support a model in which OT may help restore the balance between interoceptive and exteroceptive processing, a function relevant to both ASD and ED. Quattrocki and Friston (2014) proposed that OT deficits in ASD could underlie interoceptive impairments, which in turn may contribute to disturbed body awareness—a core feature of EDs. Clinically, OT's potential to reduce cognitive rigidity could address both repetitive behaviors in ASD and rigid eating patterns in ED.

Romano et al. (2016) demonstrated that OT administration in healthy and obese individuals reduced caloric intake and altered emotional stimulus processing in anorexia nervosa, while Kim et al. (2014) confirmed modulation of negative food- and body-related attention. In ED populations, Giel et al. (2018) reviewed evidence for a paradoxical endocrine profile in anorexia nervosa, with lower fasting OT but higher postprandial OT compared to healthy controls—suggesting that exogenous OT might help normalise dysregulated physiological responses.

While converging data point to plausible neurobiological pathways linking OT dysfunction to both ASD and ED, current clinical evidence for therapeutic efficacy is inconsistent. Heterogeneity in endocrine profiles, OXTR genetic variation, and epigenetic regulation likely influences treatment response. Longitudinal, biomarker-stratified trials—ideally incorporating sex-specific analyses—are needed to clarify which patient subgroups may benefit most from OT-based interventions.

3. Applications to the sociocultural context

3.1 An integrative approach to ED with ASD comorbidity: The croix-rouge française hospital experience

At the Croix-Rouge Française Hospital, in partnership with the Rouen University Hospital, an innovative approach to EDs has been developed that goes beyond simple diagnostic categorization. This integrative vision considers patients holistically, integrating sensory-motor, cognitive, social, experiential, and affective dimensions of their experience. This approach conceptualizes these disorders as resulting from complex non-linear multi-causality, recognizing the uniqueness of each patient's trajectory. The clinical protocol includes systematic screening for autism spectrum disorder in all patients followed in the Nutrition department at Rouen University Hospital. The therapeutic approach remains attentive to the sensory and experiential dimensions in all patients, regardless of their cognitive profile. Patient testimonials presented in the following paragraphs illustrate and support this integrative clinical approach.

This integrative framework operationalizes the allocentric-egocentric theoretical model by facilitating patients' transition from external body image preoccupations toward internal embodied awareness. As Sandra describes: "I realize that at Croix-Rouge Hospital, I was entirely focused on the exterior, I had forgotten about weight and physical appearance. Today, on the contrary, I feel focused on bodily sensations." This shift from allocentric to egocentric body perception represents a key therapeutic mechanism, particularly for autistic patients who may benefit more from approaches emphasizing internal sensory integration rather than external image modification.

3.2 Implementation of the integrative approach

Adjustment of practices and communication. The approach prioritizes active listening and the establishment of a referent caregiver who transmits information to the multidisciplinary team. Particular importance is given to patient rhythm and decisional autonomy. This empowerment contrasts with the more directive approach adopted in other establishments. Matthieu confirms the importance of this autonomy: "What also seems important to me is that I was an active participant in my care and felt responsible for it." Access to emotions is often challenging for patients, particularly those with autistic comorbidity (which represents more than a quarter of the unit), due to characteristic delays in accessing internal emotional and cognitive states, combined with pragmatic language difficulties. Therefore, the therapeutic framework promotes the development of self-awareness and greater self-determination. Self-expression in autistic patients is facilitated by systematically granting them adapted response time, considering their prolonged processing time for social and emotional information, as documented by Thye et al. (2018). The clinical protocol incorporates systematic information reformulation and comprehension verification to ensure meaningful therapeutic engagement and informed decision-making.

Respect for sensory particularities. Consideration of sensory specificities constitutes a fundamental pillar of the therapeutic approach. Environmental accommodations are made according to each patient's sensory profile, including providing the quietest available rooms for patients with acoustic hypersensitivity and implementing "sensory diet" interventions prior to meals. Carole testifies: "Care was taken, during my last hospitalizations, to place me in a quiet room, as far as possible from staff work areas, [...] from dish noises, from voice bursts [...] calm is essential to my balance." Through occupational therapy expertise, environmental modifications are precisely calibrated according to specific sensory needs, including noise-reducing headphones, compartmentalized plates, and lighting adjustments. Clara describes these adaptations: "I was able to meet the occupational therapist who made some suggestions (weighted blanket, noise-canceling headphones, z-vibe, sunglasses, scarf for odors...)." The sensory diet intervention, particularly beneficial in anorexia nervosa, involves creating a transition period before meals during which sensory stimulation is deliberately reduced to allow nervous system regulation. This approach facilitates improved integration of food-related stimuli and decreases avoidance behaviors, which can be prominent features of anorexia nervosa in individuals with autism spectrum disorder. These environmental modifications directly address the exteroceptive-interoceptive-proprioceptive integration model by optimizing external sensory inputs (exteroception) to facilitate better internal signal processing (interoception) and body position awareness (proprioception), thus supporting coherent embodied experience.

Consideration of identity and lived bodily experience. Particular attention is paid to respecting each patient's values, especially regarding food choices. Food preferences are not systematically attributed to the disorder but are considered legitimate individual choices. Carole emphasizes: "I appreciated that my decision not to eat meat was accepted, and that people stopped trying to convince me that 'it's the illness speaking'." For patients with anorexia nervosa and autistic comorbidity, a sub-normal BMI that remains medically tolerable may sometimes be accepted as a treatment goal. This approach prioritizes the egocentric perspective of body experience over allocentric standards, recognizing that for patients with autism-ED comorbidity, internal bodily comfort and familiar proprioceptive landmarks may be more therapeutically relevant than externally imposed weight norms. Annie explains this complex relationship to embodied experience: "It's not the weight number, nor the image that bothers me, but just the feeling, the obsessive physical discomfort, the discomfort in a body whose landmarks are no longer familiar".

Tools and observed results. Our approach is based on various adapted therapeutic tools. We systematically use validated assessment scales to better understand and support all our patients, whether neurotypical or neurodivergent. For interoceptive awareness assessment, we employ the Multidimensional Assessment of Interoceptive Awareness Version 2 (MAIA-2; Mehling et al. 2018), which provides comprehensive evaluation of different interoceptive dimensions. Alexithymia is measured using the Toronto Alexithymia Scale (TAS-20), allowing us to identify difficulties in emotional identification and expression. For sensory profile assessment, we utilize

Dunn's Brief Sensory Profile and, when needed, Bogdashina's Sensory Profile to capture the complexity of sensory experiences. Autism screening is conducted using the Ritvo Autism Asperger Diagnostic Scale-Revised (RAADS-R), the Autism-Spectrum Quotient (AQ), and the Empathy Quotient (EQ). This comprehensive assessment battery serves a dual purpose: identifying autistic patients who may benefit from specific adaptations and providing deeper understanding of sensory and emotional processing patterns across all patients, thus enabling more personalized care regardless of neurological profile.

Beyond assessment tools, adapted physical activity plays an important role in reconnecting patients with their body. We adapt sensory conditions (light, sounds, type of activity) to facilitate access to these activities. Armelle testifies: "Practicing sports activity is important for reconciling with one's body. I really appreciate yoga." Snoezelen is modulated according to individual tolerance.

Results include significant improvement in bodily experience, even when weight remains stable. Sandra testifies: "Weight gain was rapid but not traumatic. [...] I was no longer focused on my weight."

This integrative approach has transformed the conceptualization of relapses, now considered as potentially constructive stages in the therapeutic process. Carole illustrates: "Undoubtedly, abandoning the power struggle. [...] When facing an autistic patient, any form of power relationship must absolutely be avoided."

Annie provides an important perspective: "The ED is a way of living with ASD; it allows anesthesia, a numbing of the senses and emotions. Caregivers must therefore accept this and work not to fit into a norm that doesn't suit us, but to maintain a viable course."

The long-term impact of this approach is highlighted by Matthieu: "If I didn't really experiment with the tools available at Croix-Rouge, I nevertheless left hospitalization with avenues to explore later at the sensory level. [...] All these elements combined allowed me to find a balance that allows me to live without physically endangering myself and to no longer rely on the sensory anesthesia I was seeking through not nourishing my body."

Through these testimonials, it is observed that this integrative approach improves the hospitalization experience and promotes more sustainable therapeutic outcomes. Adaptations initially designed for patients with ASD have proven beneficial for all patients, including those without ASD, creating a more therapeutic and calming environment. This transversal approach has also positively impacted the healthcare team, promoting more reflective, less standardized practice that is better attuned to the singularity of each patient's journey. Caregivers report greater professional satisfaction and decreased feelings of helplessness when facing complex cases.

Conclusion

This chapter has explored the interactions between body image, embodied cognition, and EDs with autistic comorbidity. Analysis of allocentric and egocentric perspectives demonstrated how these perceptual modalities influence ED development. The somatosensory model, integrating exteroception, interoception, and proprioception, provided a framework for understanding the sensory mechanisms involved in body image construction.

The approach developed at Croix-Rouge Française Hospital illustrates the clinical application of these principles. By considering patients holistically and adapting practices to respect their sensory specificities, this approach has significantly enhanced the therapeutic experience.

Future research on neurobiological mechanisms involved in body perception, particularly the role of oxytocin in embodiment processes and sensory regulation, will facilitate the development of more targeted therapeutic interventions, especially for patients with comorbidities.

This integrative approach, which recognizes the multidimensional complexity of EDs and the importance of subjective bodily experience, represents a major evolution in understanding and treating EDs.

Acknowledgements

I would like to thank the multidisciplinary care team at Croix-Rouge Française Hospital in Rouen for their commitment and contribution to this integrative approach to EDs. My gratitude also goes to the patients who agreed to share their experiences, considerably enriching our understanding of these disorders. I thank the Rouen University Hospital for its partnership, as well as Drs. Johana Monthuy-Blanc and Giulia Corno for their valuable guidance during the writing of this chapter. I extend my special appreciation to Professor Dechelotte for accepting to be co-author of this work, for his unwavering support of innovation and transdisciplinary approaches, and for his exemplary humanism toward both healthcare professionals and patients.

References

Adams, K.L., W. Mandy, C. Catmur and G. Bird. 2024. Potential mechanisms underlying the association between feeding and eating disorders and autism. Neurosci. Biobehav. Rev. 162: 105717.

Adamson J., J. Leppanen, M. Murin and K. Tchanturia. 2018. Effectiveness of emotional skills training for patients with anorexia nervosa with autistic symptoms in group and individual format. Eur. Eat. Disord. Rev. 26: 367–375.

Altman, S.E. and S.A. Shankman. 2009. What is the association between obsessive-compulsive disorder and eating disorders? Clin. Psychol. Rev. 29: 638–646.

Aspell, J.E., L. Heydrich, G. Marillier, T. Lavanchy, B. Herbelin and O. Blanke. 2013. Turning body and self inside out: Visualized heartbeats alter bodily self-consciousness and tactile perception. Psychol. Sci. 24: 2445–2453.

Blanke, O. 2012. Multisensory brain mechanisms of bodily self-consciousness. Nat. Rev. Neurosci. 13: 556–571.

Brede, J., C. Babb, C. Jones, M. Elliott, C. Zanker, K. Tchanturia et al. 2020. For Me, the Anorexia is just a symptom, and the cause is the autism: investigating restrictive eating disorders in autistic women. J. Autism Dev. Disord. 50: 4280–4296.

Burmester, V., D. Nicholls, A. Buckle, B. Stanojevic and M. Crous-Bou. 2021. Review of eating disorders and oxytocin receptor polymorphisms. J. Eat. Disord. 9: 85.

Caqueo-Urízar, A., M. Ferrer-García, J. Toro, J. Gutiérrez-Maldonado, C. Peñaloza, Y. Cuadros-Sosa et al. 2011. Associations between sociocultural pressures to be thin, body distress, and eating disorder symptomatology among Chilean adolescent girls. Body Image 8: 78–81.

Corno, G., S. Serino, P. Cipresso, R.M. Baños and G. Riva. 2018. Assessing the relationship between attitudinal and perceptual component of body image disturbance using virtual reality. Cyberpsychol. Behav. Soc. Netw. 21: 679–686.

Craig, A.D. 2002. How do you feel? Interoception: the sense of the physiological condition of the body. Nat. Rev. Neurosci. 3: 655–666.

Craig, A.D. 2003. Interoception: the sense of the physiological condition of the body. Curr. Opin. Neurobiol. 13: 500–505.

Crespi, B. and N. Dinsdale. 2019. Autism and psychosis as diametrical disorders of embodiment. Evol. Med. Public Health 2019: 121–138.

Dandil, Y., K. Smith, J. Adamson and K. Tchanturia. 2020. Individual cognitive remediation therapy benefits for patients with anorexia nervosa and high autistic features. Eur. Eat. Disord. Rev. 28: 87–91.

Devoe, J.D., A. Han, A. Anderson, D.K. Katzman, S.B. Patten, A. Soumbasis et al. 2023. The impact of the COVID-19 pandemic on eating disorders: A systematic review. Int. J. Eat. Disord. 56: 5–25.

Faris, P.L., S.W. Kim, W.H. Meller, R.L. Goodale, S.A. Oakman, R.D. Hofbauer et al. 2000. Effect of decreasing afferent vagal activity with ondansetron on symptoms of bulimia nervosa: a randomised, double-blind trial. Lancet 355: 792–797.

Fuchs, T. and J.E. Schlimme. 2009. Embodiment and psychopathology: a phenomenological perspective. Curr. Opin. Psychiatry 22: 570–575.

Gerbasi, M.E., L.K. Richards, J.J. Thomas, J.C. Agnew-Blais, H. Thompson-Brenner, S.E. Gilman et al. 2014. Globalization and eating disorder risk: peer influence, perceived social norms, and adolescent disordered eating in Fiji. Int. J. Eat. Disord. 47: 727–737.

Gesi, C., C. Carmassi, M. Luciano, L. Bossini, V. Ricca, A. Fagiolini et al. 2020. Autistic traits in patients with anorexia nervosa, bulimia nervosa or binge eating disorder: A pilot study. Eur. Psychiatry 41: S100.

Giel, K., S. Zipfel and M. Hallschmid. 2018. Oxytocin and eating disorders: a narrative review on emerging findings and perspectives. Curr. Neuropharmacol. 16: 1111–1121.

Giel, K.E., K. Schag, E.J. Leehr, I. Mack, L.S. Schuster, A. Wiegand et al. 2022. OXTR DNA methylation differentiates men on the obesity spectrum with and without binge eating disorder. Clin. Epigenetics 14: 108.

Godart, N.T., F. Perdereau, Z. Rein, S. Berthoz, J. Wallier, P. Jeammet et al. 2007. Comorbidity studies of eating disorders and mood disorders. Critical review of the literature. J. Affect. Disord. 97: 37–49.

Jacquemot, A.M. and R. Park. 2020. The role of interoception in the pathogenesis and treatment of anorexia nervosa: a narrative review. Front. Psychiatry 11: 281.

Jenkins, Z.M., N. Eikelis, A. Phillipou, D.J. Castle, H.E. Wilding and E.A. Lambert. 2021. Autonomic nervous system function in anorexia nervosa: a systematic review. Front. Neurosci. 15: 682208.

John, S. and A.V. Jaeggi. 2021. Oxytocin levels tend to be lower in autistic children: A meta-analysis of 31 studies. Autism 25: 2152–2161.

Khalsa, S.S., R. Adolphs, O.G. Cameron, H.D. Critchley, P.W. Davenport, J.S. Feinstein et al. 2018. Interoception and mental health: a roadmap. Biol. Psychiatry Cogn. Neurosci. Neuroimaging 3: 501–513.

Kilteni, K., R. Groten and M. Slater. 2012. The sense of embodiment in virtual reality. Presence: Teleoperators and Virtual Environments 21: 373–387.

Kim, Y.R., C.H. Kim, J.H. Park, J. Pyo and J. Treasure. 2014. The impact of intranasal oxytocin on attention to social emotional stimuli in patients with anorexia nervosa: a double blind within-subject cross-over experiment. PLoS One 9: e90721.

Kim, Y.R., J.H. Kim, M.J. Kim and J. Treasure. 2014. Differential methylation of the oxytocin receptor gene in patients with anorexia nervosa: a pilot study. PLoS One 9: e88673.

Leppanen, J., K.W. Ng, K. Tchanturia and J. Treasure. 2017. Meta-analysis of the effects of intranasal oxytocin on interpretation and expression of emotions. Neurosci. Biobehav. Rev. 78: 125–144.

Maguire, S., A. Kesby, R. Brownlow, G.E. Hunt, M. Kim, C. McAulay et al. 2024. A phase II randomised controlled trial of intranasal oxytocin in anorexia nervosa. Psychoneuroendocrinology 164: 107032.

Mazurak, N., J. Stein, S. Kipphan, E.R. Muth, M. Teufel, S. Zipfel et al. 2011. Heart rate variability in anorexia nervosa and the irritable bowel syndrome. Neurogastroenterol. Motil. 23: e470–e478.

McElroy, S.L., M.A. Frye, G. Hellemann, L. Altshuler, G.S. Leverich, T. Suppes et al. 2011. Prevalence and correlates of eating disorders in 875 patients with bipolar disorder. J. Affect. Disord. 128: 191–198.

Mehling, W.E., J. Acree, A. Stewart, J. Silas and A. Jones. 2018. The multidimensional assessment of interoceptive awareness, Version 2 (MAIA-2). PLoS One 13: e0208034.

Momen, N.C., O. Plana-Ripoll, Z. Yilmaz, L.M. Thornton, J.J. McGrath, C.M. Bulik et al. 2022. Comorbidity between eating disorders and psychiatric disorders. Int. J. Eat. Disord. 55: 505–517.

Monteleone, A.M., G. Castellini, V. Ricca, U. Volpe, F. De Riso, M. Nigro et al. 2017. Embodiment mediates the relationship between avoidant attachment and eating disorder psychopathology. Eur. Eat. Disord. Rev. 25: 461–468.

Monteleone, P. and M. Maj. 2013. Dysfunctions of leptin, ghrelin, BDNF and endocannabinoids in eating disorders: beyond the homeostatic control of food intake. Psychoneuroendocrinology 38: 312–330.

Monthuy-Blanc, J., S. Bouchard, C. Maïano and M. Séguin. 2013. Factors influencing mental health providers' intention to use telepsychotherapy in First Nations communities. Transcult. Psychiatry 50: 323–343.

Monthuy-Blanc, J., S. Bouchard, M. Ouellet, G. Corno, S. Iceta and M. Rousseau. 2020. eLoriCorps immersive body rating scale: exploring the assessment of body image disturbances from allocentric and egocentric perspectives. J. Clin. Med. 9: 2926.

Monthuy-Blanc, J., G. Corno and S. Abou Chabake. 2023. Exploring the impact of the COVID-19 pandemic on perceptual disturbances and dysfunctional eating attitudes and behaviors: A review of the literature. Front. Psychol. 14: 1139261.

Must, A., S. Phillips, C. Curtin, S.E. Anderson, M. Maslin, K. Lividini et al. 2017. Comparison of sedentary behaviors between children with autism spectrum disorders and typically developing children. Autism 18: 376–384.

Nimbley, E., L. Golds, H. Sharpe, K. Gillespie-Smith and F. Duffy. 2022. Sensory processing and eating behaviours in autism: A systematic review. Eur. Eat. Disord. Rev. 30: 538–559.

Parker, K.J., O. Oztan, R.A. Libove, R.D. Sumiyoshi, L.P. Jackson, D.S. Karhson et al. 2017. Intranasal oxytocin treatment for social deficits and biomarkers of response in children with autism. Proc. Natl. Acad. Sci. USA 114: 8119–8124.

Plemeniti Tololeski, B., A. Suhodolčan Grabner and H.G. Kumperscak. 2021. Adolescents with autism spectrum disorder and anorexia nervosa comorbidity: common features and treatment possibilities with cognitive remediation therapy and oxytocin. Front Psychiatry 12: 686030.

Proske, U. and S.C. Gandevia. 2012. The proprioceptive senses: their roles in signaling body shape, body position and movement, and muscle force. Physiol. Rev. 92: 1651–1697.

Quattrocki, E. and K. Friston. 2014. Autism, oxytocin and interoception. Neurosci. Biobehav. Rev. 47: 410–430.

Riva, G. 2017. The neuroscience of body memory: From the self through the space to the others. Cortex 104: 241–260.

Riva, G. and A. Dakanalis. 2018. Altered processing and integration of multisensory bodily representations and signals in eating disorders: a possible path toward the understanding of their underlying causes. Front. Hum. Neurosci. 12: 49.

Romano, A., B. Tempesta, M.V. Micioni Di Bonaventura and S. Gaetani. 2016. From autism to eating disorders and more: the role of oxytocin in neuropsychiatric disorders. Front. Neurosci. 9: 497.

Russell, J., S. Maguire, G.E. Hunt, A. Kesby, A. Suraev, J. Stuart et al. 2018. Intranasal oxytocin in the treatment of anorexia nervosa: Randomized controlled trial during re-feeding. Psychoneuroendocrinology 87: 83–92.

Saure, E., M. Ålgars, M. Laasonen and A. Raevuori. 2022. Cognitive behavioral and cognitive remediation strategies for managing co-occurring anorexia nervosa and elevated autism spectrum traits. Psychol. Res. Behav. Manag. 15: 1005–1016.

Serino, A. and P. Haggard. 2010. Touch and the body. Neurosci. Biobehav. Rev. 34: 224–236.

Sikich, L., A. Kolevzon, B.H. King, C.J. McDougle, K.B. Sanders, S.J. Kim et al. 2021. Intranasal oxytocin in children and adolescents with autism spectrum disorder. N. Engl. J. Med. 385: 1462–1473.

Striegel-Moore, R.H. and C.M. Bulik. 2007. Risk factors for eating disorders. Am. Psychol. 62: 181–198.

Swinbourne, J.M. and S.W. Touyz. 2007. The co-morbidity of eating disorders and anxiety disorders: a review. Eur. Eat. Disord. Rev. 15: 253–274.

Tavolacci, M.P., J. Ladner and P. Dechelotte. 2021. Sharp increase in eating disorders among university students since the COVID-19 pandemic. Nutrients 13: 3415.

Tsakiris, M., A. Tajadura-Jiménez and M. Costantini. 2011. Just a heartbeat away from one's body: interoceptive sensitivity predicts malleability of body-representations. Proc. Biol. Sci. 278: 2470–2476.

Thaler, L., S. Brassard, L. Booij, E. Kahan, K. McGregor, A. Labbe et al. 2020. Methylation of the OXTR gene in women with anorexia nervosa: Relationship to social behavior. Eur. Eat. Disord. Rev. 28: 79–86.

Thye, M.D., H.M. Bednarz, A.J. Herringshaw, E.B. Sartin and R.K. Kana. 2018. The impact of atypical sensory processing on social impairments in autism spectrum disorder. Dev. Cogn. Neurosci. 29: 151–167.

Varela, F.J., E. Thompson and E. Rosch. 1991. The Embodied Mind: Cognitive Science and Human Experience. MIT Press, Cambridge, MA.

Watanabe, T., M. Kuroda, H. Kuwabara, Y. Aoki, N. Iwashiro, N. Tatsunobu et al. 2015. Clinical and neural effects of six-week administration of oxytocin on core symptoms of autism. Brain 138: 3400–3412.

Westwood, H., W. Mandy and K. Tchanturia. 2017. The association between symptoms of autism and neuropsychological performance in females with Anorexia Nervosa. Psychiatry Res. 258: 531–537.

Xu, X., D. Mellor, M. Kiehne, L.A. Ricciardelli, M.P. McCabe and Y. Xu. 2010. Body dissatisfaction, engagement in body change behaviors and sociocultural influences on body image among Chinese adolescents. Body Image 7: 156–164.

Yao, S., B. Becker, W. Zhao, Z. Zhao, J. Kou, X. Ma et al. 2018. Oxytocin modulates attention switching between interoceptive signals and external social cues. Neuropsychopharmacology 43: 294–301.

Zucker, N.L., R.M. Merwin, C.M. Bulik, A. Moskovich, J.E. Wildes and J. Groh. 2013. Subjective experience of sensation in anorexia nervosa. Behav. Res. Ther. 51: 256–265.

Conclusion

Johana Monthuy-Blanc[1,2,*] and *Giulia Corno*[1,3,4]

1. Content of the book

This book consists of two main and complementary themes, theoretical and practical respectively, and comprises fourteen chapters offering scientific conclusions and perspectives based on evidence and current best practices regarding DEAB induced by body perception disturbances. The first seven chapters constitute the Theoretical and Empirical Support of the book. Chapter 1 examined the impact of social media on body image (e.g., selfie practices, including photo editing, manipulation, and photo investment), and underscored how photo-based social media engagement can influence self-perception (particularly body dissatisfaction) but also correlate with broader psychological outcomes such as anxiety, depression, and disordered eating. Chapter 2, a comprehensive review of self-compassion and body image, indicated that individuals with higher levels of self-compassion are more likely to respond to perceived body flaws with kindness and warmth, recognizing the unattainable nature of societal standards while maintaining a mindful awareness of their emotions and thoughts. Rather than feeling isolated in their body distress or avoiding negative emotions, self-compassion enables a more supportive and adaptive response. Chapter 3 discussed the main advantages of implementing virtual reality in the context of severe DEAB, such as eating disorders, and concluded, drawing on 30 years of scientific evidence, that virtual reality offers significant benefits as both an assessment and intervention tool in this population. Chapter 4 focusing on attentional biases in understanding body perception disturbances and their

[1] Montreal Mental Health University Institute Research Center, 7401, rue Hochelaga, H1N 3MG, Montréal, QC, Canada.

[2] Department of Education Sciences, Université du Québec à Trois-Rivières, 3351, boulverad des Forges, G9A 5H7, Trois-Rivières, QC, Canada.

[3] Department of Psychoeducation and Psychology, Université du Québec en Outaouais, 283, bouvard Alexandre-Taché Blvd, J8X 3X7, Gatineau, QC, Canada.

[4] Centre Intégré de Santé et des Services Sociaux de l'Outaouais, 909, boulevard de la Vérendrye Ouest, J8P 7H2, Gatineau, QC, Canada.

* Corresponding author: johana.monthuy-blanc@uqtr.ca

DOI: 10.1201/9781032718125-17

relationship to DEAB, positioned virtual reality-based applications as immersive, personalized, and interactive treatments for body perception-related attentional biases in eating disorders. Chapter 5, which examined the complex issues related to DEAB and body perception disturbances in sexually and gender diverse people, concluded that managing body appearance and DEAB may serve as means to attain validation, connection, belonging, and/or safety. Chapter 6, which examined the ambivalent relationship between sport, eating attitude and behaviors, and body perceptions, highlighted that negative physical self-perception among athletes with DEAB constitutes a significant issue, profoundly affecting their mental health, performance, and overall well-being. Chapter 7, an empirical and analytic synthesis on obesity, body image and societal stigma and weight bias, underlined the potential of virtual reality in the management of body image in obesity by discussing different applications: body swapping and reference frame shifting, emotion regulation, and exergames. The last seven chapters offer a landscape of sociocultural practical applications across five countries (Belgium, Canada, France, Germany, and Switzerland; listed alphabetically). Chapter 8, which examined effective prevention interventions in DEAB through body perceptions, highlighted a Switzerland's cognitive-behavioral program and the importance of focusing on individuals in their own environments, such as families and schools, to protect them from culturally prevalent DEAB-related pressures, beliefs and attitudes. Chapter 9, a synthesis of 30 years of clinical research on body-oriented therapy in eating disorders, provided practical clinical guidelines for addressing body perception disturbances. Chapter 10, which offered an innovative analysis of eating-related occupations, presented a Canadian structured framework for understanding how the occupational sequence—before, during, and after food or drink intake—can either support well-being or contribute to difficulties in DEAB, depending on the body-perceptual filter. Chapter 11, addressing the role of informal caregivers in DEAB, presented a new French psychoeducational program (named BREF) designed to ensure accessibility and inclusivity for caregivers across various contexts. Chapter 12, focusing on the integration of the patient-partner into the care team, concluded with a Canadian practical application aimed at ensuring adequate weekly follow-up of individuals with DEAB throughout the care trajectory. Chapter 13, which examined the roles of gender and sexuality in body perception disturbances and DEAB, proposed paying greater attention to gender and sexuality in DEAB treatment in Germany and discussed emerging challenges for improving medical education and care. Last but not least, Chapter 14, which explored the interaction between body perceptions (body image and bodily embodiment) and eating disorders associated with autism spectrum disorders, presented an innovative approach developed in a French Hospital to adapt clinical practices so as to respect the sensory, identity, and bodily specificities of these patients.

2. Context of book

This book highlights the need to understand, assess, and intervene in the domain of mental health as it relates to eating among individuals presenting DEAB induced by body perception disturbances, encompassing both disordered eating and eating disorders. Beyond the almost stereotypical profile of "the anorexic teenage girl," these individuals, priority populations yet often invisible, include girls/women, particularly those who are racialized or pregnant; student, athletic, or clinical populations with co-occurring disorders; and members of the LGBTQ+ community (Crossland et al. 2023, Goltz et al. 2013, Gorrell et al. 2021, Mikhail et al. 2023, Mason et al. 2018).

The relative invisibility of these issues justifies the development of both health education and health care programs centered on these individuals and their environments. These environments may be contextual (school, workplace, sports club, etc.) as well as human (practitioners, caregivers, patient-partners, and peer supporters). As reflected throughout this volume, numerous scientific writings, supported by certain governmental bodies, reaffirm the need for early and innovative interventions, including digital health (Banatvala et al. 2023a, 2023b, Gouvernement du Québec 1992). Within a preventive health framework, interventions in health education (including awareness, promotion, and prevention) and in health care (treatment and recovery) now aim to foster autonomy and empowerment (Breslow 1999, Nutbeam and Muscat 2021, Thomas et al. 2025). Historically, "intervention" in mental health has corresponded to the well-known trichotomy of primary, secondary and tertiary prevention. The primary expected outcome of a health intervention is a "state of complete physical, mental, and social well-being, rather than merely the absence of disease or infirmity" (World Health Organization 1948). Primary prevention aims to prevent illness before it occurs, whereas secondary and tertiary prevention seek to reduce the impact of existing illness. In other words, primary prevention involves educational programmes promoting healthy and safe habits, such as eating well and exercising regularly. Secondary and tertiary prevention focus on therapeutic and rehabilitation programs, providing personal strategies to prevent chronic illness and strategies for living well. As previously mentioned, the situation of the recent pandemic has affected the general population with disordered eating (primary prevention category), as well as sub-clinical and clinical populations with eating disorders (secondary and tertiary prevention categories). To contextualize the conclusions regarding interventions drawn from the fourteen chapters of this book, Figure 1 illustrates a model of continuity of intervention that is consistent with the dimensional perspective on DEAB induced by body perceptual disturbances.

This dual-ended intervention framework delineates modalities ranging from health education, aligned with the pole of eating well-being, to health-care interventions, aligned with the pole of improved eating wellness, thereby characterizing the ultimate progression of eating attitudes and behaviors. Health-education interventions target populations exhibiting functional or partially functional eating attitudes and behaviors, whereas health-care interventions target populations presenting dysfunctional or fully nonfunctional eating attitudes and behaviors. Put differently, eating well-being corresponds to "I am doing well when I eat," while food better-being corresponds to "I am doing better when I eat" (p. 40, literal translation, Monthuy-Blanc et al. 2025). In theory, one may assign oneself to either of these eating profiles; in practice, these profiles operate more as eating states that fluctuate across the life span, consistent with the model of eating attitudes

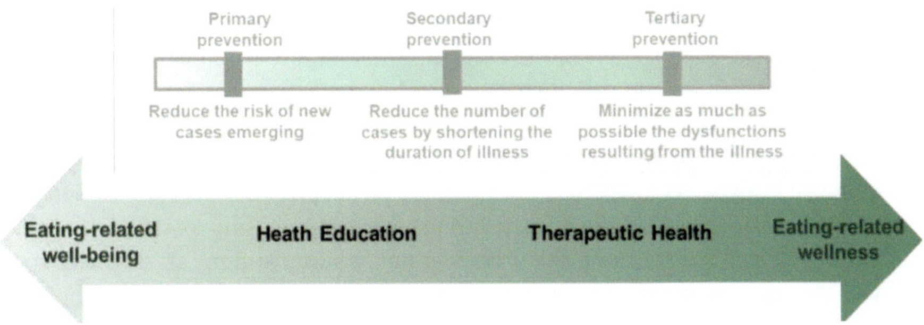

Figure 1. Continuity of interventions for dysfunctional eating attitudes and behaviours induced by body perceptual disturbances adapted from Monthuy-Blanc et al. (2023, 2025).

and behaviors. Figure 1 thus underscores that the ultimate aim is to identify one's own equilibrium in relation to one's personal conditions of alimentary health, rather than a prescribed and standardized equilibrium. This does not imply that such an equilibrium cannot be assessed by someone other than the individual concerned, such as a specialist in health education or health care using normative tools. Rather, it implies that the interpretation of assessment results must consider the individual's singularity and intrinsic functioning along the continuum.

As presented throughout the chapters in this book, positive body perceptions, including promotion of positive body image, body image flexibility over time, body-food choice congruence, interoceptive awareness/sensitivity, body acceptance and positive embodiment are the target of intervention programs on (dysfunctional) eating attitudes and behaviors focusing on different populations. These interventions can fluctuate along the model of continuity of intervention, from healthy diet education and eating-related well-being, centered on physical, intuitive and interoceptive eating at one end, to eating-related wellness, to reducing restrictive, binge and (negative) emotional eating, at the other. Indeed, through examples drawn from specific sociocultural contexts, this volume illustrates numerous prevention- and therapy-oriented interventions, empirically validated in both research and practice, that aim to support eating-related well-being or eating-related wellness (Cook-Cottone and Karwoski Anderson 2024, Holding et al. 2024, Leme et al. 2020, Lock and Pépin 2019, Stice et al. 2021). These interventions are well suited to dietary approaches aimed at maintaining or improving bodily perceptions as a lever for reducing DEAB. Increasingly, awareness and understanding of the senses, the discovery of flavors, and bodily connection through experiential situations are becoming central. Recent scientific writings confirm that these experiential situations foster a positive relationship with eating (food or drink) and the body, and contribute to beneficial changes in quality of life, body perceptions, body appreciation, and any intervention involving self-regulation, even self-management (Babbott et al. 2023).

Because the mental and physical dimensions are closely intertwined in eating attitudes and behaviors (Hou 2014), programs focused exclusively on obesity through weight reduction and "healthy eating" combined with physical activity may encourage restriction and inappropriate dieting, trigger eating-related concerns through prohibition, stigmatize individuals with higher weight (particularly youth), promote physical exercise as caloric compensation, and reduce the body to a mere object, a weight to be controlled (Irving and Neumark-Sztainer 2002, Leme et al. 2019, Monthuy-Blanc et al. 2021, Sánchez-Carracedo et al. 2012). Conversely, programs oriented solely toward eating-disorder interventions through weight-independent body acceptance may overlook the physical well-being risks associated with higher weight, particularly in preventive programs. Focusing on shared, positive, and coherent messages around body perceptions while avoiding all stigmatization constitutes the cornerstone of integrated health education. Ultimately, the body of literature in this volume leads to:

- an ethical and integrated approach, emphasizing factors that support functional eating attitudes and behaviors through positive body perceptions;
- a progressive and interactive temporal pathway, relying on dialectical techniques that foster critical thinking, informed choice, and empowerment;
- a focus on priority populations and integration into daily life contexts through mobile applications and social networks;
- the development of inter- and even transdisciplinary teams, grounding in mobilized, evidence-based data.

Acknowledgments

We wish to express our sincere gratitude to all contributing authors from the seven countries involved in this collective volume. Over more than two years, they have devoted their expertise, time, and creativity to writing these fourteen chapters on eating- and body-related mental health from an intercultural and international perspective. Their commitment to advancing knowledge on DEAB and body perceptions, and to translating this knowledge into practice, made this work possible.

References

Babbott, K.M., A. Cavadino, J. Brenton-Peters, N.S. Consedine and M. Roberts. 2023. Outcomes of intuitive eating interventions: A systematic review and meta-analysis. Eat. Disord. 31: 33–63.

Banatvala, N., S. Akselrod, P. Bovet and S. Mendis. 2023a. The WHO Global Action Plan for the Prevention and Control of NCDs 2013–2030.

Banatvala, N., S. Akselrod, P. Bovet and S. Mendis. 2023b. The WHO global action plan for the prevention and control of NCDs 2013–2030. pp. 234–239. *In*: Banatvala, N. and P. Bovet (eds.). Noncommunicable Diseases. Routledge.

Bleich, S.N., K.A. Vercammen, L.Y. Zatz, J.M. Frelier, C.B. Ebbeling and A. Peeters. 2018. Interventions to prevent global childhood overweight and obesity: a systematic review. Lancet Diabetes Endocrinol. 6: 332–346.

Breslow, L. 1999. From disease prevention to health promotion. JAMA 281: 1030–1033.

Cook-Cottone, C. and L. Karwoski Anderson. 2024. Eating disorders: the journal of treatment and prevention 2023 year in review statement from the editors celebrating 30 years and a commitment to lived experience inclusion. Eat. Disord. 32: 247–253.

Crossland, A.E., L. Munns, E. Kirk and C.E.J. Preston. 2023. Comparing body image dissatisfaction between pregnant women and non-pregnant women: a systematic review and meta-analysis. BMC Pregnancy Childbirth 23: 709.

Goltz, F.R., L.M. Stenzel and C.D. Schneider. 2013. Disordered eating behaviors and body image in male athletes. Rev. Bras. Psiquiatr. 35: 237–242.

Gorrell, S., J.M. Nagata, K.B. Hill, J.L. Carlson, A.F. Shain, J. Wilson et al. 2021. Eating behavior and reasons for exercise among competitive collegiate male athletes. Eat. Weight Disord. 26: 75–83.

Gouvernement du Québec. 1992. Ministère de la Santé et des Services sociaux. Priorités nationales de santé publique. 1997–2002. Gouvernement du Québec. https://publications.msss.gouv.qc.ca/msss/fichiers/2002/02-260-02.pdf.

Holding, A., G. Lavigne, L. Vermette and N. Carbonneau. 2024. Motivation to regulate eating behaviors, intuitive eating, and well-being: A dyadic study with mothers and adult daughters. Appetite 199: 107403.

Hou, S.I. 2014. Health education: theoretical concepts, effective strategies and core competencies. Health Promot. Pract. 15: 619–621.

Irving, L.M. and D. Neumark-Sztainer. 2002. Integrating the prevention of eating disorders and obesity: feasible or futile? Prev. Med. 34: 299–309.

Leme, A.C.B., S.T. Philippi, D. Thompson, T. Nicklas and T. Baranowski. 2019. "Healthy Habits, Healthy Girls–Brazil": an obesity prevention program with added focus on eating disorders. Eat. Weight Disord. 24: 107–119.

Leme, A.C.B., J. Haines, L. Tang, K.L. Dunker, S.T. Philippi, M. Fisberg et al. 2020. Impact of strategies for preventing obesity and risk factors for eating disorders among adolescents: a systematic review. Nutrients 12: 3134.

Lock, L. and G. Pépin. 2019. Eating disorders. pp. 154–168. *In*: Brown, C., V. Stoffel and J.P. Muñoz (eds.). Occupational Therapy in Mental Health: A Vision for Participation. 2nd ed. F.A. Davis.

Mason, T.B., R.J. Lewis and K.E. Heron. 2018. Disordered eating and body image concerns among sexual minority women: A systematic review and testable model. Psychol. Sex. Orientat. Gend. Divers. 5: 397.

Mikhail, M.E. 2023. Unheard voices: The impact of the COVID-19 pandemic on disordered eating in people with marginalized identities: Commentary on Deveci et al. (2022), Linardon et al. (2022) and Schneider et al. (2022). Int. J. Eat. Disord. 56: 68–71.

Monthuy-Blanc, J., V. Lemieux, J. Thériault and M. Rousseau. 2021. Exploratory study: A blind integrated school-based prevention program on eating disorders and obesity. Can. J. Community Mental Health 39: 61–84.

Monthuy-Blanc, J., G. Corno and S.A. Chakbe. 2023. Exploring the impact of the COVID-19 pandemic on perceptual disturbances and dysfunctional eating attitudes and behaviours: A review of the literature. Front. Psychol. 14: 1139261.

Monthuy-Blanc, J., E. Therrien and J. Harnois. 2025. Santé, boire et manger. L'alimentation en transdisciplinarité selon les perceptions. JFD éditions, QC.

Nutbeam, D. and D.M. Muscat. 2021. Health promotion glossary 2021. Health Promot. Int. 36: 1578–1598.

Sánchez-Carracedo, D., D. Neumark-Sztainer and G. López-Guimera. 2012. Integrated prevention of obesity and eating disorders: barriers, developments and opportunities. Public Health Nutr. 15: 2295–2309.

Stice, E., Z.A. Onipede and C.N. Marti. 2021. A meta-analytic review of trials that tested whether eating disorder prevention programs prevent eating disorder onset. Clin. Psychol. Rev. 87: 102046.

Thomas, S.L., I. Kickbusch, M. Kökény and O. Okan. 2025. 40 years of the Ottawa charter for health promotion—reaffirming health for all. Health Promot. Int. 40: daaf143.

Index

A

Aesthetic sports 75–79, 82, 84
Allocentric perception 188, 189, 192
Anorexia 59
Anorexia nervosa 45, 47–53, 191–194, 196
Assessment 30–32, 37–39
Athletes 73–84
Attention Bias Modification Training 44, 51–53
Attentional Bias 44–54
Autism spectrum disorder 191, 193, 195, 196
Awareness 117, 121–123, 125, 126, 128

B

Beauty ideal internalization 104
Binge Eating 89, 90, 94
Binge-eating disorder 175, 179, 181
Bisexual 58, 59, 62–64, 67, 68
Body 87–97
Body compassion 19
Body dissatisfaction 4, 5, 8–12, 44–46, 49–51, 53, 75, 76, 78–83, 103, 104, 178, 179, 184
Body dysmorphia 58, 66, 157, 191
Body experience 196
Body Illusion 93
Body image 3–12, 16, 18–26, 30–32, 34–39, 62, 64, 67, 68, 74–84, 103–111, 177, 180, 181, 188–191, 195, 197, 198
Body image disturbances 31, 32, 34, 35, 37–39
Body perception disturbance 16, 103
Body perceptions 16, 22, 23, 44, 45, 48–54
Body Surveillance 5, 7, 10
Body Swapping Illusion 91, 93
Body-oriented therapy 120–122, 127–129
BP 116–128
Breathing exercises 121, 122, 125, 127
BREF-ED program 156, 157
Bulimia 59, 94, 95
Bulimia nervosa 11, 31, 41, 55, 57, 70, 94, 98, 130, 164, 191, 199

C

Caregiver burden 154
Cognitive behavioural therapy (CBT) 120
Cognitive dissonance 106, 107
Collaborative practices 170
Compassion-based interventions 19, 26
Continuum of care 163, 164, 166, 168–170, 172, 173

D

dark side of occupation 133, 134
Dehumanization 68, 69
Digital Interventions 24
Digital tools in caregiving 154, 158
Disordered eating 63, 103
Dysfunctional eating attitudes 73–76, 80–83
Dysfunctional Eating Attitudes and Behaviors 44, 132, 133, 135, 148, 150, 157

E

Eating disorder 16, 25, 30, 31, 59, 64, 90, 94, 97, 148, 155, 156, 179–183, 188, 191, 193, 194
eating-related occupation 132–136, 139–143, 145
Efficiency 144
Egocentric perception 189
Embodiment 191, 192, 198
Estimation exercise 118, 123
Experiential knowledge 162, 163, 167, 168
Exteroception 189–191, 196, 197
Eye-Tracking 44, 47, 48, 50–53

F

Female athletes 75, 76, 79
Food Exposure 93, 94
Full Body Illusion 50, 52

G

Gay 58–60, 62–64, 66–68
Gender diversity 60
Guided imagery 122, 124, 125

H

Health education 164
Healthy Weight Program 108, 112
Homophobia 60, 63

I

Informal caregivers 148, 149, 154, 157
Instagram 3–5
Integrated conceptual map 166, 169
Integrated health 169
Integrated prevention 103, 111
Integrative approach 192, 195, 197, 198
Internalization 75, 77, 78, 84
Interoception 189–191, 196, 197
Intersectionality 65

L

Lesbian 58, 59, 62, 64, 65, 67, 68

M

meaningful occupation 132, 134–137, 139, 145
Media literacy 106, 107
Mental health 162, 164
Mental health support 148, 155
Minority stress 59–62, 64, 66, 67, 176–179, 182
Mirror exercises 121, 123, 127
Mirror Exposure Therapy 48, 52
Montreal model 163, 165
Multisensory Body 88, 89, 91
Multisensory Integration 88, 89, 91

N

Negative Body Image 16, 20, 23
Nonbinary 58, 65

O

Obesity 87–91, 93–95, 97
Objectification 68
Occupation analysis 133, 136, 137, 139, 141, 143, 145
occupational investment continuum 135
Online Self-Presentation 6, 8, 9
Oxytocin 193, 198

P

Participatory health 162, 165, 166
Partner patient 162, 163, 173
Patient partnership 162, 163, 173
Peer support 157, 158
perceptual disturbances 132–134, 136, 144, 145
PER-intake 140–142
Person–Environment–Occupation–Performance Model 139
Photo Investment 3, 6, 12
Physical standards 77
Physiotherapy 130, 131
Positive body image 16, 19, 21, 24, 26, 105, 106, 108–111
POST-intake 140–142
PRE-intake 140–142
Prevention intervention 103, 105, 106, 111
Preventive programs 206
Proprioception 189–191, 196, 197
Psychoeducation 125
Psychoeducational interventions 149, 153, 156
Psychotherapy 175

R

Recovery 164, 165, 167, 170, 171
Rejection sensitivity 60–62, 68

S

Self-Compassion 16–26
Selfie 3–12
Self-Objectification 3–5, 7–9
Sensory adaptation 197
Sensory processing 191, 193
Severe mental disorders 148
Sexual orientation 69, 70, 71, 176, 181, 183
Social Comparison 3–6, 8, 10, 12
Social Networks 3, 4
Societal pressures 81
Sociocultural model 104, 111
Socio-ecological model 104, 107, 112
Sport-specific interventions 75, 76, 78, 79
Stigma 60, 67, 68, 176, 182–184
Support pathways 151, 153, 155

T

temporal sequences of eating-related occupations 139, 141
Thin-ideal internalization 20, 25
Transdisciplinarity 164, 165, 167, 170, 171
Transgender 58, 65, 68
Transphobia 60, 65
Treatment 30–32, 34–36

V

Virtual Reality 30, 31, 38, 44, 53, 54, 90, 91, 93, 95–97
Visual Attention 45, 48, 49